PREGNANCY AND BIRTH
SOURCEBOOK
FIFTH EDITION

Health Reference Series

PREGNANCY AND BIRTH
SOURCEBOOK

FIFTH EDITION

Basic Consumer Health Information about Pregnancy and Fetal Development, Including Facts about Fertility and Conception, Physical and Emotional Changes during Pregnancy, Prenatal Care and Diagnostic Tests, High-Risk Pregnancies and Complications, Labor, Delivery, and the Postpartum Period

Along with Tips for Maintaining Health and Wellness during Pregnancy and Caring for Newborn Infants, a Glossary of Related Terms, and a Directory of Resources for Additional Help and Information

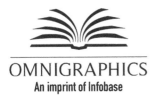

OMNIGRAPHICS
An imprint of Infobase

Bibliographic Note

Because this page cannot legibly accommodate all the copyright notices,
the Bibliographic Note portion of the Preface constitutes an extension
of the copyright notice.

* * *

OMNIGRAPHICS
An imprint of Infobase
132 W. 31st St.
New York, NY 10001
www.infobase.com
James Chambers, *Editorial Director*

* * *

Copyright © 2023 Infobase
ISBN 978-0-7808-2066-1
E-ISBN 978-0-7808-2067-8

Library of Congress Cataloging-in-Publication Data

Names: Chambers, James (Editor), editor.

Title: Pregnancy and birth sourcebook / edited by James Chambers.

Description: Fifth edition. | New York, NY: Omnigraphics, An imprint of Infobase, [2023] | Series: Health reference series | Includes index. | Summary: "Provides basic health information about pregnancy and fetal development, including facts about fertility, conception, prenatal care and diagnostic tests, pregnancy complications, labor, delivery, and postpartum care, along with tips for maintaining health and wellness during pregnancy and caring for newborns. Includes index, glossary of related terms, and other resources"-- Provided by publisher.

Identifiers: LCCN 2023023445 (print) | LCCN 2023023446 (ebook) | ISBN 9780780820661 (library binding) | ISBN 9780780820678 (ebook)

Subjects: LCSH: Pregnancy--Popular works. | Childbirth--Popular works. | Pregnancy--Complications--Popular works.

Classification: LCC RG525 .P675 2023 (print) | LCC RG525 (ebook) | DDC 618.2--dc23/eng/20230706

LC record available at https://lccn.loc.gov/2023023445

LC ebook record available at https://lccn.loc.gov/2023023446

Table of Contents

Part 3. Healthy Choices during Pregnancy

Preface

ABOUT THIS BOOK

Although the months of anticipation before a woman becomes a mother can be joyous and fulfilling, they can also mark a time filled with uncertainty and worry over potential birth defects, pregnancy complications, and chronic health conditions. Women in the United States are more likely to die from childbirth than those in other developed countries. Some women have health problems that start during pregnancy, and others have health problems before they get pregnant that could lead to complications during pregnancy. Strategies to help women adopt healthy habits and get health care before and during pregnancy can help prevent pregnancy complications. In addition, interventions to prevent unintended pregnancies can help reduce negative outcomes for women and infants. Women's health before, during, and after pregnancy can significantly impact infants' health and well-being. Women who get recommended health-care services before they get pregnant are more likely to be healthy during pregnancy and to have healthy babies.

Pregnancy and Birth Sourcebook, Fifth Edition provides health information about the reproductive process—from preconception through the postpartum period. It offers information about fertility, infertility, and pregnancy prevention. The book's chapters explain the physical and emotional changes that occur during pregnancy and discuss topics related to maintaining health during pregnancy, including eating nutritiously, exercising regularly, obtaining prenatal care, and avoiding harmful substances. Facts about high-risk pregnancies—such as those in women with chronic medical conditions, advanced maternal age, or weight concerns—are included. Finally, the book addresses common questions about labor and delivery, postpartum recovery, newborn screening, and infant care. A glossary of terms and a directory of resources for information and support are also provided.

HOW TO USE THIS BOOK

This book is divided into parts and chapters. Parts focus on broad areas of interest. Chapters are devoted to single topics within a part.

Part 1: Preparing for Pregnancy provides information about health habits, screenings, and interventions women may need before conception. This part also addresses factors that influence fertility, details common causes of infertility, and identifies methods of preventing unintended pregnancies. Additionally, it offers insights into health insurance during pregnancy for individuals.

Part 2: Pregnancy-Related Changes and Fetal Development offers trimester-by-trimester insights into the evolving physical changes in the fetus. The part also helps identify early signs of pregnancy, provides strategies for determining conception and due dates, and addresses emotional concerns and potential physical changes that may occur during pregnancy, including depression, back pain, pelvic floor and bladder problems, and vision and oral changes.

Part 3: Healthy Choices during Pregnancy highlights proactive measures that women can adopt to have a healthy pregnancy. These include obtaining regular prenatal care, undergoing necessary medical tests, using medication safely, eating nutritiously, exercising, managing weight gain, and avoiding exposure to toxic substances. This part provides valuable guidance on how pregnant women can ensure their safety in work settings and while traveling.

Part 4: High-Risk Pregnancies discusses pregnancies at high risk due to factors like maternal age, multiple fetuses, or chronic health conditions such as allergies, asthma, cancer, diabetes, epilepsy, lupus, sickle cell disease, thyroid disease, eating disorders, alpha thalassemia, sickle cell disease, and obesity.

Part 5: Pregnancy Complications explores potential diseases and disorders that can impact a pregnancy's outcome, such as amniotic fluid abnormalities, birth defects, bleeding, blood clots, gestational diabetes, hypertension, severe nausea and vomiting, placental complications, Rh incompatibility, umbilical cord abnormalities, sexually transmitted diseases, and other infections. This part also offers information about preterm labor and other related complications.

Part 6: Labor and Delivery offers information about preparing for labor and delivery, guiding through key decisions including selecting a birthing center or hospital, choosing a birth partner or doula, and creating a birth plan. This part also provides details on the pain relief options during labor, vaginal and cesarean births, strategies for handling emergency situations that may arise during childbirth.

Part 7: Postpartum and Newborn Care addresses common postpartum concerns, including recovery expectations for new mothers, newborn care and screening tests, tips about breastfeeding and formula-feeding, strategies for fostering a strong bond with a new baby, and considerations for work after a child's birth.

Part 8: Additional Help and Information includes a glossary of important terms and a directory of organizations that provide help, information, and support to low-income pregnant women and their partners.

BIBLIOGRAPHIC NOTE

This volume contains documents and excerpts from publications issued by the following U.S. government agencies: Centers for Disease Control and Prevention (CDC); Centers for Medicare & Medicaid Services (CMS); Child Welfare Information Gateway; ChildCare.gov; *Eunice Kennedy Shriver* National Institute of Child Health and Human Development (NICHD); Food and Nutrition Service (FNS); girlshealth.gov; HIV.gov; HIVinfo; MedlinePlus; National Cancer Institute (NCI); National Center on Birth Defects and Developmental Disabilities (NCBDDD); National Heart, Lung, and Blood Institute (NHLBI); National Institute for Occupational Safety and Health (NIOSH); National Institute of Arthritis and Musculoskeletal and Skin Diseases (NIAMS); National Institute of Diabetes and Digestive and Kidney Diseases (NIDDK); National Institute of Environmental Health Sciences (NIEHS); National Institute of Mental Health (NIMH); National Institute of Neurological Disorders and Stroke (NINDS); National Institute on Drug Abuse (NIDA); National Institutes of Health (NIH); National Responsible Fatherhood Clearinghouse (NRFC); News and Events; Office of Adolescent Health (OAH); Office of Disease Prevention and Health Promotion (ODPHP); Office of Population Affairs (OPA); Office on Women's Health (OWH); U.S. Department of Education (ED); U.S. Department of Health and Human Services (HHS); U.S. Department of Labor (DOL); U.S. Environmental Protection Agency (EPA); U.S. Food and Drug Administration (FDA); and Youth.gov.

It also contains original material prepared by Infobase and reviewed by medical consultants.

ABOUT THE *HEALTH REFERENCE SERIES*

The *Health Reference Series* is designed to provide basic medical information for patients, families, caregivers, and the general public. Each volume provides comprehensive coverage on a particular topic. This is especially important for people who may be dealing with a newly diagnosed disease or a chronic disorder in themselves or in a family member. People looking for preventive guidance, information about disease warning signs, medical statistics, and risk factors for health problems will also find answers to their questions in the *Health Reference Series*. The *Series*, however, is not intended to serve as a tool for diagnosing illness, in prescribing treatments, or as a substitute for the physician–patient relationship. All people concerned about medical symptoms or the possibility of disease are encouraged to seek professional care from an appropriate health-care provider.

A NOTE ABOUT SPELLING AND STYLE

Health Reference Series editors use *Stedman's Medical Dictionary* as an authority for questions related to the spelling of medical terms and *The Chicago Manual of Style* for questions related to grammatical structures, punctuation, and other editorial concerns. Consistent adherence is not always possible, however, because the individual volumes within the *Series* include many documents from a wide variety of different producers, and the editor's primary goal is to present material from each source as accurately as is possible. This sometimes means that information in different chapters or sections may follow other guidelines and alternate spelling authorities. For example, occasionally a copyright holder may require that eponymous terms be shown in possessive forms (Crohn's disease vs. Crohn disease) or that British spelling norms be retained (leukaemia vs. leukemia).

MEDICAL REVIEW

Infobase contracts with a team of qualified, senior medical professionals who serve as medical consultants for the *Health Reference Series*. As necessary, medical consultants review reprinted and originally written material for currency and accuracy. Medical consultation services are provided to the *Health Reference Series* editors by:

Dr. Vijayalakshmi, MBBS, DGO, MD
Dr. Senthil Selvan, MBBS, DCH, MD
Dr. K. Sivanandham, MBBS, DCH, MS (Research), PhD

HEALTH REFERENCE SERIES UPDATE POLICY

The inaugural book in the *Health Reference Series* was the first edition of *Cancer Sourcebook* published in 1989. Since then, the *Series* has been enthusiastically received by librarians and in the medical community. In order to maintain the standard of providing high-quality health information for the layperson, the editorial staff felt it was necessary to implement a policy of updating volumes when warranted.

Medical researchers have been making tremendous strides, and it is the purpose of the *Health Reference Series* to stay current with the most recent advances. Each decision to update a volume is made on an individual basis. Some of the considerations include how much new information is available and the feedback we receive from people who use the books. If there is a topic you would like to see added to the update list, or an area of medical concern you feel has not been adequately addressed, please write to: custserv@infobaselearning.com.

Part 1 | **Preparing for Pregnancy**

Chapter 1 | Overview of Reproductive Health

Reproductive health refers to the condition of male and female reproductive systems during all life stages. These systems are made of organs and hormone-producing glands, including the pituitary gland in the brain. Ovaries in females and testicles in males are reproductive organs, or gonads, that maintain the health of their respective systems. They also function as glands because they produce and release hormones.

Reproductive disorders affect millions of Americans each year. Female disorders include the following:

- early or delayed puberty
- endometriosis, a condition where the tissue that normally lines the inside of the womb, known as the "endometrium," grows outside of it
- inadequate breast milk supply
- infertility or reduced fertility (difficulty getting pregnant)
- menstrual problems, including heavy or irregular bleeding
- polycystic ovary syndrome (PCOS), ovaries producing more male hormones than normal
- problems during pregnancy
- uterine fibroids, noncancerous growths in a woman's uterus or womb

Figure 1.1. shows the female reproductive system.

3

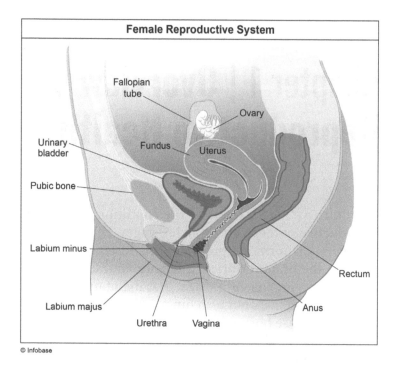

© Infobase

Figure 1.1. Female Reproductive System

Infobase

Male disorders include the following:
- impotence or erectile dysfunction (ED)
- low sperm count

Figure 1.2 shows the male reproductive system.

Scientists believe environmental factors likely play a role in some reproductive disorders. Research shows exposure to environmental factors could affect reproductive health in the following ways:
- Exposure to lead is linked to reduced fertility in both women and men.
- Mercury exposure has been linked to issues of the nervous system, such as memory, attention, and fine motor skills.

- Exposure to diethylstilbestrol (DES), a drug once prescribed to women during pregnancy, can lead to increased risks in their daughters of cancer, infertility, and pregnancy complications.
- Exposure to endocrine-disrupting compounds, chemicals that interfere with the body's hormones, may contribute to problems with puberty, fertility, and pregnancy.[1]

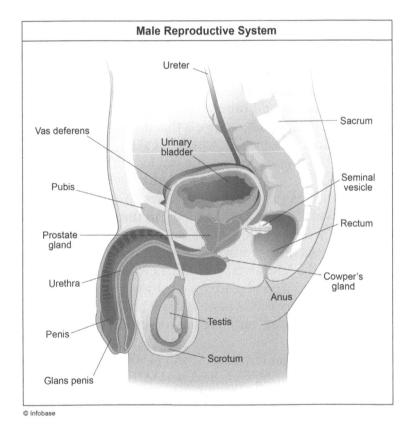

© Infobase

Figure 1.2. Male Reproductive System

Infobase

[1] "Reproductive Health," National Institute of Environmental Health Sciences (NIEHS), June 2, 2023. Available online. URL: www.niehs.nih.gov/health/topics/conditions/repro-health/index.cfm. Accessed May 11, 2023.

HOW THE FEMALE REPRODUCTIVE SYSTEM WORKS

The female reproductive system is all the parts of your body that help you reproduce or have babies. And it is quite amazing! Consider the following two fabulous facts:

- Your body likely has hundreds of thousands of eggs that could grow into a baby. And you have them from the time you are born.
- Right inside you is a perfect place for those eggs to meet with sperm and grow a whole human being!

What Is inside the Female Reproductive System?

The ovaries are two small organs. Before puberty, it is as if the ovaries are asleep. During puberty, they "wake up." The ovaries start making more estrogen and other hormones, which cause body changes. One important body change is that these hormones cause you to start getting your period, which is called "menstruating." Once a month, the ovaries release one egg (ovum). This is called "ovulation."

The fallopian tubes connect the ovaries to the uterus. The released egg moves along a fallopian tube. The uterus—or womb—is where a baby would grow. It takes several days for the egg to get to the uterus. As the egg travels, estrogen makes the lining of the uterus (called the "endometrium") thick with blood and fluid. This makes the uterus a good place for a baby to grow. You can get pregnant if you have sex with a male without birth control and his sperm joins the egg (called "fertilization") on its way to your uterus (refer to Figure 1.3).

If the egg does not get fertilized, it will be shed along with the lining of your uterus during your next period. But do not look for the egg—it is too small to see! The blood and fluid that leave your body during your period pass through your cervix and vagina. The cervix is the narrow entryway in between the vagina and the uterus. The cervix is flexible, so it can expand to let a baby pass through during childbirth.

The vagina is like a tube that can grow wider to deliver a baby that has finished growing inside the uterus. The hymen covers the opening of the vagina. It is a thin piece of tissue that has one or more holes in it. Sometimes, a hymen may be stretched or torn when you use a tampon or during a first sexual experience. If it does tear, it may bleed a little bit.

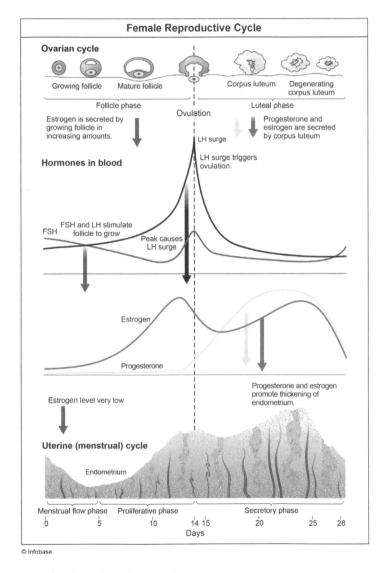

Figure 1.3. Female Reproductive Cycle

Infobase

What Is outside the Vagina?

The vulva covers the entrance to the vagina. The vulva has five parts: mons pubis, labia, clitoris, urinary opening, and vaginal opening. The mons pubis is the mound of tissue and skin above your legs, in the middle. This area becomes covered with hair when you go through puberty. The labia are the two sets of skin folds (often called "lips") on either side of the opening of the vagina.

The labia majora are the outer lips, and the labia minora are the inner lips. It is normal for the labia to look different from each other. The clitoris is a small, sensitive bump at the bottom of the mons pubis that is covered by the labia minora. The urinary opening, below the clitoris, is where your urine (pee) leaves the body. The vaginal opening is the entry to the vagina and is found below the urinary opening.[2]

WHAT ARE REPRODUCTIVE HAZARDS?

Reproductive hazards are substances that affect the reproductive health of women or men. They also include substances that affect the ability of couples to have healthy children. These substances may be chemical, physical, or biological. Some common types include the following:

- alcohol
- chemicals such as pesticides
- smoking
- legal and illegal drugs
- metals such as lead and mercury
- radiation
- some viruses

You may be exposed to reproductive hazards through contact with your skin, breathing them in, or swallowing them. This can happen anywhere, but it is more common in the workplace or at home.

---

[2] girlshealth.gov, "How the Female Reproductive System Works," Office on Women's Health (OWH), May 23, 2014. Available online. URL: www.girlshealth.gov/body/reproductive/system.html. Accessed May 11, 2023.

WHAT ARE THE HEALTH EFFECTS OF REPRODUCTIVE HAZARDS?

The possible health effects of reproductive hazards include infertility, miscarriage, birth defects, and developmental disabilities in children. What type of health effects they cause and how serious they are depend on many factors, including the following:

- What is the substance?
- How much of it are you exposed to?
- How does it enter your body?
- How long or how often are you exposed?
- How do you react to the substance?
- How can reproductive hazards affect men?

For a man, a reproductive hazard can affect the sperm. A hazard may cause a problem with the number of sperm, their shape, or the way that they swim. It could also damage the sperm's deoxyribonucleic acid (DNA). Then the sperm may not be able to fertilize an egg. Or it could cause problems with the development of the fetus.

HOW CAN REPRODUCTIVE HAZARDS AFFECT WOMEN?

For a woman, a reproductive hazard can disrupt the menstrual cycle. It can cause hormone imbalance, which can raise the risk of diseases such as osteoporosis, heart disease, and certain cancers. It can affect a woman's ability to get pregnant.

A woman who is exposed during pregnancy can have different effects, depending on when she is exposed. During the first three months of pregnancy, it might cause a birth defect or a miscarriage. During the last six months of pregnancy, it could slow the growth of the fetus, affect the development of its brain, or cause preterm labor.

HOW CAN REPRODUCTIVE HAZARDS BE AVOIDED?

To try to avoid reproductive hazards, do the following:

- Avoid alcohol and illegal drugs during pregnancy.
- If you smoke, try to quit. And, if you are not a smoker, do not start.

9

- Take precautions if you are using household chemicals or pesticides.
- Use good hygiene, including handwashing.
- If there are hazards at your job, make sure to follow safe work practices and procedures.[3]

---

[3] MedlinePlus, "Reproductive Hazards," National Institutes of Health (NIH), December 11, 2018. Available online. URL: https://medlineplus.gov/reproductivehazards.html. Accessed May 11, 2023.

Chapter 2 | **Preconception and Prenatal Care**

Chapter Contents

Section 2.1 | What Is Preconception Health?

Preconception health refers to the health of people during their reproductive years or the years they can have a child. It focuses on taking steps now to protect the health of a baby they might have some time in the future.

All people can benefit from the principles of preconception health, whether or not they plan to have a baby one day. Preconception health is about people getting and staying healthy overall across their life span. In addition, no one expects an unplanned pregnancy. But it happens often. About half of all pregnancies in the United States are not planned.

PRECONCEPTION HEALTH CARE

Preconception health care is the medical care a person receives from their doctor or other health professionals that focuses on the parts of health that have been shown to increase the chance of having a healthy baby.

Preconception health care is different for every person depending on their unique needs. Based on a person's health, the doctor or other health-care professional will suggest a course of treatment or follow-up care as needed. Ask your health-care provider about preconception health care, especially if you plan to become pregnant.

PRECONCEPTION HEALTH FOR WOMEN

Preconception health is important for every woman—not just those planning a pregnancy. It means taking control and choosing healthy habits. It means living well, being healthy, and feeling good about your life. Preconception health is about planning for the future and taking steps to get there!

PRECONCEPTION HEALTH FOR MEN

Preconception health is important for men, too. It means choosing to get and stay as healthy as possible—and helping others to do the same as well. As a partner, it means encouraging and supporting your partner's health. As a father, it means protecting your children.

Preconception health is about providing yourself and your loved ones with a bright and healthy future. Taking care of your health now will help ensure a better quality of life for yourself and your family in the coming years.[1]

WHY PRECONCEPTION HEALTH MATTERS

Every woman should be thinking about her health whether or not she is planning pregnancy. One reason is that about half of all pregnancies are not planned. Unplanned pregnancies are at a greater risk of preterm birth and low birth weight babies. Another reason is that, despite important advances in medicine and prenatal care, about one in eight babies is born too early. Researchers are trying to find out why and how to prevent preterm birth. But experts agree that women need to be healthier before becoming pregnant. By taking action on health issues and risks before pregnancy, you can prevent problems that might affect you or your baby later.

FIVE MOST IMPORTANT THINGS TO BOOST YOUR PRECONCEPTION HEALTH

Women and men should prepare for pregnancy before becoming sexually active—or at least three months before getting pregnant. Some actions, such as quitting smoking, reaching a healthy weight, or adjusting medicines you are using, should start even earlier. The following are the five most important things you can do for preconception health:

- Take 400–800 mcg (or 0.4–0.8 mg) of folic acid every day if you are planning or capable of pregnancy to lower your risk of some birth defects of the brain and spine, including spina bifida. All women need folic acid every day. Talk to your doctor about your folic acid needs. Some doctors prescribe prenatal vitamins that contain higher amounts of folic acid.
- Stop smoking and drinking alcohol.

---

[1] "Preconception Health and Health Care Is Important for All," Centers for Disease Control and Prevention (CDC), January 11, 2023. Available online. URL: www.cdc.gov/preconception/overview.html. Accessed May 11, 2023.

- If you have a medical condition, be sure it is under control. Some conditions that can affect pregnancy or be affected by it include asthma, diabetes, oral health, obesity, or epilepsy.
- Talk to your doctor about any over-the-counter (OTC) and prescription medicines you are using. These include dietary or herbal supplements. Be sure your vaccinations are up-to-date.
- Avoid contact with toxic substances or materials that could cause infection at work and at home. Stay away from chemicals and cat or rodent feces.

TALK TO YOUR DOCTOR BEFORE YOU BECOME PREGNANT

Preconception care can improve your chances of getting pregnant, having a healthy pregnancy, and having a healthy baby. If you are sexually active, talk to your doctor about your preconception health now. Preconception care should begin at least three months before you get pregnant. But some women need more time to get their bodies ready for pregnancy. Be sure to discuss your partner's health, too. Ask your doctor about the following:

- family planning and birth control
- taking folic acid
- vaccines and screenings you may need, such as a Pap test and screenings for sexually transmitted infections (STIs), including human immunodeficiency virus (HIV)
- managing health problems, such as diabetes, high blood pressure, thyroid disease, obesity, depression, eating disorders, and asthma (Find out how pregnancy may affect, or be affected by, health problems you have.)
- medicines you use, including OTC, herbal, and prescription drugs and supplements
- ways to improve your overall health, such as reaching a healthy weight, making healthy food choices, being physically active, caring for your teeth and gums, reducing stress, quitting smoking, and avoiding alcohol
- how to avoid illness
- hazards in your workplace or home that could harm you or your baby

- health problems that run in your or your partner's family
- problems you have had with prior pregnancies, including preterm birth
- family concerns that could affect your health, such as domestic violence or lack of support

YOUR PARTNER'S ROLE IN PREPARING FOR PREGNANCY

Your partner can do a lot to support and encourage you in every aspect of preparing for pregnancy. Here are some ways:

- Make the decision about pregnancy together. When both partners intend for pregnancy, a woman is more likely to get early prenatal care and avoid risky behaviors such as smoking and drinking alcohol.
- Screening for and treating STIs can help make sure infections are not passed to female partners.
- Male partners can improve their own reproductive health and overall health by limiting alcohol, quitting smoking or illegal drug use, making healthy food choices, and reducing stress. Studies show that men who drink a lot, smoke, or use drugs can have problems with their sperm. These might cause you to have problems getting pregnant. If your partner does not quit smoking, ask him not to smoke around you to avoid the harmful effects of secondhand smoke.
- Your partner should also talk to his doctor about his own health, his family health history, and any medicines he uses.
- People who work with chemicals or other toxins can be careful not to expose women to them. For example, people who work with fertilizers or pesticides should change out dirty clothes before coming near women. They should handle and wash soiled clothes separately.[2]

---

[2] Office on Women's Health (OWH), "Preconception Health," U.S. Department of Health and Human Services (HHS), February 22, 2021. Available online. URL: www.womenshealth.gov/pregnancy/you-get-pregnant/preconception-health. Accessed May 11, 2023.

Section 2.2 | Understanding Genetic Counseling and Evaluation: Is It Right for You?

WHAT IS GENETIC COUNSELING?

Genetic counseling gives you information about how genetic conditions might affect you or your family. The genetic counselor or other health-care professional will collect your personal and family health history. They can use this information to determine how likely it is that you or your family member has a genetic condition. Based on this information, the genetic counselor can help you decide whether a genetic test might be right for you or your relative.

REASONS FOR GENETIC COUNSELING

Based on your personal and family health history, your doctor can refer you for genetic counseling. There are different stages in your life when you might be referred for genetic counseling:

- **Planning for pregnancy**. Genetic counseling before you become pregnant can address concerns about factors that might affect your baby during infancy or childhood or your ability to become pregnant, including the following:
  - genetic conditions that run in your family or your partner's family
  - history of infertility, multiple miscarriages, or stillbirth
  - previous pregnancy or child affected by a birth defect or genetic condition
  - assisted reproductive technology (ART) options
- **During pregnancy.** Genetic counseling, while you are pregnant, can address certain tests that may be done during your pregnancy, any detected problems, or conditions that might affect your baby during infancy or childhood, including the following:
  - history of infertility, multiple miscarriages, or stillbirth

17

- previous pregnancy or child affected by a birth defect or genetic condition
- abnormal test results, such as a blood test, ultrasound, chorionic villus sampling (CVS), or amniocentesis
- maternal infections, such as cytomegalovirus (CMV), and other exposures, such as medicines, drugs, chemicals, and x-rays
- genetic screening that is recommended for all pregnant women, which includes cystic fibrosis, sickle cell disease (SCD), and any conditions that run in your family or your partner's family
- **Caring for children.** Genetic counseling can address concerns if your child is showing signs and symptoms of a disorder that might be genetic, including the following:
  - abnormal newborn screening results
  - birth defects
  - intellectual disability or developmental disabilities
  - autism spectrum disorder (ASD)
  - vision or hearing problems
- **Managing your health.** Genetic counseling for adults includes specialty areas such as cardiovascular genetic counseling, psychiatric genetic counseling, and cancer genetic counseling. Genetic counseling can be helpful if you have symptoms of a condition or have a family history of a condition that makes you more likely to be affected by that condition, including the following:
  - hereditary breast and ovarian cancer (HBOC) syndrome
  - Lynch syndrome (hereditary colorectal and other cancers)
  - familial hypercholesterolemia
  - muscular dystrophy and other muscle diseases

- inherited movement disorders such as Huntington disease (HD)
- inherited blood disorders such as SCD[3]

GENETIC COUNSELING AND YOUR BABY'S HEALTH

The genes your baby is born with can affect your baby's health in these ways:

- **Single-gene disorders.** These disorders are caused by a problem in a single gene. Genes contain the information your body's cells need to function. Single-gene disorders run in families. Examples of single-gene disorders are cystic fibrosis and sickle cell anemia.
- **Chromosome disorders.** These disorders occur when all or part of a chromosome is missing or extra or if the structure of one or more chromosomes is not normal. Chromosomes are structures where genes are located. Most chromosome disorders that involve whole chromosomes do not run in families.

Talk to your doctor about your and your partner's family health histories before becoming pregnant. This information can help your doctor find out any genetic risks you might have.

Depending on your genetic risk factors, your doctor might suggest you meet with a genetic professional. Some reasons a person or couple might seek genetic counseling are:

- a family history of a genetic condition, birth defect, chromosomal disorder, or cancer
- two or more pregnancy losses, a stillbirth, or a baby who died
- a child with a known inherited disorder, birth defect, or intellectual disability

---

[3] "Genetic Counseling," Centers for Disease Control and Prevention (CDC), June 24, 2022. Available online. URL: www.cdc.gov/genomics/gtesting/genetic_counseling.htm. Accessed May 11, 2023.

- a woman who is pregnant or plans to become pregnant at 35 years or older
- test results that suggest a genetic condition is present
- increased risk of getting or passing on a genetic disorder because of one's ethnic background
- people related by blood who want to have children together

During a consultation, the genetic professional meets with a person or couple to discuss genetic risks or to diagnose, confirm, or rule out a genetic condition. Sometimes, a couple chooses to have genetic testing. Some tests can help couples to know the chances that a person will get or pass on a genetic disorder. The genetic professional can help couples decide if genetic testing is the right choice for them.[4]

Section 2.3 | Genetic Testing

WHAT IS GENETIC TESTING?
Genetic testing is a type of medical test that looks for changes in your deoxyribonucleic acid (DNA). It contains the genetic instructions in all living things. Genetic tests analyze your cells or tissue to look for any changes in the following:

- **Genes.** These are parts of DNA that carry the information needed to make a protein.
- **Chromosomes.** These are thread-like structures in your cells. They contain DNA and proteins.
- **Proteins.** They do most of the work in your cells. Testing can look for changes in the amount and activity level of proteins. If it finds changes, it might be due to changes in your DNA.

---

[4] Office on Women's Health (OWH), "Preconception Health," U.S. Department of Health and Human Services (HHS), February 22, 2021. Available online. URL: www.womenshealth.gov/pregnancy/you-get-pregnant/preconception-health. Accessed May 11, 2023.

WHY IS GENETIC TESTING DONE?

Genetic testing may be done for many different reasons:

- to find genetic diseases in unborn babies, which is one type of prenatal testing
- to screen newborn babies for certain treatable conditions
- to lower the risk of genetic diseases in embryos that were created using assisted reproductive technology (ART)
- to find out if you carry a gene for a certain disease that could be passed on to your children, which is called "carrier testing"
- to see whether you are at an increased risk of developing a specific disease, which may be done for a disease that runs in your family
- to diagnose certain diseases
- to identify genetic changes that may be causing or contributing to a disease that you were already diagnosed with
- to figure out how severe a disease is
- to help guide your doctor in deciding the best medicine and dosage for you, which is called "pharmacogenomic testing"

HOW IS GENETIC TESTING DONE?

Genetic tests are often done on a blood or cheek swab sample. But they may also be done on samples of hair, saliva, skin, amniotic fluid (the fluid that surrounds a fetus during pregnancy), or other tissue. The sample is sent to a laboratory. There, a lab technician will use one of several different techniques to look for genetic changes.[5]

---

[5] MedlinePlus, "Genetic Testing," National Institutes of Health (NIH), June 11, 2021. Available online. URL: https://medlineplus.gov/genetictesting.html. Accessed May 11, 2023.

WHAT ARE THE USES OF GENETIC TESTING?

Genetic testing can provide information about a person's genetic background. The uses of genetic testing include the following.

Newborn Screening

Newborn screening is used just after birth to identify genetic disorders that can be treated early in life. Millions of babies are tested each year in the United States. The Health Resources and Services Administration (HRSA) recommends that states screen for a set of 35 conditions, which many states exceed.

Diagnostic Testing

Diagnostic testing is used to identify or rule out a specific genetic or chromosomal condition. In many cases, genetic testing is used to confirm a diagnosis when a particular condition is suspected based on physical signs and symptoms. Diagnostic testing can be performed before birth or at any time during a person's life, but it is not available for all genes or all genetic conditions. The results of a diagnostic test can influence a person's choices about health care and the management of the disorder.

Carrier Testing

Carrier testing is used to identify people who carry one copy of a gene mutation that, when present in two copies, causes a genetic disorder. This type of testing is offered to individuals who have a family history of a genetic disorder and to people in certain ethnic groups with an increased risk of specific genetic conditions. If both parents are tested, the test can provide information about a couple's risk of having a child with a genetic condition.

Prenatal Testing

Prenatal testing is used to detect changes in a fetus's genes or chromosomes before birth. This type of testing is offered during pregnancy if there is an increased risk that the baby will have a genetic or chromosomal disorder. In some cases, prenatal testing can lessen

22

a couple's uncertainty or help them make decisions about a pregnancy. It cannot identify all possible inherited disorders and birth defects, however.

Preimplantation Testing

Preimplantation testing, also called "preimplantation genetic diagnosis" (PGD), is a specialized technique that can reduce the risk of having a child with a particular genetic or chromosomal disorder. It is used to detect genetic changes in embryos that were created using assisted reproductive technology (ART), such as in vitro fertilization (IVF). IVF involves removing egg cells from a woman's ovaries and fertilizing them with sperm cells outside the body. To perform preimplantation testing, a small number of cells are taken from these embryos and tested for certain genetic changes. Only embryos without these changes are implanted in the uterus to initiate a pregnancy.

Predictive and Presymptomatic Testing

Predictive and presymptomatic types of testing are used to detect gene mutations associated with disorders that appear after birth, often later in life. These tests can be helpful to people who have a family member with a genetic disorder but who have no features of the disorder themselves at the time of testing. Predictive testing can identify mutations that increase a person's risk of developing disorders with a genetic basis, such as certain types of cancer. Presymptomatic testing can determine whether a person will develop a genetic disorder, such as hereditary hemochromatosis (an iron overload disorder), before any signs or symptoms appear. The results of predictive and presymptomatic testing can provide information about a person's risk of developing a specific disorder and help with making decisions about medical care.

Forensic Testing

Forensic testing uses DNA sequences to identify an individual for legal purposes. Unlike the tests described above, forensic testing is not used to detect gene mutations associated with the disease. This type of testing can identify crime or catastrophe victims, rule out or implicate a crime suspect, or establish biological relationships between people (e.g., paternity).[6]

WHAT ARE THE BENEFITS OF GENETIC TESTING?
The benefits of genetic testing include the following:
- helping doctors make recommendations for treatment or monitoring
- giving you more information for making decisions about your health and your family's health:
    - If you find out that you are at risk for a certain disease, you might take steps to lower that risk. For example, you may find out that you should be screened for a disease earlier and more often. Or you might decide to make healthy lifestyle changes.
    - If you find out that you are not at risk for a certain disease, then you can skip unnecessary checkups or screenings.
- a test that could give you information that helps you make decisions about having children
- identifying genetic disorders early in life so that treatment can be started as soon as possible

WHAT ARE THE DRAWBACKS OF GENETIC TESTING?
The physical risks of the different types of genetic testing are small. But there can be emotional, social, or financial drawbacks.
- Depending on the results, you may feel angry, depressed, anxious, or guilty. This can be especially true if you are diagnosed with a disease that does not have effective treatments.
- You may be worried about genetic discrimination in employment or insurance.

---

[6] MedlinePlus, "What Are the Uses of Genetic Testing?" National Institutes of Health (NIH), July 28, 2021. Available online. URL: https://medlineplus.gov/genetics/understanding/testing/uses. Accessed May 11, 2023.

- Genetic testing may give you limited information about a genetic disease. For example, it cannot tell you whether you will have symptoms, how severe a disease might be, or whether a disease will get worse over time.
- Some genetic tests are expensive, and health insurance might only cover part of the cost. Or they may not cover it at all.[7]

---

[7] See footnote [5].

Chapter 3 | **Promoting a Healthy Pregnancy**

For women who are thinking about getting pregnant, following a health-care provider's advice can reduce the risk of problems during pregnancy and after birth. A health-care provider can recommend ways to get the proper nutrition and avoid habits that can have lasting harmful effects on a fetus.

For example, taking a supplement containing at least 400 mcg of folic acid before getting pregnant can reduce the risk of complications such as neural tube defects (NTDs)—abnormalities that can occur in the brain, spine, or spinal column of a developing fetus and are present at birth. A prepregnancy care visit with your health-care provider can improve the chances of a healthy pregnancy. A health-care provider will likely recommend that you do the following.

DEVELOP A PLAN FOR YOUR REPRODUCTIVE LIFE
This plan includes your and your partner's plans for the number and timing of pregnancies based on your values and life goals. Sharing your life plan with your health-care provider can help address any potential problems before you conceive.

ADOPT A HEALTHY DIET AND LIFESTYLE
You can reduce the chance that you will be diagnosed with gestational diabetes (high blood sugar diagnosed during pregnancy) by taking steps to improve your diet and lifestyle before you get pregnant. Gestational diabetes can increase the risk to your health

as well as your infant's. In addition, prepregnancy exercise is also associated with lower risk for gestational diabetes, and the benefit increases with more vigorous levels of exercise.

Here are some specific dietary suggestions for women who are planning for a pregnancy:

- **Increase your intake of fiber.** Eating 10 more grams of fiber in the form of cereals, fruits, and vegetables is associated with 26 percent lower risk of gestational diabetes.
- **Reduce consumption of sugar-sweetened cola.** Women who drank five or more such beverages per week before they got pregnant were at a greater risk of gestational diabetes.
- **Eat less red meat, processed meats, and animal fats and cholesterol.** Eating less of these foods before pregnancy can decrease the chances of developing diabetes when you are pregnant.
- **Replace animal protein with protein from nuts to lower your risk of gestational diabetes.** Studies have shown that substituting vegetable protein for animal protein before pregnancy can decrease the risk of gestational diabetes by about half.

INCREASE YOUR INTAKE OF FOLIC ACID

Folic acid is a B vitamin (B9). It helps produce and maintain new cells. This is especially important during times when the cells are dividing and growing rapidly, such as infancy and pregnancy.

The U.S. Public Health Service recommends that all pregnant women and "women of childbearing age (15–44 years) in the United States who are capable of becoming pregnant should consume (a supplement containing) 0.4 mg of folic acid per day for the purpose of reducing their risk of having a pregnancy affected with spina bifida or other NTDs."

Although a related form of folic acid (called "folate") is present in orange juice and leafy, green vegetables (such as kale and spinach), folate is not absorbed as well as folic acid. Studies show that taking folic acid for three months before getting pregnant and for three months after conceiving can reduce the risk of NTDs such as spina bifida by up to 70 percent.

GET UP-TO-DATE ON VACCINES

Ask your health-care provider if you need a booster for any vaccines. Some vaccines can be given during pregnancy, but the rubella (German measles) and varicella (chickenpox) vaccines are recommended before you get pregnant.

TALK TO YOUR HEALTH-CARE PROVIDER ABOUT YOUR DIABETES OR OTHER MEDICAL CONDITIONS

Many health problems affect not only the pregnant woman but also the developing infant. Some examples are diabetes, hypertension (high blood pressure), infections, asthma, seizure disorders, and maternal phenylketonuria (an inherited condition in which the pregnant woman's body cannot break down the amino acid phenylalanine, resulting in high levels in her blood). Getting health problems under control before and during pregnancy reduces the risk of miscarriage and stillbirth as well as other health problems for the infant.

AVOID SMOKING, DRINKING ALCOHOL, AND TAKING DRUGS

During pregnancy, these behaviors can increase the risk of sudden infant death syndrome (SIDS), preterm birth, fetal alcohol spectrum disorders, and NTDs. If you are trying to quit smoking, drinking, or doing drugs and you need help, talk to your health-care provider about support groups or about medications.

STRIVE TO REACH A HEALTHY WEIGHT BEFORE TRYING TO GET PREGNANT

Obesity may make it more difficult to become pregnant. Being overweight or obese also puts you at risk for complications during pregnancy, such as high blood pressure, preeclampsia, gestational diabetes, and stillbirth, and increases the chances of cesarean delivery.

Eunice Kennedy Shriver National Institute of Child Health and Human Development (NICHD) researchers have found that obesity can increase your child's risk of a congenital heart defect (a problem with the heart that is present at birth) by 15 percent. Research has also uncovered a link between obesity and NTDs. Talk to your health-care provider about what a healthy weight is for you and about a plan to help you achieve it.

LEARN YOUR FAMILY'S HEALTH HISTORY

Your health-care provider will ask for information about your family's genetic and health history. You may be referred for genetic counseling if certain conditions run in your family or if a family member was born with a physical abnormality or an intellectual and developmental disability.

GET MENTALLY HEALTHY

Good mental health means you feel good about your life and value yourself. It is natural to worry or feel sad, anxious, or stressed at times. However, if these feelings do not go away and they interfere with your daily life, it is important to seek help before you get pregnant. Hormonal changes and other situations during pregnancy can worsen depression.

Many people are familiar with the phrase "postpartum depression," meaning depression that occurs after the birth of a baby. But we now know that it is not just during the postpartum period, and it is not just depression.

Women experience depression and anxiety, as well as other mental health conditions, during pregnancy and after the baby is born. These conditions can have significant effects on the health of the mother and her child. Getting mentally healthy before you get pregnant can help minimize the effects of these conditions.[1]

[1] "Can You Promote a Healthy Pregnancy before Getting Pregnant?" *Eunice Kennedy Shriver* National Institute of Child Health and Human Development (NICHD), March 28, 2019. Available online. URL: www.nichd.nih.gov/health/topics/preconceptioncare/conditioninfo/before-pregnancy. Accessed June 15, 2023.

Chapter 4 | **Understanding Fertility**

Chapter Contents

Section 4.1 | Fertility Basics

UNDERSTANDING FERTILITY: THE BASICS

It is important to understand what happens to the body during puberty and a woman's menstrual cycle, how a woman's reproductive system works, and how overall health and wellness are connected to fertility and the reproductive system.

Understanding the body and the biology of reproduction can inform decisions about preventing pregnancy and deciding whether and when to become pregnant. The next sections describe the basics of puberty, the menstrual cycle, what it means to have fertility awareness and use fertility awareness-based methods (FABMs) of family planning, and infertility in women and men.

Puberty

Puberty is the time in life when a child reaches sexual maturity. This means that the hormone levels in the body—estrogen and progesterone in girls and testosterone in boys—increase and cause physical and emotional changes to occur. Puberty usually happens between the ages of 8 and 13 for girls and the ages of 10 and 15 for boys, and the process affects boys and girls differently. When girls reach puberty, they typically start their menstrual cycle.

Menstrual Cycle

The menstrual cycle refers to the monthly process that happens in a woman's body to prepare for a possible pregnancy. It includes the release of an egg from the ovaries (called "ovulation"), changes in the cervix and thickening of the uterine wall, several hormonal changes, and shedding of the thickened uterine wall through bleeding (called "menstruation," also known as a "period" or "menses"). Hormonal fluctuations drive the changes that occur during the menstrual cycle. If pregnancy does not occur, the body sheds the extra lining of the uterus. The blood and tissue leave the uterus through the cervix and exit the body through the vagina. The length of the menstrual cycle is the number of days starting from the first day when bleeding begins until the first day of the next month when bleeding begins again.

Regular menstrual periods occurring in the years between puberty and menopause are usually a sign that the female body is working normally. Some women experience problems with menstruation, such as irregular or heavy, painful periods; this may be a sign of a health problem. Many women also experience premenstrual syndrome (PMS) symptoms. Women with period problems or PMS should talk to a health-care provider about ways to treat these issues.

In addition to the hormonal changes and the changes happening inside the body, females may also notice changes in their vaginal discharge. Vaginal discharge is a fluid—usually white or clear—that comes out of the vagina. Most females have vaginal discharge. The amount and consistency of vaginal discharge change at different points in a female's cycle. Increased vaginal discharge can be caused by normal menstrual cycle changes, vaginal infection, or cancer (rare). Unusual vaginal discharge can also be a symptom of pelvic inflammatory disease (PID), an infection of a female's reproductive organs often caused by some sexually transmitted infections (STIs). If a female has more than her usual amount of vaginal discharge, she may need to see her health-care provider.

How to Chart Menstrual Cycles

To chart her menstrual cycle, a woman can simply record the day her period starts and when it ends on a paper or electronic calendar. Smartphone and computer applications that chart menstrual cycles are also available. Over time, this tracking will help a woman see what the typical amount of time between periods is, which can help her predict when her next period will start.

Tracking the menstrual cycle can provide useful information for conversations with health-care providers. For example, a patient may want to discuss the length of her cycle or her experiences with pain or extreme bleeding during her cycle. In addition, tracking the cycle is key to predicting ovulation, which can inform decisions about when to have sex and whether the intent is to avoid pregnancy or become pregnant.

FERTILITY AWARENESS

Fertility awareness means being aware of the menstrual cycle and the changes in a woman's body that happen during this time and understanding when a woman is most likely to get pregnant. Women and couples become more familiar with the signs of ovulation and the pattern of the menstrual cycle to understand how to plan sexual activity to avoid pregnancy or become pregnant.

Fertility Awareness-Based Methods of Family Planning

FABMs involve a woman learning to recognize the signs of her fertile days, which are the days of each month in which she is most likely to become pregnant (conceive). Based on her intentions, she may plan to have unprotected sex during this time in order to conceive, or she may choose to avoid pregnancy by not having sex or by using a barrier birth control method, such as condoms, during this time.

The following are the multiple FABMs that women can use:

- natural family planning
- standard days or calendar method
- cervical mucous method
- basal body temperature method
- ovulation method
- symptothermal method (combining the other methods)

INFERTILITY

Infertility is defined as not being able to become pregnant after having regular intercourse (sex) without birth control after one year (or after six months if a woman is 35 or older). Infertility is common. Out of 100 couples in the United States, about 12–13 of them have trouble becoming pregnant.

About one-third of infertility cases are caused by fertility problems in women, and another one-third of infertility cases are due to fertility problems in men. The other cases are caused by a mixture of male and female problems or by problems that cannot be determined.

Infertility in Women

Most cases of female infertility are caused by problems with ovulation. Ovulation problems can be caused by hormone imbalances from a variety of causes. Although less common, blocked fallopian tubes can also cause female infertility. If the fallopian tube is blocked due to infection, surgery, or other problems, then sperm cannot reach the egg to fertilize it.

Other less common causes of fertility problems in women can include physical problems with the uterus or uterine fibroids, which are noncancerous tumors made of fibrous tissue and muscle cells that develop on the walls of the uterus.

Infertility in Men

There are a few different causes of male infertility. Erectile dysfunction is when a man cannot get or keep an erection (get hard) for sex. Without an erection, it is difficult for a man to release sperm inside the vagina and, therefore, difficult to get a woman pregnant.

Another problem is varicocele, which is when the veins in a man's scrotum (sac) can become too large. These big veins heat and cool the testes. When the big veins heat the testes too much, the heat damages the sperm. Sperm damage can cause male infertility.

If a man makes too few sperm or none at all, the woman cannot become pregnant. Also, if a man's sperm do not move correctly, they may not be able to meet with and fertilize an egg. Additionally, if the tubes through which sperm travel are blocked, the sperm cannot travel into and out of the penis to meet with and fertilize an egg.[1]

[1] Office of Population Affairs (OPA), "Understanding Fertility: The Basics," U.S. Department of Health and Human Services (HHS), August 17, 2020. Available online. URL: https://opa.hhs.gov/reproductive-health/understanding-fertility-basics. Accessed May 12, 2023.

Section 4.2 | Age and Infertility

WHAT IS INFERTILITY?

Infertility is the inability to achieve pregnancy after 12 months or more of regular, unprotected sexual intercourse (or after six months if the woman is older than 35). The term describes men who cannot get a woman pregnant and women who cannot get pregnant or carry a pregnancy to term.

About 7 percent of men (4.7 million) and about 11 percent of women (6.7 million) of reproductive age in the United States have experienced fertility problems. In one-third of infertile couples, the problem is with the man. In one-third of infertile couples, the problem cannot be identified or is with both men and women. In one-third of infertile couples, the problem is with the woman.

WHAT TYPES OF THINGS CAN CAUSE OR CONTRIBUTE TO INFERTILITY?

Health conditions and behaviors, age, genetics, and other factors can all cause or contribute to infertility in men and women.

Health Conditions and Behaviors

- Men:
  - certain medications, such as testosterone gels/patches to treat "low T"
  - testicular injury or overheating
- Men and women:
  - exposure to chemicals
  - cancer and/or exposure to radiation or chemotherapy
  - stress
  - conditions such as diabetes, heart disease, obesity, high blood pressure, and autoimmune disorders
  - smoking and/or alcohol and drug abuse
  - sexually transmitted infections (STIs)

- Women:
  - gynecological disorders such as polycystic ovary syndrome (PCOS), primary ovarian insufficiency (POI), endometriosis, and uterine fibroids
  - problems with the anatomy of the reproductive organs

HOW DOES AGE FACTOR INTO THIS?

People are waiting longer than ever before to start families. Women are now eight times more likely to have their first child after the age of 35 than they were in 1970. But waiting too long can cause problems.

As age increases, so does the likelihood of infertility:
- Older men produce fewer sperm and lower-quality sperm.
- Older women have fewer eggs and lower-quality eggs.
- The risk of some health conditions associated with infertility (above) increases with age.
- Age-related declines in sperm and egg quality increase the risk of health conditions, such as Down syndrome, autism, and schizophrenia, in future generations.

After the age of 30, a woman's fertility decreases rapidly every year until menopause, usually around the age of 50. In the decade before menopause, her fertility is also greatly reduced. Male fertility also declines with age but more gradually.[2]

A MOLECULAR EXPLANATION FOR AGE-RELATED FERTILITY DECLINE IN WOMEN

Scientists supported by the National Institutes of Health (NIH) have a new theory as to why a woman's fertility declines after her mid-30s. They also suggest an approach that might help slow the process, enhancing and prolonging fertility.

---

[2] "Understanding Infertility," *Eunice Kennedy Shriver* National Institute of Child Health and Human Development (NICHD), January 3, 2018. Available online. URL: www.nichd.nih.gov/sites/default/files/news/resources/links/infographics/Documents/NICHD_Infographic_Infertility.pdf. Accessed May 12, 2023.

They found that, as women age, their egg cells become riddled with deoxyribonucleic acid (DNA) damage and die off because their DNA repair systems wear out. Defects in one of the DNA repair genes—*BRCA1*—have long been linked with breast cancer and now also appear to cause early menopause.

"We all know that a woman's fertility declines in her 40s. This study provides a molecular explanation for why that happens," said Dr. Susan Taymans, Ph.D., Program Director of the Fertility and Infertility Branch of the *Eunice Kennedy Shriver* National Institute of Child Health and Human Development (NICHD), the NIH institute that funded the study. "Eventually, such insights might help us find ways to improve and extend a woman's reproductive life."

The findings appear in *Science Translational Medicine*. In general, a woman's ability to conceive and maintain a pregnancy is linked to the number and health of her egg cells. Before a baby girl is born, her ovaries contain her lifetime supply of egg cells (known as "primordial follicle oocytes") until they are more mature. As she enters her late 30s, the number of oocytes—and fertility—dips precipitously. By the time she reaches her early 50s, her original ovarian supply of about 1 million cells drops virtually to zero.

Only a small proportion of oocytes—about 500—are released via ovulation during the woman's reproductive life. The remaining 99.9 percent are eliminated by the woman's body, primarily through cellular suicide, a normal process that prevents the spread or inheritance of damaged cells. Scientists suspect that most aging oocytes self-destruct because they have accumulated a dangerous type of DNA damage called "double-stranded breaks." According to the study, older oocytes have more of this sort of damage than younger ones. The researchers also found that older oocytes are less able to fix DNA breaks due to their dwindling supply of repair molecules.

Examining oocytes from mice, as well as from women 24–41 years old, the researchers found that the activity of four DNA repair genes (*BRCA1*, *MRE11*, *Rad51*, and *ATM*) declined with age. When the research team experimentally turned off these genes in mouse oocytes, the cells had more DNA breaks and higher death rates than oocytes with properly working repair systems. The research team's findings stemmed from their initial focus on *BRCA1*, a DNA repair gene that has been closely studied for nearly 20 years because defective versions of it dramatically increase a woman's risk of breast cancer. Using mice bred to lack the *BRCA1* gene, the NICHD-supported scientists confirmed that a healthy version of *BRCA1* is vital to reproductive health. *BRCA1*-deficient mice were less fertile, had fewer oocytes, and had more double-stranded DNA breaks in their remaining oocytes than normal mice.

Abnormal *BRCA1* appears to cause the same problems in humans—the team's studies suggest that if a woman's oocytes contain mutant versions of *BRCA1*, she will exhaust her ovarian supply sooner than women whose oocytes carry the healthy version of *BRCA1*. Together, these findings show that the ability of oocytes to repair double-stranded DNA breaks is closely linked with ovarian aging and, by extension, a woman's fertility. This molecular-level understanding points to new reproductive therapies. Specifically, the scientists suggest that finding ways to bolster DNA repair systems in the ovaries might lead to treatments that can improve or prolong fertility.[3]

Section 4.3 | Fertility Preservation

WHAT IS FERTILITY PRESERVATION?

Fertility preservation is the process of saving or protecting eggs, sperm, or reproductive tissue so that a person can use them to have biological children in the future.

WHO CAN BENEFIT FROM FERTILITY PRESERVATION?

People with certain diseases, disorders, and life events that affect fertility may benefit from fertility preservation. They include people who:

[3] News and Events, "A Molecular Explanation for Age-Related Fertility Decline in Women," National Institutes of Health (NIH), May 21, 2013. Available online. URL: www.nih.gov/news-events/news-releases/molecular-explanation-age-related-fertility-decline-women. Accessed May 12, 2023.

- have been exposed to toxic chemicals in the workplace or during military duty
- have endometriosis
- have uterine fibroids
- are about to be treated for cancer
- are about to be treated for an autoimmune disease, such as lupus
- have a genetic disease that affects future fertility
- delay having children

WHAT FERTILITY-PRESERVING OPTIONS ARE AVAILABLE?

A number of fertility-preserving options are available.

Fertility-preserving options for males include the following:

- **Sperm cryopreservation.** In this process, a male provides samples of his semen. The semen is then frozen and stored for future use in a process called "cryopreservation."
- **Gonadal shielding.** Radiation treatment for cancer and other conditions can harm fertility, especially if it is used in the pelvic area. Some radiation treatments use modern techniques to aim the rays at a very small area. The testicles can also be protected with a lead shield.

Fertility-preserving options for females include the following:

- **Embryo cryopreservation.** This method, also called "embryo freezing," is the most common and successful option for preserving a female's fertility. First, a health-care provider removes eggs from the ovaries. The eggs are then fertilized with sperm from her partner or a donor in a lab in a process called "in vitro fertilization" (IVF). The resulting embryos are frozen and stored for future use.
- **Oocyte cryopreservation.** This option is similar to embryo cryopreservation, except that unfertilized eggs are frozen and stored.
- **Gonadal shielding.** This process is similar to gonadal shielding for males. Steps are taken, such as aiming rays

at a small area or covering the pelvic area with a lead shield, to protect the ovaries from radiation.

- **Ovarian transposition.** A health-care provider performs minor surgery to move the ovaries and sometimes the fallopian tubes from the area that will receive radiation to an area that will not receive radiation. For example, they may be relocated to an area of the abdomen wall that will not receive radiation.

Some of these options, such as sperm, oocyte, and embryo cryopreservation, are available only to males and females who have gone through puberty and have mature sperm and eggs. However, gonadal shielding and ovarian transposition can be used to preserve fertility in children who have not gone through puberty.[4]

---

[4] "What Is Fertility Preservation?" *Eunice Kennedy Shriver* National Institute of Child Health and Human Development (NICHD), January 31, 2017. Available online. URL: www.nichd.nih.gov/health/topics/infertility/conditioninfo/fertilitypreservation. Accessed May 12, 2023.

Chapter 5 | Trying to Conceive

Chapter Contents

Section 5.1 | **Steps to Conceive**

If you are trying to have a baby or are just thinking about it, it is not too early to start getting ready for pregnancy. Preconception health and health care focus on things you can do before and between pregnancies to increase the chances of having a healthy baby. For some people, getting their bodies ready for pregnancy takes a few months. For other people, it might take longer. Whether this is your first, second, or sixth baby, the following are important steps to help you get ready for the healthiest pregnancy possible.

MAKE A PLAN AND TAKE ACTION

Whether or not you have written them down, you have probably thought about your goals for having or not having children and how to achieve those goals. For example, when you did not want to have a baby, you used effective birth control methods. Now that you are thinking about getting pregnant, it is important to take steps to achieve your goal—getting pregnant and having a healthy baby!

SEE YOUR DOCTOR

Before getting pregnant, talk to your health-care provider about preconception health care. Your provider will want to discuss your health history and any medical conditions you currently have that could affect a pregnancy. They may want to discuss any previous pregnancy problems, medicines you are currently taking, vaccinations you might need, and steps you can take before pregnancy to help prevent certain birth defects.

Take a list of talking points, so you do not forget anything. Be sure to talk to your doctor about the following conditions.

Medical Conditions

If you currently have any medical conditions, be sure they are under control and being treated. Some of these conditions include the following:

- sexually transmitted diseases (STDs)
- diabetes
- thyroid disease
- high blood pressure
- other chronic diseases

Lifestyle and Behaviors

Talk with your health-care provider if you:

- smoke, drink alcohol, or use certain drugs
- live in a stressful or abusive environment
- work with or live around toxic substances

Health-care professionals can help you with counseling, treatment, and other support services.

Medications

Almost every pregnant person will face a decision about taking medicines before and during pregnancy. Talk to your health-care providers before starting or stopping any medicines. Be sure to discuss the following with your health-care providers:

- all medicines you take, including prescriptions, over-the-counter (OTC) medicines, herbal and dietary supplements, and vitamins
- best ways to keep any health conditions you have under control
- your personal goals and preferences for the health of you and your baby

Vaccinations (Shots)

Most vaccines are safe during pregnancy, and some, such as the flu vaccine and Tdap (adult tetanus, diphtheria, and acellular pertussis vaccine), are specifically recommended during pregnancy. Having the right vaccinations at the right time can help keep you healthy and help protect your baby from some diseases during the first few months of life.

GET 400 MICROGRAMS OF FOLIC ACID EVERY DAY

Folic acid is a B vitamin. Having enough folic acid in your body at least one month before and during pregnancy can help prevent major birth defects of the developing baby's brain and spine (anencephaly and spina bifida). The Centers for Disease Control and Prevention (CDC) urges all people who can become pregnant to get 400 mcg of folic acid each day from fortified foods or supplements or a combination of the two, in addition to a varied diet rich in folate.

STOP DRINKING ALCOHOL, SMOKING, AND USING CERTAIN DRUGS

Smoking, drinking alcohol, and using certain drugs can cause many problems during pregnancy, such as premature birth, birth defects, and infant death.

If you are trying to get pregnant and cannot stop drinking, smoking, or using drugs, contact your health-care provider, local Alcoholics Anonymous, or local alcohol treatment center.

AVOID TOXIC SUBSTANCES AND ENVIRONMENTAL CONTAMINANTS

Avoid harmful chemicals, environmental contaminants, and other toxic substances such as synthetic chemicals, some metals, fertilizer, bug spray, and cat or rodent feces around the home and in the workplace. These substances can hurt the reproductive systems of men and women. They can make it more difficult to get pregnant. Exposure to even small amounts during pregnancy, infancy, childhood, or puberty can lead to diseases.

REACH AND MAINTAIN A HEALTHY WEIGHT

People who are overweight or obese have a higher risk of many serious conditions, including complications during pregnancy, heart disease, type 2 diabetes, and certain cancers (endometrial, breast, and colon). People who are underweight are also at risk for serious health problems.

The key to achieving and maintaining a healthy weight is not about short-term dietary changes. It is about a lifestyle that includes healthy eating and regular physical activity.

If you are underweight, overweight, or obese, talk with your doctor about ways to reach and maintain a healthy weight before you get pregnant.

LEARN YOUR FAMILY HISTORY

Collecting your family's health history can help you identify factors that might affect your baby during infancy or childhood or your ability to become pregnant. You might not realize that your sister's heart defect or your cousin's sickle cell disease could affect your baby, but sharing this family history information with your doctor can be important.

Based on your family health history, your doctor might refer you for genetic counseling. Other reasons for genetic counseling include having had several miscarriages, infant deaths, or trouble getting pregnant (infertility) or having a genetic condition or birth defect that occurred during a previous pregnancy.

GET MENTALLY HEALTHY

Mental health is how we think, feel, and act as we cope with life. To be at your best, you need to feel good about your life and value yourself. Everyone feels worried, anxious, sad, or stressed sometimes. However, if these feelings do not go away and they interfere with your daily life, get help. Talk with your health-care provider about your feelings and treatment options.[1]

---

[1] "Planning for Pregnancy," Centers for Disease Control and Prevention (CDC), February 15, 2023. Available online. URL: www.cdc.gov/preconception/planning.html. Accessed May 12, 2023.

Section 5.2 | Using Ovulation Predictor Kits

FERTILITY AWARENESS: THE MENSTRUAL CYCLE

Being aware of your menstrual cycle and the changes in your body that happen during this time can help you know when you are most likely to get pregnant.

The average menstrual cycle lasts 28 days. But normal cycles can vary from 21 to 35 days. The amount of time before ovulation occurs is different in every woman and even can be different from month to month in the same woman, varying from 13 to 20 days long. Learning about this part of the cycle is important because it is when ovulation and pregnancy can occur. After ovulation, every woman (unless she has a health problem that affects her periods or becomes pregnant) will have a period within 14–16 days.

CHARTING YOUR FERTILITY PATTERN

Knowing when you are most fertile will help you plan pregnancy. The following are the three ways you can keep track of your fertile times:

- **Basal body temperature method.** Basal body temperature is your temperature at rest as soon as you awake in the morning. A woman's basal body temperature rises slightly with ovulation. So, by recording this temperature daily for several months, you will be able to predict your most fertile days. Basal body temperature differs slightly from woman to woman. Anywhere from 96 °F (35.56 °C) to 98 °F (36.67 °C) orally is average before ovulation. After ovulation, most women have an oral temperature between 97 °F (36.1 °C) and 99 °F (37.2 °C). The rise in temperature can be a sudden jump or a gradual climb over a few days.

  Usually, a woman's basal body temperature rises by only 0.4–0.8 °F (−17.56 to −17.33 °C). To detect this tiny change, women must use a basal body thermometer. These thermometers are very sensitive. Most pharmacies sell them for about $10.

The rise in temperature does not show exactly when the egg is released. But almost all women have ovulated within three days after their temperatures spike. Body temperature stays at a higher level until your period starts. You are most fertile and most likely to get pregnant:

- 2–3 days before your temperature hits the highest point (ovulation)
- 12–24 hours after ovulation

  A man's sperm can live for up to three days in a woman's body. The sperm can fertilize an egg at any point during that time. Therefore, if you have unprotected sex a few days before ovulation, you could get pregnant.

  Many things can affect basal body temperature. For your chart to be useful, make sure to take your temperature every morning at about the same time. Things that can alter your temperature include the following:

  - drinking alcohol the night before
  - smoking cigarettes the night before
  - getting a poor night's sleep
  - having a fever
  - doing anything in the morning before you take your temperature—including going to the bathroom and talking on the phone

- **Calendar method**. This involves recording your menstrual cycle on a calendar for 8–12 months. The first day of your period is day one. Circle day one on the calendar. The length of your cycle may vary from month to month. So write down the total number of days it lasts each time. Using this record, you can find the days you are most fertile in the months ahead:

  - To find out the first day when you are most fertile, subtract 18 from the total number of days in your shortest cycle. Take this new number and count ahead that many days from the first day of your next period. Draw an X through this date on your calendar. The X marks the first day you are likely to be fertile.

- To find out the last day when you are most fertile, subtract 11 from the total number of days in your longest cycle. Take this new number and count ahead that many days from the first day of your next period. Draw an X through this date on your calendar. The time between the two Xs is your most fertile window.

  This method should always be used along with other fertility awareness methods, especially if your cycles are not always the same length.

- **Cervical mucus method (also known as the "ovulation method").** This involves being aware of the changes in your cervical mucus throughout the month. The hormones that control the menstrual cycle also change the kind and amount of mucus you have before and during ovulation. Right after your period, there are usually a few days when there is no mucus present or "dry days." As the egg starts to mature, mucus increases in the vagina, appears at the vaginal opening, and is white or yellow and cloudy and sticky. The greatest amount of mucus appears just before ovulation. During these "wet days," it becomes clear and slippery, such as raw egg whites. Sometimes, it can be stretched apart. This is when you are most fertile. About four days after the wet days begin, the mucus changes again. There will be much less, and it becomes sticky and cloudy. You might have a few more dry days before your period returns. Describe changes in your mucus on a calendar. Label the days "Sticky," "Dry," or "Wet." You are most fertile at the first sign of wetness after your period or a day or two before wetness begins.

  The cervical mucus method is less reliable for some women. Women who are breastfeeding, are taking hormonal birth control (such as the pill), are using

feminine hygiene products, have vaginitis or sexually transmitted infections (STIs), or have had surgery on the cervix should not rely on this method.
To most accurately track your fertility, use a combination of all three methods. This is called the "symptothermal method." You can also purchase over-the-counter ovulation kits or fertility monitors to help find the best time to conceive. These kits work by detecting surges in a specific hormone called "luteinizing hormone," which triggers ovulation.

WHEN TO SEE YOUR DOCTOR

You should talk to your doctor about your fertility if:

- you are younger than 35 and have not been able to conceive after one year of frequent sex without birth control
- you are aged 35 or older and have not been able to conceive after six months of frequent sex without birth control
- you believe you or your partner might have fertility problems in the future (even before you begin trying to get pregnant)
- you or your partner has a problem with sexual function or libido

Happily, doctors are able to help many infertile couples go on to have babies.[2]

OVULATION SALIVA TEST
What Does This Test Do?

This is a home-use test kit to predict ovulation by looking at patterns formed by your saliva. When your estrogen increases near your time of ovulation, your dried saliva may form a fern-shaped pattern.

---

[2] Office on Women's Health (OWH), "Trying to Conceive," U.S. Department of Health and Human Services (HHS), February 22, 2021. Available online. URL: www.womenshealth.gov/pregnancy/you-get-pregnant/trying-conceive. Accessed May 12, 2023.

What Type of Test Is This?

This is a qualitative test—you find out whether or not you may be near your ovulation time, not if you will definitely become pregnant.

Why Should You Do This Test?

You should do this test if you want to know when you expect to ovulate and are in the most fertile part of your menstrual cycle. This test can be used to help you plan to become pregnant. You should not use this test to help prevent pregnancy because it is not reliable for that purpose.

How Accurate Is This Test?

This test may not work well for you. Some of the reasons are as follows:
- Not all women may show a fern-shaped pattern in the test.
- You may not be able to see the fern.
- Women who show the fern pattern on some days of their fertile period do not necessarily show the pattern on all of their fertile days.
- Formation of the fern pattern may be disrupted by:
  - smoking
  - eating
  - drinking
  - brushing your teeth
  - how you put your saliva on the slide
  - where you were when you did the test

How Do You Do This Test?

In this test, you get a small microscope with built-in or removable slides. You put some of your saliva on a glass slide, allow it to dry, and look at the pattern it makes. You will see dots and circles, a fern (full or partial), or a combination depending on where you are in your monthly cycle.

You will get your best results when you use the test within the five-day period around your expected ovulation. This period includes the two days before and the two days after your expected day of ovulation. The test is not perfect, though, and you might show the fern pattern outside of this time period or when you are pregnant. Even some men will show the fern pattern.

Is This Test Similar to the One Your Doctor Uses?

The fertility tests your doctor uses are automated, and they may give more consistent results. Your doctor may use other tests that are not yet available for home use (i.e., blood and urine laboratory tests) and information about your history to get a better view of your fertility status.

Does a Positive Test Mean You Are Ovulating?

A positive test indicates that you may be near ovulation. It does not mean that you will definitely become pregnant.

Do Negative Test Results Mean That You Are Not Ovulating?

No, there may be many reasons why you did not detect your time of ovulation. You should not use this test to help prevent pregnancy because it is not reliable for that purpose.[3]

---

[3] "Ovulation (Saliva Test)," U.S. Food and Drug Administration (FDA), February 4, 2018. Available online. URL: www.fda.gov/medical-devices/home-use-tests/ovulation-saliva-test. Accessed May 12, 2023.

Chapter 6 | Preventing Unintended Pregnancies

Chapter Contents

UNINTENDED PREGNANCY

An unintended pregnancy is a pregnancy that is either unwanted, such as pregnancy that occurs when no children or no more children are desired, or the pregnancy is mistimed (the pregnancy occurred earlier than desired). The concept of unintended pregnancy helps in understanding the fertility of populations and the unmet need for contraception, also known as "birth control," and "family planning." Most unintended pregnancies result from not using contraception or from not using it consistently or correctly.

To help women, men, and couples prevent or achieve pregnancy, it is essential to understand their pregnancy intentions or reproductive life plan. A reproductive life plan may include personal goals about becoming pregnant, such as whether they want to have any or more children and the desired timing and spacing of those children. A reproductive life plan may help identify reproductive health-care needs that include contraceptive services, pregnancy testing, and counseling to help become pregnant or manage a pregnancy with prenatal and delivery care.

PREGNANCY PREVENTION

Women who choose to delay or prevent pregnancy should be offered contraceptive services that include:

- a full range of contraceptive methods approved by the U.S. Food and Drug Administration (FDA)
- a brief assessment to identify the contraceptive methods that are safe for the client
- contraceptive counseling to help a client choose a method of contraception and learn how to use it correctly and consistently
- provision of one or more selected contraceptive methods, preferably on-site but by referral if necessary

PRECONCEPTION HEALTH PROMOTION

Women of reproductive age can make choices about their health and health care that help keep themselves healthy and, if they choose to be pregnant, have a healthy baby. Adopting healthy behaviors is the first step women can take to get ready for the healthiest pregnancy possible.

Unintended pregnancy is associated with an increased risk of problems for the mom and baby. If the mom was not planning to get pregnant, she may have unhealthy behaviors or delay getting health care during the pregnancy, which could affect the health of the baby. Therefore, it is important for all women of reproductive age to adopt the following healthy behaviors:

- Take folic acid.
- Maintain a healthy diet and weight.
- Be physically active regularly.
- Quit tobacco use.
- Refrain from excessive alcohol drinking.
- Abstain from alcohol if pregnant or planning to become pregnant.
- Take only medicines prescribed by your doctor.
- Talk to your health-care provider about screening and proper management of chronic diseases.
- Visit your health-care provider to receive recommended health care for your age, learn about possible health risks, and discuss if or when you are considering becoming pregnant.
- Use effective contraception correctly and consistently if you are sexually active but choose to delay or avoid pregnancy.[1]

OPTIONS FOR UNPLANNED PREGNANCY

If you have an unplanned pregnancy, you might not know what to do next. You might worry that the father would not welcome

---

[1] "Unintended Pregnancy," Centers for Disease Control and Prevention (CDC), March 27, 2023. Available online. URL: www.cdc.gov/reproductivehealth/contraception/unintendedpregnancy/index.htm. Accessed June 29, 2023.

the news. You might not be sure you can afford to care for a baby. You might worry if past choices you have made, such as drinking or drug use, will affect your unborn baby's health. You might be concerned that having a baby will keep you from finishing school or pursuing a career. If you are pregnant after being raped, you might feel ashamed, numb, or afraid. You might wonder what options you have. Here are some next steps to help you move forward:

- Start taking care of yourself right away. Take 400–800 mcg (or 0.4–0.8 mg) of folic acid every day. Stop alcohol, tobacco, and drug use.
- Schedule a doctor's visit to confirm your pregnancy. Discuss your health and issues that could affect your pregnancy. Ask for help quitting smoking if you smoke. Find out what you can do to take care of yourself and your unborn baby.
- Ask your doctor to recommend a counselor who you can talk to about your situation.
- Seek support from someone you trust and respect.

PARTNER ABUSE AND UNPLANNED PREGNANCY

Unplanned pregnancy is common among abused women. Research has found that some abusers force their partners to have sex without birth control and/or sabotage the birth control their partners are using, leading to unplanned pregnancy. If you have an abusive partner, get help now. Violence can hurt you and your pregnancy and have long-lasting effects on your children. About one in two men who abuse their wives also abuses their children. And children who grow up with violence in the home are more likely to become abusers as adults and have physical and emotional problems.[2]

---

[2] "Unplanned Pregnancy," Office on Women's Health (OWH), February 22, 2021. Available online. URL: www. womenshealth.gov/pregnancy/you-get-pregnant/unplanned-pregnancy. Accessed June 29, 2023.

Section 6.2 | **Understanding Birth Control and Contraception**

Contraception is the prevention of pregnancy. Contraception, or birth control, also allows couples to plan the timing of pregnancy. Some methods can also protect against infections. Choosing a particular method of birth control depends on many factors, including a woman's overall health, age, frequency of sexual activity, number of sexual partners, desire to have children in the future, and family medical history. Individuals should work with their health-care provider to choose a method that is best for them. It is also important to discuss birth control methods with one's sexual partner.

General methods of contraception include the following:

- **Barrier method.** This physically interferes with conception by keeping the egg and sperm apart.
- **Hormonal method.** This regulates ovulation by changing the balance of hormones related to the development and release of the egg and changes cervical mucus to impair sperm function or transport.
- **Intrauterine devices (IUDs).** These are small devices inserted into the uterus that change the conditions in the cervix and uterus to prevent pregnancy as well as inhibit the transit of sperm from the cervix to the fallopian tubes.
- **Sterilization.** These are surgical procedures that make a woman permanently unable to get pregnant and a man unable to get a woman pregnant.

Some forms of birth control combine methods, such as IUDs, that also release hormones. Some types of birth control may carry serious risks for some individuals. For specific information about birth control, individuals should talk to their health-care providers.

WHAT ARE THE DIFFERENT TYPES OF CONTRACEPTION?

There are many different types of contraception, but not all types are appropriate for all situations. The most appropriate method of birth control depends on an individual's overall health, age, frequency of sexual activity, number of sexual partners, desire to have children in the future, and family history of certain diseases.

Long-Acting Reversible Contraception
INTRAUTERINE METHODS
An intrauterine system (IUS) is a small, T-shaped device that is inserted into the uterus to prevent pregnancy. A health-care provider inserts the device. An IUD can remain in place and function effectively for many years at a time. After the recommended length of time or when the woman no longer needs or desires contraception, a health-care provider removes or replaces the device.

- A hormonal IUD or IUS releases progestin hormone (levonorgestrel) into the uterus. The released hormone causes thickening of the cervical mucus, inhibits sperm from reaching or fertilizing the egg, thins the uterine lining, and may prevent the ovaries from releasing eggs. The failure rate of a hormonal IUS is less than 1 percent; however, a small percentage of women may experience expulsion of the device and have to have it reinserted. Some research studies also suggest that these IUDs maintain their effectiveness for up to a year beyond their recommended use period. This method may also be used to treat heavy menstrual bleeding because the hormone often reduces or eliminates uterine bleeding.
- A copper IUD prevents sperm from reaching and fertilizing the egg, and it may prevent the egg from attaching in the womb. If fertilization of the egg does occur, the physical presence of the device prevents the fertilized egg from implanting into the lining of the uterus. The failure and expulsion/reinsertion rates of a copper IUD are similar to those of a hormonal IUD. Copper IUDs may remain in the body for 10 years. A copper IUD is not recommended for women who may be pregnant, have pelvic infections, or had uterine perforations during previous IUD insertions. It is also not recommended for women who have cervical

cancer or cancer of the uterus, unexplained vaginal bleeding, or pelvic tuberculosis. The ParaGard® is the only copper IUD approved by the U.S. Food and Drug Administration (FDA).

IMPLANTS

Implants are implantable rods. Each rod is matchstick-sized, flexible, and plastic. The method has a failure rate of less than 1 percent. A physician surgically inserts the rod under the skin of the woman's upper arm.

The rod releases progestin and can remain implanted for up to five years. Implanon® and Nexplanon®, which release etonogestrel, are the only implantable rods available in the United States. A two-rod method, Jadelle®, which releases levonorgestrel, is FDA-approved but not currently distributed in America. A new levonorgestrel-releasing, two-rod method, Sino-implant (II)®, is in clinical development.

Hormonal Methods
SHORT-ACTING HORMONAL METHODS

Hormonal methods of birth control use hormones to regulate or stop ovulation and prevent pregnancy. Ovulation is the biological process in which the ovary releases an egg, making it available for fertilization. Hormones can be introduced into the body through various methods, including pills, injections, skin patches, transdermal gels, vaginal rings, IUSs, and implantable rods. Depending on the types of hormones that are used, these methods can prevent ovulation; thicken cervical mucus, which helps block sperm from reaching the egg; or thin the lining of the uterus. Health-care providers prescribe and monitor hormonal contraceptives.

Short-acting hormonal methods (e.g., injectables, pills, patches, rings) are highly effective if used perfectly, but in typical use, they have a range of failure rates.

- **Injectable birth control.** This method involves injection of progestin, Depo-Provera® (depot medroxyprogesterone acetate (DMPA)), given in the

62

arm or buttocks once every three months. This method of birth control can cause a temporary loss of bone density, particularly in adolescents. However, this bone loss is generally regained after discontinuing the use of DMPA. Most patients using injectable birth control should eat a diet rich in calcium and vitamin D or take vitamin supplements while using this medication. A new self-injectable formulation of DMPA, Sayana® Press, is approved in the United Kingdom and is expected to be approved more widely in the near future. This subcutaneous injectable product has a lower amount of hormone and may be more acceptable for some users.

- **Progestin-only pills (POPs).** A woman takes one pill daily, preferably at the same time each day. POPs may interfere with ovulation or with sperm function. POPs thicken cervical mucus, making it difficult for sperm to swim into the uterus or to enter the fallopian tube. POPs alter the normal cyclical changes in the uterine lining and may result in unscheduled or breakthrough bleeding. These hormones do not appear to be associated with an increased risk of blood clots.

COMBINED HORMONAL METHODS

Combined hormonal methods contain synthetic estrogen (ethinyl estradiol) and one of the many progestins approved in the United States. All of the products work by inhibiting ovulation and thickening cervical mucus. The combined estrogen/progestin drugs can be delivered by pills, a patch, or a vaginal ring. The combined hormonal methods have some medical risks, such as blood clots, that are associated with the synthetic estrogen in the product. These risks have not been observed with progestin-only hormonal methods, such as injectable birth control, POPs, or hormonal long-acting reversible contraception (LARC). Your health-care provider can discuss your risk factors and help you select the most appropriate contraceptive method for you.

- **Combined oral contraceptives (COCs; "the pill").** They contain synthetic estrogen and progestin, which function to inhibit ovulation. A woman takes one pill daily, preferably at the same time each day. Many types of oral contraceptives are available, and a health-care provider helps determine which type best meets a woman's needs.
- **Contraceptive patch.** This is a thin, plastic patch that sticks to the skin and releases hormones through the skin into the bloodstream. The patch is placed on the lower abdomen, buttocks, outer arm, or upper body. A new patch is applied once a week for three weeks, and no patch is used on the fourth week to enable menstruation. Ortho Evra® is the only patch that is FDA-approved.
- **Vaginal ring.** The ring is thin, flexible, and approximately 2 inches in diameter. It delivers a combination of ethinyl estradiol and progestin. The ring is inserted into the vagina, where it continually releases hormones for three weeks. The woman removes it for the fourth week and reinserts a new ring seven days later. Risks for this method of contraception are similar to those for the COC pills. A vaginal ring may not be recommended for women with certain health conditions, including high blood pressure, heart disease, or certain types of cancer. The NuvaRing® is the only FDA-approved vaginal ring. A new contraceptive vaginal ring that can be used for 13 cycles is under clinical development.

Barrier Methods

Designed to prevent sperm from entering the uterus, barrier methods are removable and may be an option for women who cannot use hormonal methods of contraception. Failure rates for barrier methods differ depending on the method.

Types of barrier methods that do not require a health-care provider visit include the following:

- **Male condoms.** This condom is a thin sheath that covers the penis to collect sperm and prevent it from entering the woman's body. Male condoms are generally made of latex or polyurethane, but a natural alternative is lambskin (made from the intestinal membrane of lambs). Latex or polyurethane condoms reduce the risk of spreading sexually transmitted diseases (STDs). Lambskin condoms do not prevent STDs. Male condoms are disposed of after a single use.
- **Female condoms.** These are thin, flexible plastic pouches. A portion of the condom is inserted into a woman's vagina before intercourse to prevent sperm from entering the uterus. The female condom also reduces the risk of STDs. Female condoms are disposed of after a single use.
- **Contraceptive sponges.** These are soft, disposable, spermicide-filled foam sponges. One is inserted into the vagina before intercourse. The sponge helps block sperm from entering the uterus, and the spermicide also kills the sperm cells. The sponge should be left in place for at least six hours after intercourse and then removed within 30 hours after intercourse. The Today® Vaginal Contraceptive Sponge is the only sponge approved by the FDA.
- **Spermicides.** A spermicide can kill sperm cells. A spermicide can be used alone or in combination with a diaphragm or cervical cap. The most common spermicidal agent is a chemical called "nonoxynol-9" (N-9). It is available in several concentrations and forms, including foam, jelly, cream, suppository, and film. A spermicide should be inserted into the vagina close to the uterus no more than 30 minutes prior to intercourse and left in place 6–8 hours after intercourse to prevent pregnancy. Spermicides do not prevent the

transmission of STDs and may cause allergic reactions or vaginitis.

Methods that require a health-care provider visit include the following:

- **Diaphragms.** Each diaphragm is a shallow, flexible cup made of latex or soft rubber that is inserted into the vagina before intercourse, blocking sperm from entering the uterus. Spermicidal cream or jelly should be used with a diaphragm. The diaphragm should remain in place for 6–8 hours after intercourse to prevent pregnancy, but it should be removed within 24 hours. Traditional latex diaphragms must be the correct size to work properly, and a health-care provider can determine the proper fit. A diaphragm should be replaced after one or two years. Women also need to be measured for a new diaphragm after giving birth, having pelvic surgery, or gaining or losing more than 15 pounds. Newer diaphragms, such as Caya®, are designed to fit most women and do not require fitting by a health-care provider.
- **Cervical caps.** These are similar to diaphragms but are smaller and more rigid. The cervical cap is a thin silicone cup that is inserted into the vagina before intercourse to block sperm from entering the uterus. As with a diaphragm, the cervical cap should be used with spermicidal cream or jelly. The cap must remain in place for 6–8 hours after intercourse to prevent pregnancy, but it should be removed within 48 hours. Cervical caps come in different sizes, and a health-care provider determines the proper fit. With proper care, a cervical cap can be used for two years before replacement. FemCap is the only cervical cap approved by the FDA.

Emergency Contraception

Emergency contraception can be used after unprotected intercourse or if a condom breaks.

- **Copper IUD.** This is the most effective method of emergency contraception. The device can be inserted within 120 hours of unprotected intercourse. The method is nearly 100 percent effective at preventing pregnancy and has the added benefit of providing a highly effective method of contraception for as long as the device remains in place. There are very few contraindications to the use of the copper IUD, and there are no issues related to weight or obesity associated with the effectiveness of the method.

- **Emergency contraceptive pills (ECPs)**. These are hormonal pills, taken either as a single dose or two doses 12 hours apart, that are intended for use in the event of unprotected intercourse. If taken prior to ovulation, the pills can delay or inhibit ovulation for at least five days to allow the sperm to become inactive. They also cause thickening of cervical mucus and may interfere with sperm function. ECPs should be taken as soon as possible after semen exposure and should not be used as a regular contraceptive method. Pregnancy can occur if the pills are taken after ovulation or if the woman has unprotected sex in the same cycle.

Sterilization

Sterilization is a permanent form of birth control that either prevents a woman from getting pregnant or prevents a man from releasing sperm. A health-care provider must perform the sterilization procedure, which usually involves surgery. These procedures are usually not reversible.

- A sterilization implant is a nonsurgical method for permanently blocking the fallopian tubes. A health-care provider threads a thin tube through the vagina and into the uterus to place a soft, flexible insert into each fallopian tube. No incisions are necessary. During the next three months, scar tissue forms around the inserts and blocks the fallopian tubes so that sperm cannot reach an egg. After three months, a health-care provider conducts tests to ensure that scar tissue has fully blocked the fallopian tubes. A backup method of contraception is used until the tests show that the tubes are fully blocked.

• Tubal ligation is a surgical procedure in which a doctor cuts, ties, or seals the fallopian tubes. This procedure blocks the path between the ovaries and the uterus. The sperm cannot reach the egg to fertilize it, and the egg cannot reach the uterus.

• Vasectomy is a surgical procedure that cuts, closes, or blocks the vas deferens. This procedure blocks the path between the testes and the urethra. The sperm cannot leave the testes and cannot reach the egg. It can take as long as three months for the procedure to be fully effective. A backup method of contraception is used until tests confirm that there is no sperm in the semen.

HOW EFFECTIVE IS CONTRACEPTION?

Different methods of contraception have different rates of effectiveness in preventing pregnancy.

Contraception is most effective when used correctly and consistently. The failure rate increases if a method of contraception is used incorrectly or inconsistently. Only male and female condoms are effective at reducing the spread of STDs.

CAN CONTRACEPTION REDUCE THE RISK OF GETTING AN INFECTION?

Only condoms have been proven to reduce the risk of getting some STDs.

According to the U.S. Department of Health and Human Services (HHS) Office on Women's Health, the male latex condom is the best method for protecting against STDs, including human immunodeficiency virus (HIV)/acquired immunodeficiency syndrome (AIDS). Polyurethane condoms are an effective alternative if either partner has a latex allergy. Natural/lambskin condoms do not prevent the spread of STDs because of the presence of tiny pores (holes) that may allow viruses, such as HIV, hepatitis B, and herpes, to spread.

The female condom has properties similar to the male condom, but researchers have not studied its effectiveness in reducing the spread of STDs as much as they have studied the male condom.

The most common STD is the human papillomavirus (HPV). No method of contraception can fully prevent the transmission of the HPV because it can infect areas not covered by a condom. However, using a condom with every sex act can lower the risk of transmission.

If you have questions about birth control and STDs, talk to your health-care provider. If you think you may have an STD, you should see your health-care provider.[3]

Section 6.3 | Mifepristone (The Morning-After Pill)

WHAT IS MIFEPRISTONE, AND HOW DOES IT WORK?

Mifepristone is a drug that blocks a hormone called "progesterone" that is needed for a pregnancy to continue. Mifepristone, when used together with another medicine called "misoprostol," is used to end a pregnancy through 10-week gestation (70 days or less since the first day of the last menstrual period). The approved mifepristone dosing regimen is as follows:

- on day one: 200 mg of mifepristone taken by mouth
- 24–48 hours after taking mifepristone: 800 mcg of misoprostol taken buccally (in the cheek pouch) at a location appropriate for the patient
- about 7–14 days after taking mifepristone: follow-up with the health-care provider

---

[3] "Contraception and Birth Control," *Eunice Kennedy Shriver* National Institute of Child Health and Human Development (NICHD), January 31, 2017. Available online. URL: www.nichd.nih.gov/health/topics/contraception. Accessed May 18, 2023.

WHEN DID THE U.S. FOOD AND DRUG ADMINISTRATION APPROVE MIFEPRISTONE FOR MEDICAL TERMINATION OF PREGNANCY?

The U.S. Food and Drug Administration (FDA) first approved Mifeprex (mifepristone) in September 2000 for medical termination of pregnancy through seven-week gestation, and this was extended to 10-week gestation in 2016. The FDA approved a generic version of Mifeprex, Mifepristone Tablets, 200 mg, in April 2019. The agency's approval of this generic reflects the FDA's determination that Mifepristone Tablets, 200 mg, are therapeutically equivalent to Mifeprex and can be safely substituted for Mifeprex. Like Mifeprex, the approved generic product is indicated for the medical termination of intrauterine pregnancy through 70-day gestation. The labeling for the approved generic version of Mifeprex is consistent with the labeling for Mifeprex.

WHO SHOULD NOT TAKE MIFEPRISTONE, IN A REGIMEN WITH MISOPROSTOL, FOR MEDICAL TERMINATION OF PREGNANCY?

An individual should not take mifepristone, in a regimen with misoprostol, for medical termination of pregnancy if it has been more than 70 days since the first day of their last menstrual period or if they:

- have an ectopic pregnancy (a pregnancy outside of the uterus)
- have problems with the adrenal glands (the glands near the kidneys)
- are currently being treated with long-term corticosteroid therapy (medications)
- have had an allergic reaction to mifepristone, misoprostol, or similar drugs
- have bleeding problems or are taking anticoagulant (blood thinning) drug products
- have inherited porphyria (a rare disorder that can affect the liver and other organs)
- have an intrauterine device (IUD) in place (It must be removed before taking mifepristone.)

IS IT SAFE TO USE MIFEPRISTONE?

Yes. Mifepristone is safe when used as indicated and directed and consistent with the Mifepristone Risk Evaluation and Mitigation Strategy (REMS) Program. The FDA approved Mifeprex more than 20 years ago based on a thorough and comprehensive review of the scientific evidence presented and determined that it was safe and effective for its indicated use. As of 2016, it can be used for medical termination of pregnancy up to 70 days of gestation. The FDA's periodic reviews of the postmarketing data for Mifeprex and its approved generic have not identified any new safety concerns with the use of mifepristone for medical termination of pregnancy through 70 days of gestation. As with all drugs, the FDA continues to closely monitor the postmarketing safety data on mifepristone for the medical termination of pregnancy.

WHAT SERIOUS ADVERSE EVENTS HAVE BEEN REPORTED AFTER THE USE OF MIFEPRISTONE FOR MEDICAL TERMINATION OF PREGNANCY THROUGH 10 WEEKS OF GESTATION?

The FDA has received reports of serious adverse events in patients who took mifepristone. As of June 30, 2022, there were 28 reports of deaths in patients associated with mifepristone since the product was approved in September 2000, including two cases of ectopic pregnancy (a pregnancy located outside the womb, such as in the fallopian tubes) resulting in death and several fatal cases of severe systemic infection (also called "sepsis"). The adverse events cannot with certainty be causally attributed to mifepristone because of concurrent use of other drugs, other medical or surgical treatments, coexisting medical conditions, and information gaps about patient health status and clinical management of the patient.

DOES THE U.S. FOOD AND DRUG ADMINISTRATION ENDORSE THIS DRUG PRODUCT?

The FDA does not endorse any drug product. The agency evaluates all drug applications submitted by sponsors to determine whether the data and information in an application support the approval of the application. The same standards are applied to the drug applications for Mifeprex and the approved generic Mifepristone Tablets, 200 mg, as are applied to all drug applications.

WHERE CAN PATIENTS GET MIFEPRISTONE FOR MEDICAL TERMINATION OF PREGNANCY THROUGH 10 WEEKS OF GESTATION?

Mifepristone must be prescribed by a certified prescriber who meets certain qualifications and agrees to follow certain guidelines for use. Under the Mifepristone REMS Program, mifepristone can be dispensed by a certified pharmacy or by or under the supervision of a certified prescriber.

IS MIFEPRISTONE AVAILABLE FOR OVER-THE-COUNTER USE?

No. Mifepristone for medical termination of a pregnancy through 10 weeks of gestation is currently only available by prescription. An applicant seeking to switch mifepristone for medical termination of pregnancy through 10 weeks of gestation from prescription to nonprescription (also referred to as over-the-counter (OTC)) status would need to submit this information to the FDA for evaluation. In order for a drug product to be approved for nonprescription use (including switching a prescription drug product to nonprescription marketing), the applicant must provide sufficient information demonstrating that the drug can be used safely and effectively by consumers without the supervision of a licensed health-care practitioner.

IS IT POSSIBLE FOR AN INDIVIDUAL TO BECOME PREGNANT AGAIN AFTER TAKING MIFEPRISTONE FOR MEDICAL TERMINATION OF PREGNANCY THROUGH 10 WEEKS OF GESTATION?

It is possible for an individual to become pregnant again soon after a pregnancy ends. A patient should consult with their health-care provider regarding any specific questions they may have.[4]

---

[4] "Questions and Answers on Mifepristone for Medical Termination of Pregnancy through Ten Weeks Gestation," U.S. Food and Drug Administration (FDA), January 4, 2023. Available online. URL: www.fda.gov/drugs/postmarket-drug-safety-information-patients-and-providers/questions-and-answers-mifepristone-medical-termination-pregnancy-through-ten-weeks-gestation. Accessed May 18, 2023.

Chapter 7 | Health Insurance and Pregnancy

All Health Insurance Marketplace® and Medicaid plans cover pregnancy and childbirth. This is true even if your pregnancy begins before your coverage starts.

Maternity care and newborn care—services provided before and after your child is born—are essential health benefits. This means all qualified health plans inside and outside the Marketplace must cover them.

IF YOU ARE PREGNANT OR PLANNING TO GET PREGNANT
If You Do Not Have Health Coverage

- Health coverage makes it easier to get medical checkups and screening tests to help keep both you and your baby healthy during pregnancy.
- If you qualify for a special enrollment period due to a life event such as moving or losing other coverage, you may be able to enroll in a Marketplace health plan right now. Being pregnant does not qualify you for a special enrollment period, but the birth of a child does.
- Create an account at www.healthcare.gov/create-account to apply for Marketplace coverage through the open enrollment period or a special enrollment period. If you select the option to get help paying for coverage on your application, you will be asked if you are pregnant. Reporting your pregnancy may help you and your family members get the most affordable coverage.

- If you do not qualify for a special enrollment period right now, you will be eligible to apply within 60 days of your child's birth. You can also enroll in coverage for the next plan year during the next open enrollment period this fall.
- If eligible for Medicaid or the Children's Health Insurance Program (CHIP), your coverage can begin at any time.

If You Currently Have Marketplace Coverage

- If you want to keep your current Marketplace coverage, do not report your pregnancy to the Marketplace. When filling out your application for Marketplace coverage, select the "Learn more" link when Marketplace asks if you are pregnant to read tips to help you best answer this question.
- If you keep your Marketplace coverage, be sure to update the application after you give birth to add the baby to the plan or enroll them in coverage through Medicaid or CHIP, if they qualify.
- If you report your pregnancy, you may be found eligible for free or low-cost coverage through Medicaid or the CHIP. If you are found eligible for Medicaid or CHIP, your information will be sent to the state agency, and you will not be given the option to keep your Marketplace plan.

If You May Qualify for Medicaid or the Children's Health Insurance Program

- Medicaid and the CHIP provide free or low-cost health coverage to millions of Americans, including some low-income people, families and children, and pregnant women.
- Eligibility for these programs depends on your household size, income, and citizenship or immigration status. Specific rules and benefits vary by state.

- You can apply for Medicaid or the CHIP any time during the year, not just during the annual open enrollment period.
  - You can apply in two ways: directly through your state agency or by filling out a Marketplace application and selecting that you want help paying for coverage.
- If found eligible during your pregnancy, you will be covered for at least 60 days after you give birth, depending on your state.
  - Some states offer coverage for a full 12 months after you give birth. Check with your state or view states (in blue) that offer extended coverage.
  - When your state's coverage period ends, you may no longer qualify.
  - Your state will notify you if your coverage is ending. If your coverage ends, you can apply and enroll in a Marketplace plan.
- If you have Medicaid when you give birth, your newborn is automatically enrolled in Medicaid coverage, and they will remain eligible for at least a year.

IF YOU RECENTLY GAVE BIRTH
If You Do Not Have Health Coverage

- It is important to have access to health-care services for both new parents and baby. Make sure you apply within 60 days after your baby's birth. Your plan can cover you, your baby, and any other household members.
- If you had Medicaid or CHIP coverage that ended after you gave birth (or if your state told you it will end soon), you can apply for Marketplace coverage. Losing other coverage qualifies you for a special enrollment period. When you fill out your application, select that you were found ineligible for Medicaid or the CHIP by the state agency.

If You Currently Have Marketplace Coverage

- If you already have Marketplace coverage when your baby is born, you can do the following:
  - Keep your current plan and add your baby to your coverage.
  - Create a separate enrollment group for your baby and enroll him or her in any plan for the remainder of the year.
- No matter when your child is born, you should report their birth to the Marketplace by updating your application as soon as possible. Your coverage options and potential savings may change as a result. You may qualify for more savings than you are getting now, which could lower what you pay in monthly premiums.
- When you update your application, Marketplace will also tell you if you or your baby may be eligible for Medicaid or the CHIP. If you are found eligible (or possibly eligible) for Medicaid or the CHIP and other household members are still eligible for Marketplace coverage, wait until you have confirmation from the Medicaid or CHIP agency about your eligibility and coverage start the date before you make updates to your Marketplace plan.
- Log into your account to "Report a Life Change" (www. healthcare.gov/login).

If You Have Medicaid or the Children's Health Insurance Program

- If found eligible during your pregnancy, you will be covered for at least 60 days after you give birth, depending on your state.
  - Some states offer coverage for a full 12 months after you give birth. Check with your state, or view states (in blue) that offer extended coverage.
  - When your coverage period ends, you may no longer qualify.

- Your state Medicaid or CHIP agency will notify you if your coverage is ending. As soon as you find out that your Medicaid coverage is ending, you can apply and enroll in a Marketplace plan.
- If you have Medicaid when you give birth, your newborn is automatically enrolled in Medicaid coverage, and they will remain eligible for at least a year.[1]

[1] "Health Coverage If You're Pregnant, Plan to Get Pregnant, or Recently Gave Birth," Centers for Medicare & Medicaid Services (CMS), June 21, 2013. Available online. URL: www.healthcare.gov/what-if-im-pregnant-or-plan-to-get-pregnant. Accessed May 18, 2023.

Part 2 | **Pregnancy-Related Changes and Fetal Development**

Chapter 8 | Are You Pregnant?

Chapter Contents

Section 8.1 | Signs of Pregnancy

WHAT ARE SOME COMMON SIGNS OF PREGNANCY?

The primary sign of pregnancy is missing a menstrual period or two or more consecutive periods, but many women experience other symptoms of pregnancy before they miss a period.

Missing a period does not always mean a woman is pregnant. Menstrual irregularities are common and can have a variety of causes, including taking birth control pills, conditions such as diabetes and polycystic ovary syndrome (PCOS), eating disorders, and certain medications. Women who miss a period should see their health-care provider to find out whether they are pregnant or whether they have another health problem.

Pregnancy symptoms vary from woman to woman. A woman may experience every common symptom, just a few, or none at all. Some signs of early pregnancy include the following:

- **Slight bleeding**. One study shows as many as 25 percent of pregnant women experience slight bleeding or spotting that is lighter in color than normal menstrual blood. This typically occurs at the time of implantation of the fertilized egg (about 6–12 days after conception) but is common in the first 12 weeks of pregnancy.

- **Tender, swollen breasts or nipples**. Women may notice this symptom as early as one to two weeks after conception. Hormonal changes can make the breasts sore or even tingly. The breasts feel fuller or heavier as well.

- **Fatigue**. Many women feel more tired early in pregnancy because their bodies are producing more of a hormone called "progesterone," which helps maintain the pregnancy and encourages the growth of milk-producing glands in the breasts. In addition, during pregnancy, the body pumps more blood to carry nutrients to the fetus. Pregnant women may notice fatigue as early as one week after conception.

- **Headaches.** The sudden rise of hormones may trigger headaches early in pregnancy.
- **Nausea and/or vomiting.** This symptom can start anywhere from two to eight weeks after conception and can continue throughout pregnancy. Commonly referred to as "morning sickness," it can actually occur at any time during the day.
- **Food cravings or aversions.** Sudden cravings and developing a dislike of favorite foods are both common throughout pregnancy. A food craving or aversion can last the entire pregnancy or vary throughout this period.
- **Mood swings.** Hormonal changes during pregnancy often cause sharp mood swings. These can occur as early as a few weeks after conception.
- **Frequent urination.** The need to empty the bladder more often is common throughout pregnancy. In the first few weeks of pregnancy, the body produces a hormone called "human chorionic gonadotropin," which increases blood flow to the pelvic region, causing women to have to urinate more often.

Many of these symptoms can also be signs of other conditions, the result of changing birth control pills, or effects of stress, so they do not always mean that a woman is pregnant. Women should see their health-care provider if they suspect they are pregnant.[1]

---

[1] "What Are Some Common Signs of Pregnancy?" *Eunice Kennedy Shriver* National Institute of Child Health and Human Development (NICHD), January 31, 2017. Available online. URL: www.nichd.nih.gov/health/topics/pregnancy/conditioninfo/signs. Accessed May 15, 2023.

Section 8.2 | Pregnancy Tests

If you think you may be pregnant, taking a pregnancy test as soon as the first day of your missed period can help you get the care and support you need. A home pregnancy test can tell whether you are pregnant with almost 99 percent accuracy, depending on how you use it. If a pregnancy test says you are pregnant, you should see your doctor for another test to confirm the pregnancy and talk about the next steps.

HOW SOON CAN YOU USE A HOME PREGNANCY TEST?

Some home pregnancy tests are more sensitive than others and can be taken before your missed period. But you may get more accurate results if you wait until after the first day of your missed period. This is because the amount of the pregnancy hormone, called "human chorionic gonadotropin" (hCG), in your urine increases with time. The earlier you take the test, the harder it is for the test to detect the hCG.

hCG is made when a fertilized egg implants in the uterus. This usually happens about 10 days after conception (when the man's sperm fertilizes the woman's egg).

YOUR PREGNANCY TEST SAYS YOU ARE PREGNANT. WHAT SHOULD YOU DO NEXT?

If a home pregnancy test shows that you are pregnant, you should call your doctor to schedule an appointment. Your doctor can use a blood test to tell for sure whether you are pregnant. Seeing your doctor early in your pregnancy also means you can begin prenatal care to help you and your baby stay healthy.

YOUR PREGNANCY TEST SAYS YOU ARE NOT PREGNANT. COULD YOU STILL BE PREGNANT?

Yes, it is possible you could still be pregnant. It is possible to be pregnant and to have a pregnancy test show that you are not pregnant.

The accuracy of home pregnancy test results varies from woman to woman because of the following reasons:

- Each woman ovulates at a different time in her menstrual cycle.
- The fertilized egg can implant in a woman's uterus at different times.
- Sometimes, women get false-negative results when they test too early in the pregnancy. False negative means the test says you are not pregnant when you are.
- Problems with the pregnancy can affect the amount of hCG in the urine.

If a test says you are not pregnant, take another pregnancy test in a few days. If you are pregnant, your hCG levels should double every 48 hours. If you think you are pregnant but more tests say you are not, call your doctor.

WHAT IF YOU CANNOT TELL WHETHER YOUR PREGNANCY TEST IS POSITIVE OR NEGATIVE?

Sometimes, it can be hard to tell whether the test is positive or negative. The line may be faint, or you may worry whether you peed too much or too little on the stick.

No matter how faint the line or plus sign, if you see it, you are most likely pregnant. The faintness of the line can mean you are early in your pregnancy and your hCG levels are still low.

Also, the pregnancy test should have a control line that tells you whether the test was done correctly. If the control line is blank, then the test did not work, and you should take another test.

WHAT SHOULD YOU CONSIDER WHEN BUYING A PREGNANCY TEST?

- Cost. Home pregnancy tests come in many different types. Most stores sell them over the counter (OTC; without a doctor's prescription). The cost varies depending on the brand and how many tests come in the box.

- **Accuracy.** Most tests can be taken as soon as you miss your period. Some newer, more expensive tests say they can be used four or five days before your period. Even so, they claim the best accuracy only after the date of your expected period.

WHAT ARE THE DIFFERENT TYPES OF PREGNANCY TESTS?

Pregnancy tests check for the hCG hormone in the following two ways:
- **Urine test.** This type of pregnancy test can be done at home or at a doctor's office.
- **Blood test.** This type of pregnancy test can only be done at a doctor's office. It takes longer than a urine test to get results, but it can detect a pregnancy earlier than a urine test (about 10 days after conception, compared to typically two weeks or more for a urine test). Your doctor may use one or both types of blood tests:
  - **A quantitative blood test.** Also called a "beta hCG test," this test measures the exact amount of hCG in your blood. It can find even tiny amounts of hCG. It can also tell you and your doctor how many weeks you are pregnant.
  - **A qualitative hCG blood test.** This test checks to see whether the pregnancy hormone is present or not. The qualitative hCG blood test is about as accurate as a urine test.

HOW DO YOU USE A HOME PREGNANCY TEST?

All home pregnancy tests come with written instructions. Depending on the brand you buy, the instructions may vary:
- You hold a stick in your urine stream.
- You pee into a cup and dip the stick into it.
- You pee into a cup and then use a dropper to put a few drops of the urine into a special container.

Different brands tell you to wait different amounts of time although most are around two minutes. Depending on the brand of the test, you may see a line or a plus symbol or the words "pregnant" or "not pregnant." A line or plus symbol, no matter how faint, means the result is positive.

Most tests also have a "control indicator" in the result window. This control line or symbol shows whether the test is working properly. If the control line or symbol does not appear, the test is not working properly. Look for the toll-free phone number on the package to call in case of questions about use or results.

HOW ACCURATE ARE HOME PREGNANCY TESTS?

Most home pregnancy tests claim to be up to 99 percent accurate. But the accuracy depends on the following:

- **How to use them**. Be sure to check the expiration date and follow the instructions. Wait up to 10 minutes after taking the test to check the results window. Research suggests that waiting 10 minutes will give the most accurate result.
- **When to use them**. The amount of hCG or pregnancy hormone in your urine increases with time. The earlier you take the test, the harder it is for the test to detect the hCG. Most home pregnancy tests can accurately detect pregnancy after a missed period. Also, testing your urine first thing in the morning can boost the accuracy.
- **Who uses them?** Each woman ovulates at a different time in her menstrual cycle. Plus, the fertilized egg can implant in a woman's uterus at different times. Your body makes hCG after implantation occurs. In up to 10 percent of women, implantation does not occur until after the first day of a missed period. This means home pregnancy tests can be accurate as soon as one day after a missed period for some women but not for others.
- **The brand of the test**. Some home pregnancy tests are more sensitive than others. For that reason, some tests

are better than others at detecting hCG early on. Talk to your pharmacist about which brand may be best for you.

YOU HAVE IRREGULAR PERIODS AND DO NOT KNOW WHEN YOUR NEXT PERIOD WILL START. WHEN SHOULD YOU TAKE A PREGNANCY TEST?

Most pregnancy tests claim to be the most accurate after a missed period. But irregular periods can make it hard to predict when to take the test.

Periods are considered irregular if:

- the number of days between periods is either shorter than 21 days or longer than 35 days
- the number of days in the menstrual cycle varies from month to month (e.g., your cycle may be 22 days one month and 33 days the next month)

If you have irregular periods, try counting 36 days from the start of your last menstrual cycle or four weeks from the time you had sex. At this point, if you are pregnant, your levels of hCG should be high enough to detect the pregnancy.

If your test says you are not pregnant, but you still think you may be pregnant, wait a few more days and take another pregnancy test. Or call your doctor for a blood test.

CAN ANYTHING AFFECT HOME PREGNANCY TEST RESULTS?

Yes. If you take medicine with the pregnancy hormone hCG as an active ingredient, you may get a false-positive test result. A false positive is when a test says you are pregnant when you are not.

Some examples of medicines with hCG include certain medicines for infertility. If you are taking medicine to help you get pregnant, you may want to see your doctor for a pregnancy test.

Most medicines should not affect the results of a home pregnancy test. This includes OTC and prescription medicines such as birth control and antibiotics. Also, alcohol and illegal drugs do not affect pregnancy test results.

HOW DO PREGNANCY TESTS WORK?

All pregnancy tests work by detecting the pregnancy hormone, hCG, in the urine or blood. This hormone is present only when a woman is pregnant. If the pregnancy test detects hCG, it will say you are pregnant.

hCG is made when a fertilized egg implants in the uterus. This usually happens about 10 days after conception (when the man's sperm fertilizes the woman's egg). The amount of hCG builds up quickly in your body with each passing day you are pregnant.

So, if you take a home pregnancy test too soon after implantation, your hCG level may not be high enough to detect the pregnancy. If the test says you are not pregnant, take another pregnancy test in a few days.[2]

---

[2] Office on Women's Health (OWH), "Pregnancy Tests," U.S. Department of Health and Human Services (HHS), February 22, 2021. Available online. URL: www.womenshealth.gov/a-z-topics/pregnancy-tests. Accessed May 15, 2023.

Chapter 9 | The Three Trimesters of Pregnancy: You and Your Baby

Pregnancy lasts about 40 weeks, counting from the first day of your last normal period. The weeks are grouped into three trimesters. Find out what is happening with you and your baby in these three stages.

FIRST TRIMESTER (WEEKS 1–12)

During the first trimester, your body undergoes many changes. Hormonal changes affect almost every organ system in your body. These changes can trigger symptoms even in the very first weeks of pregnancy. Your period stopping is a clear sign that you are pregnant. Other changes may include:

- extreme tiredness
- tender, swollen breasts (Your nipples might also stick out.)
- upset stomach with or without throwing up (morning sickness)
- cravings or distaste for certain foods
- mood swings
- constipation (trouble having bowel movements)
- need to pass urine more often
- headache
- heartburn
- weight gain or loss

As your body changes, you might need to make changes to your daily routine, such as going to bed earlier or eating frequent, small meals. Fortunately, most of these discomforts will go away as your pregnancy progresses. And some women might not feel any discomfort at all. If you have been pregnant before, you might feel differently this time around. Just as each woman is different, so is each pregnancy.

From Four to Five Weeks
- Your baby's brain and spinal cord have begun to form.
- The heart begins to form.
- Arm and leg buds appear.
- Your baby is now an embryo and one twenty-fifth inch long.

At Eight Weeks
- All major organs and external body structures have begun to form.
- Your baby's heart beats with a regular rhythm.
- The arms and legs grow longer, and fingers and toes have begun to form.
- The sex organs begin to form.
- The eyes have moved forward on the face, and eyelids have formed.
- The umbilical cord is clearly visible.
- At the end of eight weeks, your baby is a fetus and looks more like a human. Your baby is nearly 1 inch long and weighs less than one-eighth ounce.

At 12 Weeks
- The nerves and muscles begin to work together. Your baby can make a fist.
- The external sex organs show if your baby is a boy or a girl. A woman who has an ultrasound in the second trimester or later might be able to find out the baby's sex.

- Eyelids close to protect the developing eyes. They will not open again until the 28th week.
- Head growth has slowed, and your baby is much longer. Now, at about 3 inches long, your baby weighs almost an ounce.

SECOND TRIMESTER (WEEKS 13–28)

Most women find the second trimester of pregnancy easier than the first. But it is just as important to stay informed about your pregnancy during these months.

You might notice that symptoms such as nausea and fatigue are going away. But other new, more noticeable changes to your body are now happening. Your abdomen will expand as the baby continues to grow. And, before this trimester is over, you will feel your baby beginning to move.

As your body changes to make room for your growing baby, you may have:

- body aches, such as back, abdomen, groin, or thigh pain
- stretch marks on your abdomen, breasts, thighs, or buttocks
- darkening of the skin around your nipples
- a line on the skin running from the belly button to the pubic hairline
- patches of darker skin, usually over the cheeks, forehead, nose, or upper lip (Patches often match on both sides of the face. This is sometimes called the "mask of pregnancy.")
- numb or tingling hands, called "carpal tunnel syndrome" (CTS)
- itching on the abdomen, palms, and soles of the feet. (Call your doctor if you have nausea, loss of appetite, vomiting, jaundice, or fatigue combined with itching. These can be signs of a serious liver problem.)
- swelling of the ankles, fingers, and face (If you notice any sudden or extreme swelling or if you gain a lot of weight really quickly, call your doctor right away. This could be a sign of preeclampsia.)

At 16 Weeks

- Muscle tissue and bone continue to form, creating a more complete skeleton.
- Skin begins to form. You can nearly see through it.
- Meconium develops in your baby's intestinal tract. This will be your baby's first bowel movement.
- Your baby makes sucking motions with the mouth (sucking reflex).
- Your baby reaches a length of about 4–5 inches and weighs almost 3 ounces.

At 20 Weeks

- Your baby is more active. You might feel slight fluttering.
- Your baby is covered by fine, downy hair called "lanugo" and a waxy coating called "vernix." This protects the forming skin underneath.
- Eyebrows, eyelashes, fingernails, and toenails have formed. Your baby can even scratch itself.
- Your baby can hear and swallow.
- Now halfway through your pregnancy, your baby is about 6 inches long and weighs about 9 ounces.

At 24 Weeks

- The bone marrow begins to make blood cells.
- Taste buds form on your baby's tongue.
- Footprints and fingerprints have formed.
- Real hair begins to grow on your baby's head.
- The lungs are formed but do not work.
- The hands and startle reflex develop.
- Your baby sleeps and wakes regularly.
- If your baby is a boy, his testicles begin to move from the abdomen into the scrotum. If your baby is a girl, her uterus and ovaries are in place, and a lifetime supply of eggs has formed in the ovaries.
- Your baby stores fat and has gained quite a bit of weight. Now, at about 12 inches long, your baby weighs about 1½ pounds.

THIRD TRIMESTER (WEEKS 29–40)

You are in the home stretch. Some of the same discomforts you had in your second trimester will continue. Plus, many women find breathing difficult and notice they have to go to the bathroom even more often. This is because the baby is getting bigger, and it is putting more pressure on your organs. Do not worry, your baby is fine, and these problems will lessen once you give birth.

Some new body changes you might notice in the third trimester include:

- shortness of breath
- heartburn
- swelling of the ankles, fingers, and face (If you notice any sudden or extreme swelling or if you gain a lot of weight really quickly, call your doctor right away. This could be a sign of preeclampsia.)
- hemorrhoids
- tender breasts, which may leak a watery premilk called "colostrum"
- stuck-out belly button
- trouble sleeping
- the baby "dropping" or moving lower in your abdomen
- contractions, which can be a sign of real or false labor

As you near your due date, your cervix becomes thinner and softer (called "effacing"). This is a normal, natural process that helps the birth canal (vagina) to open during the birthing process. Your doctor will check your progress with a vaginal exam as you near your due date.

At 32 Weeks

- Your baby's bones are fully formed but still soft.
- Your baby's kicks and jabs are forceful.
- The eyes can open and close and sense changes in light.
- Lungs are not fully formed, but practice "breathing" movements occur.
- Your baby's body begins to store vital minerals, such as iron and calcium.

- Lanugo begins to fall off.
- Your baby is gaining weight quickly, about one-half pounds a week. Now, your baby is about 15–17 inches long and weighs about 4–4½ pounds.

At 36 Weeks

- The protective waxy coating called "vernix" gets thicker.
- Body fat increases. Your baby is getting bigger and bigger and has less space to move around. Movements are less forceful, but you will feel stretches and wiggles.
- Your baby is about 16–19 inches long and weighs about 6–6½ pounds.

During Weeks 37–40

- At 39 weeks, your baby is considered full-term. Your baby's organs are ready to function on their own.
- As you near your due date, your baby may turn into a head-down position for birth. Most babies "present" head down.
- At birth, your baby may weigh somewhere between 6 pounds 2 ounces and 9 pounds 2 ounces and be 19–21 inches long. Most full-term babies fall within these ranges. But healthy babies come in many different sizes.[1]

---

[1] Office on Women's Health (OWH), "Stages of Pregnancy," U.S. Department of Health and Human Services (HHS), February 22, 2021. Available online. URL: www.womenshealth.gov/pregnancy/youre-pregnant-now-what/stages-pregnancy. Accessed May 15, 2023.

Chapter 10 | Physical Changes during Pregnancy

Chapter Contents

Section 10.1 | Common Pregnancy Discomforts

Everyone expects pregnancy to bring an expanding waistline. But many women are surprised by the other body changes that pop up. Get the lowdown on stretch marks, weight gain, heartburn, and other "joys" of pregnancy. It is important to find out what you can do to feel better.

BODY ACHES

As your uterus expands, you may feel aches and pains in the back, abdomen, groin area, and thighs. Many women also have back-aches and aching near the pelvic bone due to the pressure of the baby's head, increased weight, and loosening joints. Some pregnant women complain of pain that runs from the lower back, down the back of one leg, to the knee or foot. This is called "sciatica." It is thought to occur when the uterus puts pressure on the sciatic nerve.

What Might Help?

- lying down
- taking rest
- applying heat

Call the doctor if the pain does not get better.

BREAST CHANGES

A woman's breasts increase in size and fullness during pregnancy. As the due date approaches, hormone changes will cause your breasts to get even bigger to prepare for breastfeeding. Your breasts may feel full, heavy, or tender.

In the third trimester, some pregnant women begin to leak colostrum from their breasts. Colostrum is the first milk that your breasts produce for the baby. It is a thick, yellowish fluid containing antibodies that protect newborns from infection.

What Might Help?
- wearing a maternity bra with good support
- putting pads in bra to absorb leakage

Tell your doctor if you feel a lump or have nipple changes or discharge (that is not colostrum) or skin changes.

CONSTIPATION

Many pregnant women complain of constipation. Signs of constipation include having hard, dry stools; fewer than three bowel movements per week; and painful bowel movements.

Higher levels of hormones due to pregnancy slow down digestion and relax muscles in the bowels, leaving many women constipated. Plus, the pressure of the expanding uterus on the bowels can contribute to constipation.

What Might Help?
- drinking 8–10 glasses of water daily
- not drinking caffeine
- eating fiber-rich foods, such as fresh or dried fruit, raw vegetables, and whole-grain cereals and breads
- trying mild physical activity

Tell your doctor if constipation does not go away.

DIZZINESS

Many pregnant women complain of dizziness and light-headedness throughout their pregnancies. Fainting is rare but does happen even in some healthy pregnant women. There are many reasons for these symptoms. The growth of more blood vessels in early pregnancy, the pressure of the expanding uterus on blood vessels, and the body's increased need for food can all make a pregnant woman feel light-headed and dizzy.

What Might Help?
- standing up slowly
- avoiding standing for too long
- not skipping meals
- lying on your left side
- wearing loose clothing

Call your doctor if you feel faint and have vaginal bleeding or abdominal pain.

FATIGUE AND SLEEP PROBLEMS

During your pregnancy, you might feel tired even after you have had a lot of sleep. Many women find they are exhausted in the first trimester. Do not worry. This is normal! This is your body's way of telling you that you need more rest. In the second trimester, tiredness is usually replaced with a feeling of well-being and energy. But, in the third trimester, exhaustion often sets in again. As you get larger, sleeping may become more difficult. The baby's movements, bathroom runs, and an increase in the body's metabolism might interrupt or disturb your sleep. Leg cramping can also interfere with a good night's sleep.

What Might Help?
- lying on your left side
- using pillows for support, such as behind your back, tucked between your knees, and under your tummy
- practicing good sleep habits, such as going to bed and getting up at the same time each day and using your bed only for sleep and sex
- going to bed a little earlier
- napping if you are not able to get enough sleep at night
- drinking needed fluids earlier in the day, so you can drink less in the hours before bed

HEARTBURN AND INDIGESTION

Hormones and the pressure of the growing uterus cause indigestion and heartburn. Pregnancy hormones slow down the muscles of the digestive tract. So food tends to move more slowly, and digestion is sluggish. This causes many pregnant women to feel bloated.

Hormones also relax the valve that separates the esophagus from the stomach. This allows food and acids to come back up from the stomach to the esophagus. The food and acid cause the burning feeling of heartburn. As your baby gets bigger, the uterus pushes on the stomach, making heartburn more common in later pregnancy.

What Might Help?

- eating several small meals instead of three large meals—eat slowly
- drinking fluids between meals—not with meals
- not eating greasy and fried foods
- avoiding citrus fruits or juices and spicy foods
- not eating or drinking within a few hours of bedtime
- not lying down right after meals

Call your doctor if symptoms do not improve after trying these suggestions. Ask your doctor about using an antacid.

HEMORRHOIDS

Hemorrhoids are swollen and bulging veins in the rectum. They can cause itching, pain, and bleeding. Up to 50 percent of pregnant women get hemorrhoids. Hemorrhoids are common during pregnancy for many reasons. During pregnancy, blood volume increases greatly, which can cause veins to enlarge. The expanding uterus also puts pressure on the veins in the rectum. Plus, constipation can worsen hemorrhoids. Hemorrhoids usually improve after delivery.

What Might Help?

- drinking lots of fluids
- eating fiber-rich foods, such as whole grains, raw or cooked leafy green vegetables, and fruits

- trying not to strain with bowel movements
- talking to your doctor about using products such as witch hazel to soothe hemorrhoids

ITCHING
About 20 percent of pregnant women feel itchy during pregnancy. Usually, women feel itchy in the abdomen. But red, itchy palms and soles of the feet are also common complaints. Pregnancy hormones and stretching skin are probably to blame for most of your discomfort. Usually, the itchy feeling goes away after delivery.

What Might Help?
- using gentle soaps and moisturizing creams
- avoiding hot showers and baths
- avoiding itchy fabrics

Call your doctor if symptoms do not improve after a week of self-care.

LEG CRAMPS
At different times during your pregnancy, you might have sudden muscle spasms in your legs or feet. They usually occur at night. This is due to a change in the way your body processes calcium.

What Might Help?
- gently stretching muscles
- getting mild exercise
- flexing your foot forward for sudden cramps
- eating calcium-rich foods
- asking your doctor about calcium supplements

MORNING SICKNESS
In the first trimester, hormone changes can cause nausea and vomiting. This is called "morning sickness" although it can occur at any time of day. Morning sickness usually tapers off by the second trimester.

What Might Help?

- eating several small meals instead of three large meals to keep your stomach from being empty
- not lying down after meals
- eating dry toast, saltines, or dry cereals before getting out of bed in the morning
- eating bland foods that are low in fat and easy to digest, such as cereal, rice, and bananas
- sipping on water, weak tea, or clear soft drinks or eating ice chips
- avoiding smells that upset your stomach

Call your doctor if you have flu-like symptoms, which may signal a more serious condition, or if you have severe, constant nausea and/or vomiting several times every day.

NASAL PROBLEMS

Nosebleeds and nasal stuffiness are common during pregnancy. They are caused by the increased amount of blood in your body and hormones acting on the tissues of your nose.

What Might Help?

- blowing your nose gently
- drinking fluids and using a cool mist humidifier
- squeezing your nose between your thumb and forefinger for a few minutes to stop a nosebleed

Call your doctor if nosebleeds are frequent and do not stop after a few minutes.

NUMB OR TINGLING HANDS

Feelings of swelling, tingling, and numbness in fingers and hands, called "carpal tunnel syndrome" (CTS), can occur during pregnancy. These symptoms are due to swelling of tissues in the narrow passages in your wrists, and they should disappear after delivery.

What Might Help?

• taking frequent breaks to rest hands
• asking your doctor about fitting you for a splint to keep your wrists straight

STRETCH MARKS AND SKIN CHANGES

Stretch marks are red, pink, or brown streaks on the skin. Most often, they appear on the thighs, buttocks, abdomen, and breasts. These scars are caused by the stretching of the skin and usually appear in the second half of pregnancy.

Some women notice other skin changes during pregnancy. For many women, the nipples become darker and browner during pregnancy. Many pregnant women also develop a dark line (called the "linea nigra") on the skin that runs from the belly button down to the pubic hairline. Patches of darker skin, usually over the cheeks, forehead, nose, or upper lip, are also common. Patches often match on both sides of the face. These spots are called "melasma" or "chloasma" and are more common in darker-skinned women.

What Might Help?

• being patient—stretch marks and other changes usually fade after delivery

SWELLING

Many women develop mild swelling in the face, hands, or ankles at some point in their pregnancies. As the due date approaches, swelling often becomes more noticeable.

What Might Help?

• drinking 8–10 glasses of fluids daily
• not drinking caffeine or eating salty foods
• taking rest and elevating your feet
• asking your doctor about support hose

Call your doctor if your hands or feet swell suddenly or you rapidly gain weight—it may be preeclampsia.

URINARY FREQUENCY AND LEAKING

Temporary bladder control problems are common in pregnancy. Your unborn baby pushes down on the bladder, urethra, and pelvic floor muscles. This pressure can lead to the more frequent need to urinate, as well as the leaking of urine when sneezing, coughing, or laughing.

What Might Help?

- taking frequent bathroom breaks
- drinking plenty of fluids to avoid dehydration
- doing Kegel exercises to tone pelvic muscles

Call your doctor if you experience burning along with the frequency of urination—it may be an infection.

VARICOSE VEINS

During pregnancy, blood volume increases greatly. This can cause veins to enlarge. Plus, pressure on the large veins behind the uterus causes the blood to slow in its return to the heart. For these reasons, varicose veins in the legs and anus (hemorrhoids) are more common in pregnancy.

Varicose veins look like swollen veins raised above the surface of the skin. They can be twisted or bulging and are dark purple or blue in color. They are found most often on the backs of the calves or on the inside of the leg.

What Might Help?

- avoiding tight knee-highs
- sitting with your legs and feet raised[1]

[1] Office on Women's Health (OWH), "Body Changes and Discomforts," U.S. Department of Health and Human Services (HHS), February 22, 2021. Available online. URL: www.womenshealth.gov/pregnancy/youre-pregnant-now-what/body-changes-and-discomforts. Accessed May 24, 2023.

Section 10.2 | Back Pain during Pregnancy

During pregnancy, a woman can expect some degree of discomfort in her back. Back pain is prevalent in almost 50–70 percent of all pregnant women and can be experienced at any point of the pregnancy. However, it occurs most commonly in the later stages of pregnancy. This pain may persist after delivery (postpartum)—but usually resolves after some months—and can sometimes be intense enough to disrupt daily activities and interfere with a good night's sleep.

The types of back pain that occur during pregnancy are as follows:

- **Lumbar or lower-back pain**. This pain generally occurs in the center of the back, at and above the waist. It is similar to the lower-back pain experienced by nonpregnant women. Lumbar or lower-back pain that radiates into the legs or feet is called "sciatica." Lower-back pain during pregnancy may or may not be concurrent with sciatica.

- **Posterior pelvic pain**. It is a deep pain felt below and at the side of the waistline and across the tailbone on either side. This kind of pain in the back or pelvis can sometimes radiate down to the buttocks region and further down to the upper posterior portion of the thighs (the back of the thighs) but does not extend below the knees. Posterior pelvic pain can sometimes be associated with pubic pain and morning stiffness.

Risk factors for back pain during pregnancy include obesity and a prior history of back pain. Some of the potential causes of back pain or discomfort during pregnancy are as follows:

- **Hormonal changes**. Hormones released during pregnancy allow the softening and relaxation of ligaments attached to the pelvic bones and spine and loosen the joints in preparation for birth. These changes affect back support and cause pain while walking, climbing stairs, sitting for prolonged periods of time, rolling over in bed, getting out of a low chair or the tub, bending, and lifting.

- **Muscle separation.** As the uterus expands during pregnancy, rectal abdominis muscles (two parallel sheets of muscles that run from the rib cage to the pubic bone) separate to create space for the fetus to grow. This can worsen back pain or discomfort.
- **Center of gravity.** An expectant mother's center of gravity shifts forward as a result of significant weight gain in the abdominal region. This postural change can trigger back pain.
- **Additional weight.** As the fetus grows, the back is responsible for managing the additional weight, which can contribute to some amount of discomfort.
- **Posture or position.** Poor posture while walking, sitting for prolonged periods of time, excessive standing, and inappropriate bending can escalate back pain.
- **Increased stress.** Stress increases muscle stiffness, especially in weak areas, which contributes to pain.

TIPS FOR REDUCING BACK PAIN THROUGHOUT THE PREGNANCY

- Avoid excessive weight gain. Gain a healthy amount of weight by maintaining a healthy diet.
- Maintain good posture. Stand straight with a high chest and relaxed shoulders and back.
- Avoid standing for long periods of time.
- Wear supportive footwear and avoid high heels. Move your feet while turning to avoid twisting your spine. Balance your weight on both sides when completing activities.
- Ensure that the chairs that you sit in provide good back support and use a lumbar pillow for additional support.
- Elevate your feet while resting.
- When bending down, bend at your knees and try to keep your back straight (squat) as you pick things up.
- Avoid heavy lifting.
- Avoid sleeping on your back. Try to sleep on your side instead, with pillows tucked under your abdomen and between your knees for support.

- Avoid tight clothing. Wearing comfortable, loose garments may relieve back pressure to some extent.
- Include pregnancy-safe exercise in your daily routine. Pregnancy-safe exercise includes swimming, relaxed walking, and pelvic tilts and is designed to support and strengthen the abdomen and back.
- If the back pain seems to be related to stress, then prenatal yoga, meditation, and extra rest may be helpful.
- Use cold compresses (ice packs) and prenatal massage to relax and soothe an aching back.
- Get plenty of rest.
- Contact a local chiropractor who specializes in pregnancy-related care and learn how small adjustments can help ease back pain.
- If the pain is unbearable, then contact your doctor. Do not take any pain-relief medication without prior approval from your doctor.

References

"Back Pain during Pregnancy," Mayoclinic, April 5, 2016. Available online. URL: www.mayoclinic.org/healthy-lifestyle/pregnancy-week-by-week/in-depth/pregnancy/art-20046080. Accessed May 29, 2023.

"Back Pain in Pregnancy," WebMD, August 4, 2018. Available online. URL: www.webmd.com/baby/guide/back-pain-in-pregnancy#1. Accessed May 29, 2023.

"Types of Back Pain in Pregnancy," SPINE-health, May 28, 2008. Available online. URL: www.spine-health.com/conditions/pregnancy-and-back-pain/types-back-pain-pregnancy. Accessed May 29, 2023.

Section 10.3 | Carpal Tunnel Syndrome

WHAT IS CARPAL TUNNEL SYNDROME?

Carpal tunnel syndrome (CTS) is the name for a group of problems that includes swelling, pain, tingling, and loss of strength in your wrist and hand. Your wrist is made of small bones that form a narrow groove or carpal tunnel. Tendons and a nerve called the "median nerve" must pass through this tunnel from your forearm into your hand. The median nerve controls the feelings and sensations in the palm side of your thumb and fingers. Sometimes, swelling and irritation of the tendons can put pressure on the wrist nerve, causing the symptoms of CTS. A person's dominant hand is the one that is usually affected. However, nearly half of CTS sufferers have symptoms in both hands.

CTS has become more common in the United States and is quite costly in terms of time lost from work and expensive medical treatment. The U.S. Department of Labor (DOL) reported that in 2015, the average number of missed days of work due to CTS was 28 days.

WHAT CAUSES CARPAL TUNNEL SYNDROME, AND WHO IS MORE LIKELY TO DEVELOP IT?

Women are three times more likely to have CTS than men. Although there is limited research on why this is the case, scientists have several ideas. It may be that the wrist bones are naturally smaller in most women, creating a tighter space through which the nerves and tendons must pass. Other researchers are looking at genetic links that make it more likely for women to have musculoskeletal injuries such as CTS. Women also deal with strong hormonal changes during pregnancy and menopause that make them more likely to suffer from CTS. Generally, women are at higher risk of CTS between the ages of 45 and 54. Then the risk increases for both men and women as they age.

There are other factors that can cause CTS, including certain health problems, and in some cases, the cause is unknown. The following are a few risk factors that might increase your chances of developing CTS:

- **Genetic predisposition.** The carpal tunnel is smaller in some people than in others.
- **Repetitive movements.** People who do the same movements with their wrists and hands over and over may be more likely to develop CTS. People with certain types of jobs are more likely to have CTS, including manufacturing and assembly-line workers, grocery store checkers, violinists, and carpenters. Some hobbies and sports that use repetitive hand movements can also cause CTS, such as golfing, knitting, and gardening. Whether or not long-term typing or computer use causes CTS is still being debated. Limited research points to a weak link, but more research is needed.
- **Injury or trauma.** A sprain or a fracture of the wrist can cause swelling and pressure on the nerve, increasing the risk of CTS. Forceful and stressful movements of the hand and wrist can also cause trauma, such as strong vibrations caused by heavy machinery or power tools.
- **Pregnancy.** Hormonal changes during pregnancy and buildup of fluid can put pregnant women at greater risk of getting CTS, especially during the last few months. Most doctors treat CTS in pregnant women with wrist splints or rest rather than surgery, as CTS almost always goes away following childbirth.
- **Menopause.** Hormonal changes during menopause can put women at greater risk of getting CTS. Also, in some postmenopausal women, the wrist structures become enlarged and can press on the wrist nerve.
- **Breast cancer.** Some women who have a mastectomy get lymphedema, the buildup of fluids that go beyond the lymph system's ability to drain it. In mastectomy patients, this causes pain and swelling of the arm. Although rare, some of these women will get CTS due to pressure on the nerve from this swelling.

- **Medical conditions.** People who have diabetes, hypothyroidism, lupus, obesity, and rheumatoid arthritis are more likely to get CTS. In some of these patients, the normal structures in the wrist can become enlarged and lead to CTS.

Also, smokers with CTS usually have worse symptoms and recover more slowly than nonsmokers.

WHAT ARE THE SYMPTOMS OF CARPAL TUNNEL SYNDROME?

Typically, CTS begins slowly with feelings of burning, tingling, and numbness in the wrist and hand. The areas most affected are the thumb and index and middle fingers. At first, symptoms may happen more often at night. Many CTS sufferers do not make the connection between a daytime activity that might be causing the CTS and the delayed symptoms. Also, many people sleep with their wrist bent, which may cause more pain and symptoms at night. As CTS gets worse, the tingling may be felt during the daytime, too, along with pain moving from the wrist to your arm or down to your fingers. Pain is usually felt more on the palm side of the hand.

Another symptom of CTS is the weakness of the hands that gets worse over time. Some people with CTS find it difficult to grasp an object, make a fist, or hold onto something small. The fingers may even feel like they are swollen even though they are not. Over time, this feeling will usually happen more often.

If left untreated, those with CTS can have a loss of feeling in some fingers and permanent weakness of the thumb. Thumb muscles can actually waste away over time. Eventually, CTS sufferers may have trouble telling the difference between hot and cold temperatures by touch.

HOW IS CARPAL TUNNEL SYNDROME TREATED?

It is important to be treated by a doctor for CTS in order to avoid permanent damage to the wrist nerve and muscles of the hand and thumb. Underlying causes, such as diabetes or a thyroid problem, should be addressed first. Left untreated, CTS can cause nerve damage that leads to loss of feeling and hand strength. Over time, the muscles of the thumb can become weak and damaged. You can even lose the ability to feel hot and cold by touch. Permanent injury occurs in about 1 percent of those with CTS.

CTS is much easier to treat early on. Most CTS patients get better after first-step treatments and the following tips for protecting the wrist. Treatments for CTS include the following:

- **Wrist splint.** A splint can be worn to support and brace your wrist in a neutral position so that the nerves and tendons can recover. A splint can be worn 24 hours a day or only at night. Sometimes, wearing a splint at night helps to reduce the pain. Splinting can work best when done within three months of having any symptoms of CTS.
- **Rest.** For people with mild CTS, stopping or doing less of a repetitive movement may be all that is needed. Your doctor will likely talk to you about steps that you should take to prevent CTS from coming back.
- **Medication.** The short-term use of nonsteroidal anti-inflammatory drugs (NSAIDs) may be helpful in controlling CTS pain. NSAIDs include aspirin, ibuprofen, and other nonprescription pain relievers. In severe cases, an injection of cortisone may help reduce swelling. Your doctor may also give you corticosteroids in pill form. But these treatments only relieve symptoms temporarily. If CTS is caused by another health problem, your doctor will probably treat that problem first. If you have diabetes, it is important to know that long-term corticosteroid use can make it hard to control insulin levels.
- **Physical therapy.** A physical therapist can help you do special exercises to make your wrist and hand stronger. There are also many different kinds of treatments that can make CTS better and help relieve symptoms. Massage, yoga, ultrasound, chiropractic manipulation, and acupuncture are just a few such options that have

been found to be helpful. You should talk with your doctor before trying these alternative treatments.

- **Surgery.** CTS surgery is one of the most common surgeries done in the United States. Generally, surgery is only an option for severe cases of CTS and/or after other treatments have failed for a period of at least six months. Open release surgery is a common approach to CTS surgery and involves making a small incision in the wrist or palm and cutting the ligament to enlarge the carpal tunnel. This surgery is done under a local anesthetic to numb the wrist and hand area and is an outpatient procedure.

WHAT IS THE BEST WAY TO PREVENT CARPAL TUNNEL SYNDROME?

Research is focused on figuring out what causes CTS and how to prevent it. The National Institute of Neurological Disorders and Stroke (NINDS) and the National Institute of Arthritis and Musculoskeletal and Skin Diseases (NIAMS) support research on work-related factors that may cause CTS. Scientists are also researching better ways to detect and treat CTS, including alternative treatments such as acupuncture.

The following steps can help prevent CTS:

- **Prevent workplace musculoskeletal injury.** Make sure that your workspace and equipment are at the right height and distance for your hands and wrist to work with less strain. If you are working on a computer, the keyboard should be at a height that allows your wrist to rest comfortably without having to bend at an angle. Desk or table workspace should be about 27–29 inches above the floor for most people. It also helps keep your elbows close to your sides as you type to reduce the strain on your forearm. Keeping good posture and wrist position can lower your risk of getting CTS.
- **Take breaks.** Allowing your hand and wrist to rest and recover every so often will lower your risk of swelling. Experts believe that taking a 10- to 15-minute break every hour is a good way to prevent CTS.

- **Vary tasks**. Avoid repetitive movements without changing up your routine. Try to do tasks that use different muscle movements during each hour. Break up tasks that require repetitive wrist and hand motion with those that do not.
- **Relax your grip**. Sometimes, people get into a habit of tensing muscles without needing to. Practice doing hand and wrist motion tasks more gently and less tightly. Stress and tension play a role in muscle strain and irritation.
- **Do exercises**. After doing repetitive movements for a while, you can sometimes cancel out the effects of those movements by flexing and bending your wrists and hands in the opposite direction. For example, after typing with your wrist and hand extended, it is helpful to make a tight fist and hold it for a second and then stretch out the fingers and hold for a few seconds. Try repeating this several times.
- **Stay warm**. Muscles that are warm are less likely to get hurt, and the risk of getting CTS is greater in a cold environment. It is important to keep your hands warm while you work, even if you must wear fingerless gloves.[2]

---

[2] Office on Women's Health (OWH), "Carpal Tunnel Syndrome," U.S. Department of Health and Human Services (HHS), February 22, 2021. Available online. URL: www.womenshealth.gov/a-z-topics/carpal-tunnel-syndrome. Accessed May 24, 2023.

Chapter 11 | Pregnancy, Pelvic Floor Disorders, and Bladder Control

Chapter Contents

Section 11.1 | Pregnancy and Pelvic Floor Disorders

WHAT IS THE PELVIC FLOOR?

The "pelvic floor" is the group of muscles that form a sling or hammock across the floor of the pelvis. Together with surrounding tissues, these muscles hold the pelvic organs in place, so they can function correctly. The pelvic organs include the bladder, urethra, intestines, and rectum. A woman's pelvic organs also include the uterus, cervix, and vagina.

WHAT IS A PELVIC FLOOR DISORDER?

A pelvic floor disorder (PFD) occurs when the pelvic muscles and connective tissue weaken or are injured. The most common types of PFDs are as follows:

- **Pelvic organ prolapse.** "Prolapse" happens in women when the pelvic muscles and tissue can no longer support one or more pelvic organs, causing them to drop or press into the vagina. For instance, in uterine prolapse, the cervix and uterus can descend into the vagina and may even come out of the vaginal opening. In vaginal prolapse, the top of the vagina loses support and can drop toward or through the vaginal opening. Prolapse can also cause a kink in the urethra, the tube that brings urine from the bladder to the outside of the body.

- **Bladder problems.** Urinary symptoms can include urinating too often in the day or night, strong urgency to urinate, or urinary leakage. The leaking of urine, a problem called "urinary incontinence," can occur in women or men. This leakage may occur as a result of exertion (such as a cough or sneeze) or other factors involving the bladder muscles. The National Institute of Diabetes and Digestive and Kidney Diseases (NIDDK) offers information about different types of bladder control problems, including these common types:

- stress incontinence
- urge or urgency incontinence (also called "overactive bladder")
- overflow incontinence
- **Bowel control problems**. The leaking of liquid or solid stool from the rectum, called "fecal incontinence," can occur in women and men. It can result from damage to or weakening of the anal sphincter, the ring of muscles that keeps the anus closed, or from other causes.

WHAT CAUSES PELVIC FLOOR DISORDERS?

The complete picture about what contributes to the development of pelvic floor problems is not clear and is quite complex, but the following conditions are being studied as risk factors for the development of PFDs:

- **Childbirth**. Pregnancy, childbirth, and their link to pelvic floor problems have been an active area of research, but the connection is not clear. In some studies, the risk increases with the number of children a woman has delivered. The risk may be greater if forceps or a vacuum device is used during delivery. However, because pelvic problems also affect women who have never been pregnant and because delivering via cesarean section only reduces but does not eliminate the risk of pelvic floor problems, the relationship among pregnancy, childbirth, and PFDs remains unclear.
- **Factors that put pressure on the pelvic floor**. These factors include overweight or obesity, chronic constipation or chronic straining to have a bowel movement, heavy lifting, and chronic coughing from smoking or health problems.
- **Getting older**. The pelvic floor muscles can weaken as women age and during menopause.

- **Having weaker tissues.** Genes influence the strength of a woman's bones, muscles, and connective tissues. Some women are born with conditions that affect the strength of connective tissues, and they are more likely to have pelvic organ prolapse.
- **Surgery.** Previous hysterectomy and prior surgery to correct prolapse are associated with higher risks of PFDs.
- **Race.** Certain groups of women, such as White or Latina women, appear to be at higher risk of some forms of PFDs.

WHAT ARE THE SYMPTOMS OF PELVIC FLOOR DISORDERS?

Because there are different types of PFDs, symptoms of different PFDs can vary or overlap. For example, women with PFDs may:

- feel heaviness, fullness, pulling, or aching in the vagina that gets worse by the end of the day or is related to a bowel movement
- see or feel a "bulge" or "something coming out" of the vagina
- have difficulty starting to urinate or emptying the bladder completely
- leak urine when coughing, laughing, or exercising
- feel an urgent or frequent need to urinate
- feel pain while urinating
- leak stool or have difficulty controlling gas
- have constipation
- have difficulty making it to the bathroom in time

Some women with pelvic floor problems do not have symptoms at first. Many women are reluctant to tell their health-care provider about symptoms because they may feel embarrassed. In addition, many women think that problems with bladder control are normal and live with their symptoms. However, bladder control problems are treatable, and these treatments can help women with pelvic floor problems.

HOW ARE PELVIC FLOOR DISORDERS DIAGNOSED?

A health-care provider may be able to diagnose a PFD with a physical exam. In some cases, a woman's health-care provider will see or feel a bulge during a routine pelvic exam that suggests a prolapse. In other cases, a woman may see her doctor about symptoms she is experiencing, such as problems with bladder or bowel control. In addition to a physical exam, a doctor will also ask about medical history, including whether a woman has been pregnant, has had surgery, and takes any medicines.

Depending on the findings from the exam or the severity of the symptoms, a health-care provider may do tests. Some tests used to help with the diagnosis or with treatment planning are as follows.

Bladder Control Problems

- **Cystoscopy**. This test examines the insides of the bladder to look for problems, such as bladder stones, tumors, or inflammation.
- **Urinalysis**. This urine test can detect if you have a bladder infection, kidney problems, or diabetes.
- **Urodynamics**. This test is used to evaluate how the bladder and urethra are working. It can help determine the plan for surgery to treat certain forms of bladder control problems.

Bowel Control Problems

- **Anal manometry**. This test evaluates the strength of the anal sphincter muscles.
- **Colonoscopy or sigmoidoscopy**. This procedure examines the inside of the colon or the sigmoid (the part of the bowel near the rectum) to look for signs of disease or inflammation that may be causing symptoms.
- **Dynamic defecography**. This test is used to evaluate the pelvic floor and rectum while the patient is having a bowel movement.

HOW ARE PELVIC FLOOR DISORDERS TREATED?

Treatment can often help when symptoms are bothersome or restrict a woman's activities. Some types of treatments include the following.

Lifestyle Changes

Talk to your health-care provider about ways to reduce or ease symptoms. Your health-care provider may recommend the following actions:

- **Limit foods and drinks that stimulate the bladder.** Some foods and drinks, such as caffeinated beverages, carbonated beverages, citrus fruits and drinks, artificial sweeteners, and alcoholic beverages, can stimulate the bladder and make you need to use the bathroom.
- **For certain bowel problems, eat a high-fiber diet**. Fiber helps your body to digest food. It helps make stool the right consistency, which can also prevent constipation and the chronic straining associated with having a bowel movement when constipated. Fiber is found in fruits, vegetables, legumes (such as beans and lentils), and whole grains. Fiber supplements are also available.
- **Lose weight**. For women who are overweight or obese, losing weight may reduce bladder control and pelvic organ prolapse symptoms by relieving pressure on pelvic organs.

Nonsurgical Treatment

Nonsurgical treatments commonly used for PFDs include the following:

- **Bladder training**. This involves using the bathroom on a set schedule to regain bladder control and applying techniques to overcome inappropriate urges to urinate. A woman starts by using the bathroom at a specific interval and slowly, over many months, increases that time, with a goal of using the bathroom only every 2.5–3 hours.

- **Pelvic floor muscle training (PFMT).** Often referred to as Kegel exercises, PFMT involves squeezing and relaxing the pelvic floor muscles. If performed correctly and routinely, PFMT may improve the symptoms of urinary incontinence and prolapse. However, PFMT cannot correct prolapse. Women can do the exercises on their own or with the help of a pelvic floor physical therapist. Biofeedback during pelvic floor physical therapy is sometimes used to help teach women which muscle group to squeeze.
- **Medicine.** Medicine is sometimes prescribed to treat certain bladder control problems or to prevent loose stools or frequent bowel movements.
- **Vaginal pessary.** This plastic device is used to treat prolapse. It can sometimes be used to improve bladder control. A woman or her health-care provider inserts the pessary into the vagina to help support the pelvic organs. A woman's doctor will fit her for a pessary that is of a comfortable shape and size and instruct her on how to use and care for it.

Surgical Treatment

In some cases, surgery is the best treatment option, especially when other treatments are not helpful. Some surgical treatments can be performed as outpatient procedures, which means the patient can usually go home the same day as the procedure.

- **For prolapse.** Surgery involves repairing the prolapse and attempting to restore well-supported anatomy. There are many ways to do this, depending on the type of prolapse and other factors. Women with uterine prolapse may also have the uterus removed (hysterectomy). Women who have surgery to repair prolapse may need surgery at the same time to correct or prevent bladder control problems. Some women choose to have a surgery called "colpocleisis." This surgery treats prolapse by narrowing and shortening the vagina. It works well and carries a low risk, but it is not a good choice for women who want to be able to have vaginal intercourse.

- **For bladder control problems**. Surgery works well to treat problems with urinary leakage that occur as a result of an activity such as sneezing, coughing, laughing, or exercising (stress incontinence). Stress incontinence occurs when the exertion squeezes the bladder and urine leaks out because the support around the urethra has weakened. The type of surgery used most often is a mid-urethral sling. The surgeon places material under the urethra to support it and prevent urine leakage during activity. In another procedure, "bulking agents" can be injected near the bladder neck and urethra to make the tissues thicker and close the bladder opening. Repeat injections may be needed over time.
- **For bowel control problems**. Surgery may be needed to repair a damaged anal sphincter muscle, inject medications into the sphincter, or implant a stimulator for the nerves that control bowel function.

Not all women are good candidates for surgery. In general, women who want to have children should not have these types of surgery. Also, prolapse can recur even after surgery is performed to correct it. Researchers are working to develop low-risk procedures and devices that work well to treat pelvic floor problems. Researchers are also comparing treatment methods to see what works best. For example, the Study of Uterine Prolapse Procedures—Randomized Trial (SUPeR) found comparable effectiveness in two types of surgery to treat vaginal prolapse. The Extended Operations and Pelvic Muscle Training in the Management of Apical Support Loss (E-OPTIMAL) study found that two other surgical treatments had comparable effectiveness. The Effects of Surgical Treatment Enhanced with Exercise for Mixed Urinary Incontinence (ESTEEM) study found that surgery may benefit women who have both stress and urge incontinence.

Combination Treatment

"Combination" can mean a woman is getting treated for more than one type of PFD, such as a treatment for both uterine prolapse and urinary incontinence. It can also mean using different treatments together to address PFDs, such as using PFMT and surgery to treat symptoms.

Researchers are studying combination treatments to find out how to get the best outcomes for women with PFDs. For instance, the Outcomes Following Vaginal Prolapse Repair and Mid-Urethral Sling (OPUS) study evaluated whether adding a procedure to treat stress incontinence at the time of surgery for pelvic organ prolapse in women who do not have symptoms of stress incontinence can help prevent stress incontinence from happening after surgery and without increasing risk. The Controlling Anal Incontinence by Performing Anal Exercises with Biofeedback or Loperamide (CAPABLe) study compared different combinations of treatments for anal incontinence.[1]

Section 11.2 | Pregnancy and Bladder Control

WHAT IS URINARY INCONTINENCE?

Urinary incontinence is the loss of bladder control, or leaking urine. Urine is made by the kidneys and stored in the bladder. The bladder has muscles that tighten when you need to urinate. When the bladder muscles tighten, urine is forced out of your bladder through a tube called the "urethra." At the same time, sphincter muscles around the urethra relax to let the urine out of your body.

Incontinence can happen when the bladder muscles suddenly tighten and the sphincter muscles are not strong enough to pinch the urethra shut. This causes a sudden, strong urge to urinate that you may not be able to control. Pressure caused by laughing, sneezing,

---

[1] "About Pelvic Floor Disorders (PFDs)," *Eunice Kennedy Shriver* National Institute of Child Health and Human Development (NICHD), January 8, 2020. Available online. URL: www.nichd.nih.gov/health/topics/pelvicfloor/conditioninfo. Accessed May 16, 2023.

or exercising can cause you to leak urine. Urinary incontinence may also happen if there is a problem with the nerves that control the bladder muscles and urethra. Urinary incontinence can mean you leak a small amount of urine or release a lot of urine all at once.

WHO GETS URINARY INCONTINENCE?

Urinary incontinence affects twice as many women as men. This is because reproductive health events unique to women, such as pregnancy, childbirth, and menopause, affect the bladder, urethra, and other muscles that support these organs.

Urinary incontinence can happen to women at any age, but it is more common in older women. This is probably because of hormonal changes during menopause. More than 4 in 10 women aged 65 and older have urinary incontinence.

WHY DOES URINARY INCONTINENCE AFFECT MORE WOMEN THAN MEN?

Women have unique health events, such as pregnancy, childbirth, and menopause, that may affect the urinary tract and the surrounding muscles. The pelvic floor muscles that support the bladder, urethra, uterus (womb), and bowels may become weaker or damaged. When the muscles that support the urinary tract are weak, the muscles in the urinary tract must work harder to hold urine until you are ready to urinate. This extra stress or pressure on the bladder and urethra can cause urinary incontinence or leakage.

Also, the female urethra is shorter than the male urethra. Any weakness or damage to the urethra in a woman is more likely to cause urinary incontinence. This is because there is less muscle keeping the urine in until you are ready to urinate.

WHAT ARE THE TYPES OF URINARY INCONTINENCE THAT AFFECT WOMEN?

The two most common types of urinary incontinence in women are as follows:

- **Stress incontinence**. This is the most common type of incontinence. It is also the most common type of incontinence that affects younger women. Stress incontinence happens when there is stress or pressure on the bladder. Stress incontinence can happen when weak pelvic floor muscles put pressure on the bladder and urethra by making them work harder. With stress incontinence, everyday actions that use the pelvic floor muscles, such as coughing, sneezing, or laughing, can cause you to leak urine. Sudden movements and physical activity can also cause you to leak urine.

- **Urge incontinence.** With urge incontinence, urine leakage usually happens after a strong, sudden urge to urinate and before you can get to a bathroom. Some women with urge incontinence are able to get to a bathroom in time but feel the urge to urinate more than eight times a day. They also do not urinate much once they get to the bathroom. Urge incontinence is sometimes called "overactive bladder." Urge incontinence is more common in older women. It can happen when you do not expect it, such as during sleep, after drinking water, or when you hear or touch running water.

Many women with urinary incontinence have both stress and urge incontinence. This is called "mixed incontinence."

WHAT CAUSES URINARY INCONTINENCE?

Urinary incontinence is usually caused by problems with the muscles and nerves that help the bladder hold or pass urine. Certain health events unique to women, such as pregnancy, childbirth, and menopause, can cause problems with these muscles and nerves.

Other causes of urinary incontinence are as follows:

- **Overweight.** Having overweight puts pressure on the bladder, which can weaken the muscles over time. A weak bladder cannot hold as much urine.
- **Constipation.** Problems with bladder control can happen to people with long-term (chronic)

constipation. Constipation, or straining to have a bowel movement, can put stress or pressure on the bladder and pelvic floor muscles. This weakens the muscles and can cause urinary incontinence or leaking.

- **Nerve damage**. Damaged nerves may send signals to the bladder at the wrong time or not at all. Childbirth and health problems such as diabetes and multiple sclerosis can cause nerve damage in the bladder, urethra, or pelvic floor muscles.
- **Surgery**. Any surgery that involves a woman's reproductive organs, such as a hysterectomy, can damage the supporting pelvic floor muscles, especially if the uterus is removed. If the pelvic floor muscles are damaged, a woman's bladder muscles may not work as they should. This can cause urinary incontinence.

Sometimes, urinary incontinence lasts only for a short time and happens because of other reasons, including the following:

- **Certain medicines**. Urinary incontinence may be a side effect of medicines such as diuretics ("water pills" used to treat heart failure, liver cirrhosis, hypertension, and certain kidney diseases). The incontinence often goes away when you stop taking the medicine.
- **Caffeine**. Drinks with caffeine can cause the bladder to fill quickly, which can cause you to leak urine. Studies suggest that women who drink more than two cups of drinks with caffeine per day may be more likely to have problems with incontinence. Limiting caffeine may help with incontinence because there is less strain on your bladder.
- **Infection**. Infections of the urinary tract and bladder may cause incontinence for a short time. Bladder control often returns when the infection goes away.

WHAT ARE THE SYMPTOMS OF URINARY INCONTINENCE?

Urinary incontinence is not a disease by itself. Urinary incontinence is a symptom of another health problem, usually weak pelvic floor muscles. In addition to urinary incontinence, some women have other urinary symptoms:

- pressure or spasms in the pelvic area that cause a strong urge to urinate
- going to the bathroom more than usual (more than eight times a day or more than twice at night)
- urinating while sleeping (bed-wetting)

HOW DOES PREGNANCY CAUSE URINARY INCONTINENCE?

As many as 4 in 10 women get urinary incontinence during pregnancy. During pregnancy, as your unborn baby grows, he or she pushes down on your bladder, urethra, and pelvic floor muscles. Over time, this pressure may weaken the pelvic floor muscles and lead to leaks or problems passing urine.

Most problems with bladder control during pregnancy go away after childbirth when the muscles have had some time to heal. If you are still having bladder problems six weeks after childbirth, talk to your doctor, nurse, or midwife.

HOW DOES CHILDBIRTH CAUSE URINARY INCONTINENCE?

Problems during labor and childbirth, especially vaginal birth, can weaken pelvic floor muscles and damage the nerves that control the bladder. Most problems with bladder control that happen as a result of labor and delivery go away after the muscles have had some time to heal. If you are still having bladder problems six weeks after childbirth, talk to your doctor, nurse, or midwife.

WHAT TYPE OF DOCTOR OR NURSE SHOULD YOU GO TO FOR HELP WITH URINARY INCONTINENCE?

If you have urinary incontinence, you can make an appointment with your primary care provider, your obstetrician/gynecologist (OB/GYN), or a nurse practitioner. Your doctor or nurse will work with you to treat your urinary incontinence or refer you to a specialist if you need a different treatment.

The specialist may be a urologist, who treats urinary problems in both men and women, or a urogynecologist, who has special training in the female urinary system. You might also need to see a pelvic floor specialist, a type of physical therapist, who will work with you to strengthen your pelvic floor muscles that support the urinary tract.

HOW IS URINARY INCONTINENCE DIAGNOSED?

Your doctor or nurse will ask you about your symptoms and your medical history, including:

- how often you empty your bladder
- how and when you leak urine
- how much urine you leak
- when your symptoms started
- what medicines you take
- if you have ever been pregnant and what your labor and delivery experience was like

Your doctor or nurse will do a physical exam to look for signs of health problems that can cause incontinence.

Your doctor or nurse may also do the following tests:

- **Urine test**. After you urinate into a cup, the doctor or nurse will send your urine to a lab. At the lab, your urine will be checked for infection or other causes of incontinence.
- **Ultrasound**. Your doctor will use an ultrasound wand on the outside of your abdomen to take pictures of the kidneys, bladder, and urethra. Your doctor will look for anything unusual that may be causing urinary incontinence.
- **Bladder stress test**. During this test, you will cough or bear down as if pushing during childbirth as your doctor watches for loss of urine.
- **Cystoscopy**. Your doctor inserts a thin tube with a tiny camera into your urethra and bladder to look for damaged tissue. Depending on the type of cystoscopy

you need, your doctor may use medicine to numb your skin and urinary organs while you are still awake, or you may be fully sedated.

- **Urodynamics.** Your doctor inserts a thin tube into your bladder and fills your bladder with water. This allows your doctor to measure the pressure in your bladder to see how much fluid your bladder can hold.

Your doctor or nurse may ask you to keep a diary for two to three days to track when you empty your bladder or leak urine. The diary may help your doctor or nurse see patterns in the incontinence that give clues about the possible cause and treatments that might work for you.

HOW IS URINARY INCONTINENCE TREATED?

You and your doctor or nurse will work together to create a treatment plan. You may start with steps you can take at home. If these steps do not improve your symptoms, your doctor or nurse may recommend other treatments depending on whether you have stress incontinence or urge incontinence or both.

Be patient as you work with your doctor or nurse on a treatment plan. It may take a month or longer for different treatments to begin working.

WHAT STEPS CAN YOU TAKE AT HOME TO TREAT URINARY INCONTINENCE?

Your doctor or nurse may suggest some things you can do at home to help treat urinary incontinence. Some people do not think that such simple actions can treat urinary incontinence. But, for many women, these steps make urinary incontinence go away entirely or help leak less urine. These steps may include the following:

- **Doing Kegel exercises.** If you have stress incontinence, Kegel exercises to strengthen your pelvic floor muscles may help. Some women have urinary symptoms because the pelvic floor muscles are always tightened.

In this situation, Kegel exercises will not help your urinary symptoms and may cause more problems. Talk to your doctor or nurse about your urinary symptoms before doing Kegel exercises.

- **Training your bladder.** You can help control an overactive bladder or urge incontinence by going to the bathroom at set times. Start by tracking how often you go to the bathroom each day in a bladder diary. Then slowly add about 15 minutes between bathroom visits. Urinate each time, even if you do not feel the urge to go. By gradually increasing the amount of time between visits, your bladder learns to hold more urine before it signals the need to go again.
- **Losing weight.** Extra weight puts more pressure on your bladder and nearby muscles, which can lead to problems with bladder control. If you have overweight, your doctor or nurse can help you create a plan to lose weight by choosing healthy foods and getting regular physical activity. Your doctor or nurse may refer you to a dietitian or physical therapist to create a healthy eating and exercise plan.
- **Changing your eating habits.** Drinks with caffeine, carbonation (such as sodas), or alcohol may make bladder leakage or urinary incontinence worse. Your doctor might suggest that you stop drinking these drinks for a while to see if that helps.
- **Quitting smoking.** Smoking can make many health problems, including urinary incontinence, worse.
- **Treating constipation.** Your doctor might recommend that you eat more fiber since constipation can make urinary incontinence worse. Eating foods with a lot of fiber can make you less constipated.

You can also buy pads or protective underwear while you take other steps to treat urinary incontinence. These are sold in many stores that also sell feminine hygiene products such as tampons and pads.

WHAT ARE KEGEL EXERCISES?

Kegel exercises, also called "Kegels" or "pelvic floor muscle training," are exercises for your pelvic floor muscles to help prevent or reduce stress urinary incontinence. Your pelvic floor muscles support your uterus, bladder, small intestine, and rectum.

Four in ten women improved their symptoms after trying Kegels. Kegels can be done daily and may be especially helpful during pregnancy. They can help prevent the weakening of pelvic floor muscles, which often happens during pregnancy and childbirth. Your pelvic floor muscles may also weaken with age and less physical activity.

Some women have urinary symptoms because the pelvic floor muscles are always tightened. In this situation, Kegel exercises will not help your urinary symptoms and may cause more problems. Talk to your doctor or nurse about your urinary symptoms before doing Kegel exercises.

HOW DO YOU DO KEGEL EXERCISES?

The following is the procedure for doing Kegels:

- **Lie down**. It may be easier to learn how to do Kegels correctly while lying down. You do not have to lie down once you learn to do Kegels correctly.
- **Squeeze**. Squeeze the muscles in your genital area as if you were trying to stop the flow of urine or passing gas. Try not to squeeze the muscles in your belly or legs at the same time. Try to squeeze only the pelvic muscles. Be extra careful not to tighten your stomach, legs, or buttocks (because then you will not be using your pelvic floor muscles).
- **Relax**. Squeeze the muscles again and hold for three seconds. Then relax for three seconds. Work up to 3 sets of 10 each day.
- **Practice Kegels anywhere**. When your muscles get stronger, try doing Kegels while sitting or standing. You can do these exercises at any time, such as while sitting at your desk or in the car, waiting in line, or doing the

dishes. Do not do Kegel exercises at the same time you are urinating. This can weaken your pelvic floor muscles over time.

If you are uncomfortable or uncertain about doing Kegel exercises on your own, a doctor or nurse can also teach you how to do Kegels. A pelvic floor physical therapist or other specialist may also be available in your area to help teach you how to strengthen these muscles.

HOW SOON AFTER STARTING KEGEL EXERCISES WILL URINARY INCONTINENCE GET BETTER?

It may take four to six weeks before you notice any improvement in your symptoms. Kegel exercises work differently for each person. Your symptoms may go away totally, you may notice an improvement in your symptoms but still have some leakage, or you may not see any improvement at all. But, even if your symptoms do not get better, Kegel exercises can help prevent your incontinence from getting worse.

You may need to continue doing Kegel exercises for the rest of your life. Even if your symptoms improve, urinary incontinence can come back if you stop doing the exercises.

SHOULD YOU DRINK LESS WATER OR OTHER FLUIDS IF YOU HAVE URINARY INCONTINENCE?

No. Many people with urinary incontinence think they need to drink less to reduce how much urine leaks out. But you need fluids, especially water, for good health. (But alcohol and caffeine can irritate or stress the bladder and make urinary incontinence worse.)

Women need 91 ounces (about 11 cups) of fluids a day from food and drinks. Getting enough fluids helps keep your kidneys and bladder healthy, prevents urinary tract infections, and prevents constipation, which may make urinary incontinence worse. After age 60, people are less likely to get enough water, putting them at risk for dehydration and conditions that make urinary incontinence worse.

WHAT ARE SOME MEDICAL TREATMENTS FOR STRESS INCONTINENCE?

If steps you can take at home do not work to improve your stress incontinence, your doctor may talk to you about other options:

- **Medicine.** After menopause, applying vaginal creams, rings, or patches with estrogen (called "topical estrogen") can help strengthen the muscles and tissues in the urethra and vaginal areas. A stronger urethra will help with bladder control.

- **Vaginal pessary**. A reusable pessary is a small plastic or silicone device (shaped like a ring or small donuts) that you put into your vagina. The pessary pushes up against the wall of the vagina and the urethra to support the pelvic floor muscles and help reduce stress incontinence. Pessaries come in different sizes, so your doctor or nurse must write a prescription for the size that will fit you. Another type of pessary looks like a tampon and is used once and then thrown away. You can get this type of pessary at a store that also sells feminine hygiene products.

- **Bulking agents**. Your doctor can inject a bulking agent, such as collagen, into tissues around the bladder and urethra to cause them to thicken. This helps keep the bladder opening closed and reduces the amount of urine that can leak out.

- **Surgery**. Surgery for urinary incontinence is not recommended if you plan to get pregnant in the future. Pregnancy and childbirth can cause leakage to happen again. The two most common types of surgery for urinary incontinence are as follows:

  - **Sling procedures**. The mid-urethral sling is the most common type of surgery to treat stress incontinence. The sling is either a narrow piece of synthetic (man-made) mesh or a piece of tissue from your own body that your doctor places under your urethra. The sling acts like a hammock to support the urethra and hold the bladder in place. Serious complications from the sling procedure include pain, infection, pain during sex, and damage to nearby organs, such as the bladder. The U.S. Food and Drug Administration (FDA) reports that in 1 out of every 50 patients who have synthetic mesh for urinary incontinence, the mesh moves after surgery and sticks out, into the vagina, causing pain. The FDA recommends discussing treatment options with your doctor before surgery and asking specific questions about side effects.

- **Colposuspension.** This surgery also helps hold the bladder in place with stitches on either side of the urethra. This is often referred to as a Burch procedure.

WHAT ARE SOME NONSURGICAL TREATMENTS FOR URGE INCONTINENCE?

If steps you can take at home do not work to improve your urge incontinence, your doctor may suggest one or more of the following treatments:

- **Medicines.** Medicines to treat urge incontinence help relax the bladder muscle and increase the amount of urine your bladder can hold. Common side effects of these medicines include constipation and dry eyes and mouth.
- **Botox.** Botox injections in the bladder can help if other treatments do not work. Botox helps relax the bladder and increases the amount of urine your bladder can hold. You may need to get Botox treatments about once every three months.
- **Nerve stimulation.** This treatment uses mild electric pulses to stimulate nerves in the bladder. The pulses may increase blood flow to the bladder and strengthen the muscles that help control the bladder. Talk to your doctor about the different types of nerve stimulation.
- **Biofeedback.** Biofeedback helps you see how your bladder responds on a screen. A therapist puts an

electrical patch on the skin over your bladder and urethral muscles. A wire connected to the patch is linked to a screen. You and your therapist watch the screen to see when these muscles contract, so you can learn to control them.

- **Surgery.** If you have severe urge incontinence, your doctor may recommend surgery to help increase the amount of urine your bladder can hold or to remove your bladder. Removing your bladder is a serious surgery and is an option only when no other treatments work and the quality of your life is seriously affected.

HOW CAN YOU PREVENT URINARY INCONTINENCE?

Although you cannot always prevent urinary incontinence, you can take steps to lower your risk:

- Practice Kegels daily, especially during pregnancy and after talking to your doctor, nurse, or midwife.
- Reach or stay at a healthy weight.
- Eat foods with fiber to help prevent constipation.[2]

---

[2] Office on Women's Health (OWH), "Urinary Incontinence," U.S. Department of Health and Human Services (HHS), February 22, 2021. Available online. URL: www.womenshealth.gov/a-z-topics/urinary-incontinence. Accessed May 16, 2023.

Chapter 12 | **Pregnancy, Breastfeeding, and Bone Health**

HOW DO PREGNANCY AND BREASTFEEDING AFFECT A WOMAN'S BONES?

Calcium is in high demand during both pregnancy and breastfeeding—since it is needed to support the baby's growth and development in the mother's womb and after birth.

Some of these calcium needs are met by the movement of calcium out of the mother's bones through a process called "remodeling," especially during the third trimester and during breastfeeding.

HOW MUCH CALCIUM DO PREGNANT AND BREASTFEEDING WOMEN NEED TO KEEP THEIR BONES HEALTHY?

The amounts of calcium that women need do not change when they are pregnant or nursing. The recommended amount for teen girls aged 14–18 is 1,300 mg a day. Women who are older than age 18 should get 1,000 mg of calcium a day. Getting more than the recommended amount of calcium from food or supplements does not prevent the loss of calcium from bones during pregnancy or nursing. So extra calcium does not have much effect on how much bone mass a woman loses at this time of life.

Pregnant and nursing women who are thinking about taking a calcium supplement should talk to their health-care provider. Although decreases in bone density are a normal part of pregnancy and lactation, in very rare cases, pregnant and nursing women can develop osteoporosis. Osteoporosis causes bones to become weak and brittle, which increases the risk of fractures (broken bones).

Fractures in these women may occur spontaneously or as the result of normal activities, with minimal trauma or stress. Spine fractures are most common in pregnant or nursing women with osteoporosis, but other types of fractures may happen. In some cases, the mother has a known medical condition or is taking medication that increases her risk of osteoporosis and fracture.

WHAT ARE THE LONG-TERM EFFECTS OF PREGNANCY AND BREASTFEEDING ON BONES?

Temporary decreases in bone density are a normal part of pregnancy and breastfeeding. However, bone density is typically restored after pregnancy and during/after weaning. Large studies show that pregnancy and breastfeeding are not associated with an increased risk of osteoporosis or fractures later in life.[1]

[1] "Pregnancy, Breastfeeding, and Bone Health," National Institute of Arthritis and Musculoskeletal and Skin Diseases (NIAMS), May 1, 2023. Available online. URL: www.niams.nih.gov/health-topics/pregnancy-breastfeeding-and-bone-health. Accessed May 25, 2023.

Chapter 13 | Vision and Oral Changes during Pregnancy

Chapter Contents

Section 13.1 | Pregnancy and Your Vision

During pregnancy, a woman's body undergoes many physical changes in order to support a growing fetus. Natural fluctuations in hormone levels, metabolism, circulation, and fluid retention can affect the eyes just as they affect other organs. As a result, many pregnant women experience changes in their eyes or vision. Although most pregnancy-related eye issues are minor and disappear on their own after delivery, a few types of vision changes can indicate a health condition that requires medical attention. Experts recommend that expectant mothers check with their doctors if they experience any of the following symptoms:

- double vision
- temporary loss of vision
- sensitivity to light
- seeing spots, auras, or blinking lights

VISION CHANGES DURING PREGNANCY

Most of the vision changes that occur during pregnancy are temporary. Although they can be annoying, they are usually not a cause for concern. They occur due to changing hormone levels and fluid retention, which are a normal part of pregnancy. Some of the common eye changes that occur during pregnancy include blurry vision, dry eyes, and puffy eyelids.

Blurry Vision

The fluid retention that most women experience during pregnancy can temporarily change the thickness and shape of the cornea, the transparent layer that helps focus light as it enters the eye. These changes can affect the power of corrective lenses the woman needs, resulting in blurry vision. Since the cornea will likely return to normal following delivery, experts generally recommend against getting a new prescription for corrective lenses during pregnancy. Many eye doctors can provide a temporary lens if the blurry vision makes it difficult to drive a car or perform other everyday tasks safely.

Dry Eyes

Many expectant mothers find that their eyes become dry and irritated during pregnancy and breastfeeding. This problem can be uncomfortable and make it difficult to wear contact lenses. Experts suggest using over-the-counter (OTC) lubricating or rewetting eye drops to soothe dry eyes and relieve discomfort. Pregnant women may switch to glasses temporarily and take frequent breaks while working at a computer to avoid eyestrain.

Puffy Eyelids

Many women experience swollen ankles during pregnancy as a result of water retention. A lesser-known effect of pregnancy hormones is swelling around the eyes and puffy eyelids, which can interfere with peripheral vision. To limit fluid retention, experts recommend drinking lots of water and eating a healthy diet low in sodium and caffeine.

VISION CHANGES OF CONCERN DURING PREGNANCY

A few vision changes that may occur during pregnancy can be symptoms of a serious medical condition, such as preeclampsia or gestational diabetes. Expectant mothers who experience sudden or severe vision disruptions should seek medical attention.

Preeclampsia

Preeclampsia is a complication that occurs in 5–8 percent of all pregnancies. The main symptoms are high blood pressure, swelling of the hands and feet, and protein in the urine. Many women who develop preeclampsia experience vision problems, such as double vision, temporary loss of vision, sensitivity to light, or seeing spots, auras, or blinking lights. Preeclampsia can progress quickly to cause bleeding, organ damage, and detachment of the retinas in the eyes. Expectant mothers who experience symptoms of preeclampsia should seek medical attention and have their blood pressure checked immediately.

Diabetes and Gestational Diabetes

Diabetes is a disease that affects the body's ability to metabolize carbohydrates, resulting in high levels of sugar in the blood. High blood sugar can damage the blood vessels in the retina, causing a serious eye condition called "diabetic retinopathy." Women who are diabetic need to monitor their blood sugar closely and get regular eye screenings to check for damage to the retina. This is especially important during pregnancy, which increases the risk of vision loss associated with diabetes.

Gestational diabetes is a form of diabetes that develops during pregnancy. Expectant mothers who develop the condition should be examined by an eye doctor for signs of retinopathy. Pregnant women with either form of diabetes should also seek medical attention if they experience blurry vision, which can be a sign of elevated blood sugar levels.

References

"Can Pregnancy Affect Your Eyes?" WebMD, 2017. Available online. URL: www.webmd.com/eye-health/pregnancy-and-vision. Accessed June 7, 2023.

"Pregnancy and Your Vision," Prevent Blindness, 2017. Available online. URL: www.preventblindness.org/pregnancy-and-your-vision. Accessed June 7, 2023.

"Vision Changes during Pregnancy," BabyCenter, 2017. Available online. URL: www.babycenter.com/0_vision-changes-during-pregnancy_1456567.bc?showAll=true. Accessed June 7, 2023.

Section 13.2 | **Pregnancy and Oral Health**

WHAT IS ORAL HEALTH?

Oral health is the health of your mouth, including your teeth, gums, throat, and the bones around the mouth. Oral health problems, such as gum disease, might be a sign that you have other health problems. Gum diseases are infections caused by plaque, which is a sticky film of bacteria that forms on your teeth. If left untreated, the bacteria in plaque can destroy the tissue and bone around your teeth, leading to tooth loss. The bacteria can travel throughout your body and make you sick. Infections in your mouth can also affect your unborn baby if you are pregnant.

HOW OFTEN SHOULD YOU BRUSH AND FLOSS YOUR TEETH?

Dentists recommend that everyone brush their teeth at least twice a day with fluoride toothpaste and floss once a day. Flossing removes plaque between your teeth, a place that you cannot reach by brushing. You can also remove this plaque with tools other than floss. These tools, called "interdental cleaners," include wooden or plastic picks and water flossers.

HOW OFTEN SHOULD YOU VISIT THE DENTIST?

Most people should go to the dentist once or twice a year. Your dentist may suggest that you come more often if you have a health problem such as diabetes or a weakened immune system. These health problems can make you more likely to develop gum disease or other dental diseases.

Women are also at higher risk of gum disease during pregnancy. And gum problems and bone loss may happen more quickly in women after menopause. Talk to your dentist about how often you should visit.

HOW DO WOMEN'S HORMONES AFFECT ORAL HEALTH?

Changing hormone levels at different stages of a woman's life can affect oral health. When your hormone levels change, your gums can get swollen and irritated. Your gums may also bleed, especially during pregnancy, when your body's immune system is more sensitive than usual. This can cause inflammation (redness, swelling, and sometimes pain) in the gums. Regular, careful brushing and flossing can lessen gum irritation and bleeding.

Other causes of changing hormone levels that may affect your oral health include:

- your menstrual cycle
- hormonal birth control
- menopause

HOW DOES PREGNANCY AFFECT ORAL HEALTH?

Pregnancy can make brushing difficult. Some women experience nausea from strongly flavored toothpaste. Switching to a neutral-flavored toothpaste may help.

During pregnancy, your hormone levels also go up and down. This raises your risk for several oral health problems:

- **Severe gum disease (periodontitis)**. Changing hormone levels during pregnancy can make gum disease worse or lead to severe gum disease in as many as two in five pregnant women. Periodontitis is an infection of the tissues that hold your teeth in place. It is usually caused by not brushing and flossing or brushing and flossing in a way that allows plaque—a sticky film of bacteria—to build up on the teeth and harden. Periodontitis can cause sore, bleeding gums, painful chewing, and tooth loss. Women who do not get regular dental care and women who smoke are more likely to have periodontitis.
- **Loose teeth**. The tissue supporting your teeth may loosen during pregnancy since many of your joints and tissues loosen in preparation for childbirth. Taking good care of your mouth can help prevent tooth loss.
- **Wearing down of your tooth enamel**. If you have morning sickness that causes vomiting, the stomach acid that comes up during vomiting can erode tooth

enamel (the hard, protective coating on the outside of your teeth). Heartburn, another common pregnancy discomfort, can also wear down your tooth enamel over time if stomach acid is coming up into your throat and mouth. To prevent this erosion, the American Dental Association (ADA) recommends rinsing your mouth with one teaspoon of baking soda mixed in a cup of water 30 minutes before brushing your teeth.

YOU ARE PREGNANT. IS IT SAFE FOR YOU TO GET A DENTAL CHECKUP?

Yes. You need to continue your regular dentist visits to help protect your teeth during pregnancy.

- **Tell your doctor you are pregnant**. Because you are pregnant, your dentist might not take routine x-rays. But the health risk to your unborn baby is very small. If you need emergency treatment or specific dental x-rays to treat a serious problem, your doctor can take extra care to protect your baby.
- **Schedule your dental exam early in your pregnancy**. After your 20th week of pregnancy, you may be uncomfortable sitting in a dental chair.
- **Have all needed dental treatments**. If you avoid treatment, you may risk your own health and your baby's health.

HOW CAN YOU PREVENT ORAL HEALTH PROBLEMS?

You can help prevent oral health problems by taking the following steps:

- **Visit your dentist once or twice a year**. Your dentist may recommend more or fewer visits depending on your oral health. At most routine visits, the dentist and a dental hygienist (assistant) will treat you. During regular checkups, dentists look for signs of disease, infections, and injuries.

- **Choose healthy foods**. Limit the amount of sugary foods and drinks you have. Lower your risk for tooth decay by brushing after meals and flossing once a day.
- **Do not smoke**. Smoking raises your risk of gum disease and mouth and throat cancers. It can also stain your teeth and cause bad breath.
- **Drink less soda**. If you drink soda, try to drink less and replace it with water. Even diet soda has acids that can erode tooth enamel.

WHAT IF YOU ARE AFRAID TO GO TO THE DENTIST?

Some people avoid the dentist because they are afraid of the physical pain. Women who experienced trauma or violence may also have trouble sitting or lying in a dentist's chair because of post-traumatic stress or fear.

Talk with your dentist about your concerns and ways to make you more comfortable before the exam begins. For example, you may prefer to see a female dentist or to have a female assistant in the room during the visit. It may also help bring a friend or loved one to the dentist with you.

Your dentist can also make you feel more in control by:

- explaining what will happen next throughout the visit
- agreeing to stop at any time if you signal to do so (You may want to decide upon a signal beforehand. You can tap your leg or raise your hand.)

Your dentist can also help you relax by playing music, having a TV in the room, or using other relaxation techniques. Some dentists may suggest giving you medicine to help you relax. One common type of medicine is nitrous oxide, also known as "laughing gas." Nitrous oxide can help relieve pain and anxiety, but it may not be a good option if you worry about losing control.

If anxiety prevents you from going to the dentist, you may want to talk to a mental health professional, such as a psychologist. Therapy may help reduce your fear. Oral health is a vital part of overall health, so removing fear or anxiety about the dentist is worth the time and effort.

HOW CAN YOU GET HELP TO PAY FOR DENTAL CARE?

Sometimes, dental insurance is included in your health insurance plan. Sometimes, dental coverage comes from a separate, stand-alone dental plan. Low-cost options may also be available in your area.

- In the Health Insurance Marketplace, you can get dental coverage as part of a health plan or as a separate, stand-alone dental plan.
- If you have insurance that is not part of the Marketplace, check with your insurance provider to find out whether dental care is included or whether you can purchase more dental coverage.
- Most Medicare plans (Parts A, B, and D) do not cover dental care, but Medicare Advantage plans (also called "Part C") usually do. Check with your Medicare insurance provider to find out if dental care is included.
- If you have Medicaid, the benefits are different in each state, but dental care must be covered for children under 18 and in many states for people under 21. With Medicaid, dental visits may also be covered during pregnancy. Check with your state's program to find out what coverage is available.
- For low-cost options in your area, contact your state dental association.[1]

---

[1] Office on Women's Health (OWH), "Oral Health," U.S. Department of Health and Human Services (HHS), February 22, 2021. Available online. URL: www.womenshealth.gov/a-z-topics/oral-health. Accessed May 16, 2023.

Chapter 14 | Emotional Concerns and Pregnancy

Chapter Contents

Section 14.1 | Perinatal Depression

Perinatal depression is a depression that occurs during or after pregnancy. The symptoms can range from mild to severe. In rare cases, the symptoms are severe enough that the health of the mother and baby may be at risk. Perinatal depression can be treated. This section describes perinatal depression and how you or a loved one can get help.

WHAT IS PERINATAL DEPRESSION?

Perinatal depression is a mood disorder that can affect women during pregnancy and after childbirth. The word "perinatal" refers to the time before and after the birth of a child. Perinatal depression includes depression that begins during pregnancy (called "prenatal depression") and depression that begins after the baby is born (called "postpartum depression"). Mothers with perinatal depression experience feelings of extreme sadness, anxiety, and fatigue that may make it difficult for them to carry out daily tasks, including caring for themselves or others.

WHAT CAUSES PERINATAL DEPRESSION?

Perinatal depression is a real medical illness and can affect any mother—regardless of age, race, income, culture, or education. Women are not to blame or at fault for having perinatal depression: It is not brought on by anything a mother has or has not done. Perinatal depression does not have a single cause. Research suggests that perinatal depression is caused by a combination of genetic and environmental factors. Life stress (e.g., demands at work or experiences of past trauma), the physical and emotional demands of childbearing and caring for a new baby, and changes in hormones that occur during and after pregnancy can contribute to the development of perinatal depression. In addition, women are at greater risk of developing perinatal depression if they have a personal or family history of depression or bipolar disorder or if they have experienced perinatal depression with a previous pregnancy.

SIGNS AND SYMPTOMS OF PERINATAL DEPRESSION

Some women may experience a few symptoms of perinatal depression; others may experience several symptoms. Some of the more common symptoms of perinatal depression include:

- persistent sad, anxious, or "empty" mood
- irritability
- feelings of guilt, worthlessness, hopelessness, or helplessness
- loss of interest or pleasure in hobbies and activities
- fatigue or abnormal decrease in energy
- feeling restless or having trouble sitting still
- difficulty concentrating, remembering, or making decisions
- difficulty sleeping (even when the baby is sleeping), awakening early in the morning, or oversleeping
- abnormal appetite, weight changes, or both
- aches or pains, headaches, cramps, or digestive problems that do not have a clear physical cause or do not ease even with treatment
- trouble bonding or forming an emotional attachment with the new baby
- persistent doubts about the ability to care for the new baby
- thoughts about death, suicide, or harming oneself or the baby

Only a health-care provider can help a woman determine whether the symptoms she is feeling are due to perinatal depression or something else. It is important for women who experience any of these symptoms to see a health-care provider.

TREATMENT FOR PERINATAL DEPRESSION

Treatment for perinatal depression is important for the health of both the mother and the baby, as perinatal depression can have serious health effects on both. With proper treatment, most women feel better, and their symptoms improve. Treatment for perinatal depression often includes therapy, medications, or a combination of the two. If these treatments do not reduce symptoms, brain stimulation therapies, such as electroconvulsive therapy (ECT), may be an option to explore.

Psychotherapy

Several types of psychotherapy (sometimes called "talk therapy" or "counseling") can help women with perinatal depression. Two examples of evidence-based approaches that have been used to treat perinatal depression include cognitive-behavioral therapy (CBT) and interpersonal therapy (IPT).

Cognitive-Behavioral Therapy

CBT is a type of psychotherapy that can help people with depression and anxiety. It teaches people different ways of thinking, behaving, and reacting to situations. People learn to challenge and change unhelpful patterns of thinking and behavior as a way of improving their depressive and anxious feelings and emotions. CBT can be conducted individually or with a group of people who have similar concerns.

Interpersonal Therapy

IPT is an evidence-based therapy that has been used to treat depression, including perinatal depression. It is based on the idea that interpersonal and life events impact mood and vice versa. The goal of IPT is to help people improve their communication skills within relationships, develop social support networks, and develop realistic expectations that allow them to deal with crises or other issues that may be contributing to their depression.

Medication

Women with perinatal depression are most commonly treated with antidepressants, which are medications used to treat depression. They may help improve the way the brain uses certain chemicals that control mood or stress. Women who are pregnant or breastfeeding should notify their health-care provider before starting antidepressants, so their health-care provider can work to minimize the baby's exposure to the medication during pregnancy or breast-feeding. The risk of birth defects and other problems for babies of mothers who take antidepressants during pregnancy is very low; however, women should work with their health-care provider to weigh the risks and benefits of treatment and to find the best solution for their situation. Women may need to try several different medications before finding the one that improves their symptoms and has manageable side effects.

Antidepressants take time—usually six to eight weeks—to work, and symptoms such as sleep, appetite, and concentration problems often improve before mood lifts. It is important to give medication a chance before deciding whether or not it works.

Do not stop taking antidepressants without the help of a health-care provider. Sometimes, people taking antidepressants feel better and then stop taking the medication on their own, and the depression returns. Stopping medications abruptly can cause withdrawal symptoms. When a woman and her health-care provider have decided it is time to stop the medication, the health-care provider will help her decrease the dose slowly and safely.

After the birth of a child, many women experience a drop in certain hormones, which can lead to feelings of depression. The U.S. Food and Drug Administration (FDA) has approved one medication, called "brexanolone," specifically to treat severe postpartum depression. Administered in a hospital, this drug works to relieve depression by restoring the levels of these hormones.

HOW CAN FAMILY AND FRIENDS HELP?

It is important to understand that depression is a medical condition that impacts the mother, the child, and the family. Spouses, partners, family members, and friends may be the first to recognize symptoms of perinatal depression in a new mother. Treatment is central to recovery. Family members can encourage the mother to talk with a health-care provider, offer emotional support, and assist with daily tasks such as caring for the baby or the home.

Support or advocacy groups can offer a good source of support and information. One example of this type of group is Postpartum

Support International (www.postpartum.net); others can be found through online searches.[1]

Section 14.2 | Postpartum Depression

Your body and mind go through many changes during and after pregnancy. If you feel empty, emotionless, or sad all or most of the time for longer than two weeks during or after pregnancy, reach out for help. If you feel like you do not love or care for your baby, you might have postpartum depression. Treatment for depression, such as therapy or medicine, works and will help you and your baby be as healthy as possible in the future.

WHAT IS POSTPARTUM DEPRESSION?

"Postpartum" means the time after childbirth. Most women get the "baby blues" or feel sad or empty within a few days of giving birth. For many women, the baby blues go away in three to five days. If your baby blues do not go away or you feel sad, hopeless, or empty for longer than two weeks, you may have postpartum depression. Feeling hopeless or empty after childbirth is not a regular or expected part of being a mother.

Postpartum depression is a serious mental illness that involves the brain and affects your behavior and physical health. If you have depression, then sad, flat, or empty feelings do not go away and can interfere with your day-to-day life. You might feel unconnected to your baby as if you are not the baby's mother, or you might not love or care for the baby. These feelings can be mild to severe.

Mothers can also experience anxiety disorders during or after pregnancy.

---

[1] "Perinatal Depression," National Institute of Mental Health (NIMH), February 19, 2014. Available online. URL: www.nimh.nih.gov/health/publications/perinatal-depression. Accessed May 25, 2023.

HOW COMMON IS POSTPARTUM DEPRESSION?

Depression is a common problem after pregnancy. One in nine new mothers has postpartum depression.

HOW DO YOU KNOW IF YOU HAVE POSTPARTUM DEPRESSION?

Some normal changes after pregnancy can cause symptoms similar to those of depression. Many mothers feel overwhelmed when a new baby comes home. But, if you have any of the following symptoms of depression for more than two weeks, call your doctor, nurse, or midwife:

- feeling restless or moody
- feeling sad, hopeless, or overwhelmed
- crying a lot
- having thoughts of hurting the baby
- having thoughts of hurting yourself
- not having any interest in the baby, not feeling connected to the baby, or feeling as if your baby is someone else's baby
- having no energy or motivation
- eating too little or too much
- sleeping too little or too much
- having trouble focusing or making decisions
- having memory problems
- feeling worthless, guilty, or like a bad mother
- losing interest or pleasure in activities you used to enjoy
- withdrawing from friends and family
- having headaches, aches, pains, or stomach problems that do not go away

Some women do not tell anyone about their symptoms. New mothers may feel embarrassed, ashamed, or guilty about feeling depressed when they are supposed to be happy. They may also worry they will be seen as bad mothers. Any woman can become depressed during pregnancy or after having a baby. It does not mean you are a bad mom. You and your baby do not have to suffer.

There is help. Your doctor can help you figure out whether your symptoms are caused by depression or something else.

WHAT CAUSES POSTPARTUM DEPRESSION?

Hormonal changes may trigger symptoms of postpartum depression. When you are pregnant, levels of the female hormones estrogen and progesterone are the highest they will ever be. In the first 24 hours after childbirth, hormone levels quickly drop back to normal prepregnancy levels. Researchers think this sudden change in hormone levels may lead to depression. This is similar to hormone changes before a woman's period but involves much more extreme swings in hormone levels.

Levels of thyroid hormones may also drop after giving birth. The thyroid is a small gland in the neck that helps regulate how your body uses and stores energy from food. Low levels of thyroid hormones can cause symptoms of depression. A simple blood test can tell whether this condition is causing your symptoms. If so, your doctor can prescribe thyroid medicine.

Other feelings may contribute to postpartum depression. Many new mothers say they:

- feel tired after labor and delivery
- feel tired from a lack of sleep or broken sleep
- feel overwhelmed with a new baby
- have doubts about their ability to be a good mother
- feel stressed from changes in work and home routines
- feel an unrealistic need to be a perfect mom
- grieve about the loss of who they were before having the baby
- feel less attractive
- do not have free time

These feelings are common among new mothers. But postpartum depression is a serious health condition and can be treated. Postpartum depression is not a regular or expected part of being a new mother.

ARE SOME WOMEN MORE AT RISK OF POSTPARTUM DEPRESSION?

Yes. You may be more at risk of postpartum depression if you:
- have a personal history of depression or bipolar disorder
- have a family history of depression or bipolar disorder
- do not have support from family and friends
- were depressed during pregnancy
- had problems with a previous pregnancy or birth
- have relationship or money problems
- are younger than 20
- have alcoholism, use illegal drugs, or have some other problem with drugs
- have a baby with special needs
- have difficulty breastfeeding
- had an unplanned or unwanted pregnancy

The U.S. Preventive Services Task Force (USPSTF) recommends that doctors look for and ask about symptoms of depression during and after pregnancy, regardless of a woman's risk of depression.

WHAT IS THE DIFFERENCE BETWEEN "BABY BLUES" AND POSTPARTUM DEPRESSION?

Many women have baby blues in the days after childbirth. If you have baby blues, you may:
- have mood swings
- feel sad, anxious, or overwhelmed
- have crying spells
- lose your appetite
- have trouble sleeping

The baby blues usually go away in three to five days after they start. The symptoms of postpartum depression last longer and are more severe. Postpartum depression usually begins within the first month after childbirth, but it can begin during pregnancy or for up to a year after birth. Postpartum depression needs to be treated by a doctor or nurse.

WHAT IS POSTPARTUM PSYCHOSIS?

Postpartum psychosis is rare. It happens in up to four new mothers out of every 1,000 births. It usually begins in the first two weeks after childbirth. It is a medical emergency. Women who have bipolar disorder or another mental health condition called "schizoaffective disorder" have a higher risk of postpartum psychosis. Symptoms may include:

- seeing or hearing things that are not there
- feeling confused most of the time
- having rapid mood swings within several minutes (e.g., crying hysterically, then laughing a lot, followed by extreme sadness)
- trying to hurt yourself or your baby
- paranoia (thinking that others are focused on harming you)
- restlessness or agitation
- behaving recklessly or in a way that is not normal for you

WHAT SHOULD YOU DO IF YOU HAVE SYMPTOMS OF POSTPARTUM DEPRESSION?

Call your doctor, nurse, midwife, or pediatrician if:

- your baby blues do not go away after two weeks
- symptoms of depression get more and more intense
- symptoms of depression begin within one year of delivery and last more than two weeks
- it is difficult to work or get things done at home
- you cannot care for yourself or your baby (e.g., eating, sleeping, bathing)
- you have thoughts about hurting yourself or your baby

Ask your partner or a loved one to call for you if necessary. Your doctor, nurse, or midwife can ask you questions to test for depression. They can also refer you to a mental health professional for help and treatment.

WHAT CAN YOU DO AT HOME TO FEEL BETTER WHILE SEEING A DOCTOR FOR POSTPARTUM DEPRESSION?

Here are some ways to begin feeling better or getting more rest, in addition to talking to a health-care professional:

- Rest as much as you can. Sleep when the baby is sleeping.
- Do not try to do too much or to do everything by yourself. Ask your partner, family, and friends for help.
- Make time to go out, visit friends, or spend time alone with your partner.
- Talk about your feelings with your partner, supportive family members, and friends.
- Talk with other mothers so that you can learn from their experiences.
- Join a support group. Ask your doctor or nurse about groups in your area.
- Do not make any major life changes right after giving birth. More major life changes in addition to a new baby can cause unneeded stress. Sometimes, big changes cannot be avoided. When that happens, try to arrange support and help in your new situation ahead of time.

It can also help you have a partner, a friend, or another caregiver who can help take care of the baby while you are depressed. If you are feeling depressed during pregnancy or after having a baby, do not suffer alone. Tell a loved one and call your doctor right away.

HOW IS POSTPARTUM DEPRESSION TREATED?

The common types of treatment for postpartum depression are as follows:

- **Therapy.** During therapy, you talk to a therapist, psychologist, or social worker to learn strategies to change how depression makes you think, feel, and act.
- **Medicine.** There are different types of medicines for postpartum depression. All of them must be prescribed by your doctor or nurse. The most common type is

antidepressants. Antidepressants can help relieve symptoms of depression, and some can be taken while you are breastfeeding. Antidepressants may take several weeks to start working.

The U.S. Food and Drug Administration (FDA) has also approved a medicine called "brexanolone" to treat postpartum depression in adult women. Brexanolone is given by a doctor or nurse through an IV for two and a half days (60 hours). Because of the risk of side effects, this medicine can only be given in a clinic or office while you are under the care of a doctor or nurse. Brexanolone may not be safe to take while pregnant or breastfeeding.

Another type of medicine called "esketamine" can treat depression and is given as a nasal (nose) spray in a doctor's office or clinic. Esketamine can hurt an unborn baby. You should not take esketamine if you are pregnant or breastfeeding.

- **Electroconvulsive therapy (ECT).** This can be used in extreme cases to treat postpartum depression.

These treatments can be used alone or together. Talk with your doctor or nurse about the benefits and risks of taking medicine to treat depression when you are pregnant or breastfeeding.

Having depression can affect your baby. Getting treatment is important for you and your baby. Taking medicines for depression or going to therapy does not make you a bad mother or a failure. Getting help is a sign of strength.

WHAT CAN HAPPEN IF POSTPARTUM DEPRESSION IS NOT TREATED?

Untreated postpartum depression can affect your ability to parent. You may:
- not have enough energy
- have trouble focusing on the baby's needs and your own needs
- feel moody

- not be able to care for your baby
- have a higher risk of attempting suicide

Feeling like a bad mother can make depression worse. It is important to reach out for help if you feel depressed.

Researchers believe postpartum depression in a mother can affect her child throughout childhood, causing:

- delays in language development and problems learning
- problems with mother–child bonding
- behavior problems
- more crying or agitation
- shorter height and higher risk of obesity in preschoolers
- problems dealing with stress and adjusting to school and other social situations[2]

[2] Office on Women's Health (OWH), "Postpartum Depression," U.S. Department of Health and Human Services (HHS), February 17, 2021. Available online. URL: www.womenshealth.gov/mental-health/mental-health-conditions/postpartum-depression. Accessed May 25, 2023.

Part 3 | Healthy Choices during Pregnancy

Chapter 15 | Choosing a Pregnancy Health-Care Provider

You will see your prenatal care provider many times before you have your baby. So you want to be sure that the person you choose has a good reputation and listens to and respects you. You will want to find out if the doctor or midwife can deliver your baby in the place you want to give birth, such as a specific hospital or birthing center. Your provider should also be willing and able to give you the information and support you need to make an informed choice about whether to breastfeed or bottle-feed.

Health-care providers who care for women during pregnancy include the following:

- **Obstetricians (OBs)**. OBs are medical doctors who specialize in the care of pregnant women and in delivering babies. OBs also have special training in surgery, so they are also able to do a cesarean delivery. Women who have health problems or are at risk of pregnancy complications should see an OB. Women with the highest-risk pregnancies might need special care from a maternal–fetal medicine specialist.
- **Family practice doctors**. These are medical doctors who provide care for the whole family through all stages of life. This includes care during pregnancy and delivery and following birth. Most family practice doctors cannot perform cesarean deliveries.

- **Certified nurse-midwife (CNM) and certified professional midwife (CPM).** CNM and CPM are trained to provide pregnancy and postpartum care. Midwives can be a good option for healthy women at low risk of problems during pregnancy, labor, or delivery. A CNM is educated in both nursing and midwifery. Most CNMs practice in hospitals and birth centers. A CPM is required to have experience delivering babies in home settings because most CPMs practice in homes and birthing centers. All midwives should have a backup plan with an OB in case of a problem or emergency.

Ask your primary care doctor, friends, and family members for provider recommendations. When making your choice, think about:
- reputation
- personality and bedside manner
- the provider's gender and age
- office location and hours
- whether you always will be seen by the same provider during office checkups and delivery
- who covers for the provider when he or she is not available
- where you want to deliver
- how the provider handles phone consultations and after-hours calls

WHAT IS A DOULA?

A doula is a professional labor coach, who gives physical and emotional support to women during labor and delivery. They offer advice on breathing, relaxation, movement, and positioning. Doulas also give emotional support and comfort to women and their partners during labor and birth. Doulas and midwives often work together during a woman's labor. A recent study showed that continuous doula support during labor was linked to shorter labors and much lower use of:

- pain medicines
- oxytocin (medicine to help labor progress)
- cesarean delivery

Check with your health insurance company to find out if they will cover the cost of a doula. When choosing a doula, find out if she is certified by Doulas of North America (DONA) or another professional group.

PLACES TO DELIVER YOUR BABY

Many women have strong views about where and how they would like to deliver their babies. In general, women can choose to deliver at a hospital, birth center, or home. You will need to contact your health insurance provider to find out what options are available. Also, find out if the doctor or midwife you are considering can deliver your baby in the place you want to give birth.

- **Hospitals**. This is a good choice for women with health problems, those with pregnancy complications, or those who are at risk of problems during labor and delivery. Hospitals offer the most advanced medical equipment and highly trained doctors for pregnant women and their babies. In a hospital, doctors can do a cesarean delivery if you or your baby is in danger during labor. Women can get epidurals or many other pain relief options. Also, more and more hospitals now offer on-site birth centers, which aim to offer a style of care similar to standalone birth centers.

The following are a few questions to ask when choosing a hospital:

- Is it close to your home?
- Will the doctor who can give pain relief, such as an epidural, be at the hospital 24 hours a day?

- Will the labor and delivery rooms be comfortable for you?
- Are private rooms available?
- How many support people can you invite into the room with you?
- Does it have a neonatal intensive care unit (NICU) in case of serious problems with the baby?
- Can the baby stay in the room with you?
- Does the hospital have the staff and setup to support successful breastfeeding?
- Does it have an on-site birth center?
- **Birth or birthing centers**. These centers give women a "homey" environment in which to labor and give birth. They try to make labor and delivery a natural and personal process by doing away with most high-tech equipment and routine procedures. So you will not automatically be hooked up to an IV. Likewise, you will not have an electronic fetal monitor around your belly the whole time. Instead, the midwife or nurse will check in on your baby from time to time with a handheld machine. Once the baby is born, all exams and care will occur in your room. Usually, CNMs, not OBs, deliver babies at birth centers. Healthy women who are at low risk of problems during pregnancy, labor, and delivery may choose to deliver at a birth center

  Women cannot receive epidurals at a birth center, although some pain medicines may be available. If a cesarean delivery becomes necessary, women must be moved to a hospital for the procedure. After delivery, babies with problems can receive basic emergency care while being moved to a hospital.

  Many birthing centers have showers or tubs in their rooms for laboring women. They also tend to have comforts of home such as large beds and rocking chairs. In general, birth centers allow more people in the delivery room than hospitals.

Birth centers can be inside of hospitals, a part of a hospital, or completely separate facilities. If you want to deliver at a birth center, make sure it meets the standards of the Accreditation Association for Ambulatory Healthcare (AAAHC), the Joint Commission, or the American Association of Birth Centers (AABC). Accredited birth centers must have doctors who can work at a nearby hospital in case of problems with the mom or baby. Also, make sure the birth center has the staff and setup to support successful breastfeeding.

- **Home birth.** This is an option for healthy pregnant women with no risk factors for complications during pregnancy, labor, or delivery. It is also important that women have a strong aftercare support system at home. Some CNMs and doctors will deliver babies at home. Many health insurance companies do not cover the cost of care for home births. So check with your plan if you would like to deliver at home.

Home births are common in many countries in Europe. However, in the United States, planned home births are not supported by the American Congress of Obstetricians and Gynecologists (ACOG). The ACOG states that hospitals are the safest place to deliver a baby. In case of an emergency, says the ACOG, a hospital's equipment and highly trained doctors can provide the best care for a woman and her baby.

If you are thinking about a home birth, you need to weigh the pros and cons. The main advantage is that you will be able to experience labor and delivery in the privacy and comfort of your own home. Since there will be no routine medical procedures, you will have control of your experience.

The main disadvantage of a home birth is that in case of a problem, you and the baby will not have immediate hospital/medical care. It will have to wait until you are transferred to the hospital. Plus, women who deliver at home have no options for pain relief.

To ensure your safety and that of your baby, you must have a highly trained and experienced midwife along with a fail-safe backup plan. You will need fast, reliable transportation to a hospital. If you live far away from a hospital, home birth may not be the best choice. Your midwife must be experienced and have the necessary skills and supplies to start emergency care for you and your baby if need be. Your midwife should also have access to a doctor 24 hours a day.[1]

[1] Office on Women's Health (OWH), "Prenatal Care and Tests," U.S. Department of Health and Human Services (HHS), February 22, 2021. Available online. URL: www.womenshealth.gov/pregnancy/youre-pregnant-now-what/prenatal-care-and-tests. Accessed May 19, 2023.

Chapter 16 | Prenatal Medical Tests and Care during Pregnancy

Having a healthy pregnancy is one of the best ways to promote a healthy birth. Getting early and regular prenatal care improves the chances of a healthy pregnancy. This care can begin even before pregnancy with a prepregnancy care visit to a health-care provider.

PREPREGNANCY CARE

A prepregnancy care visit can help women take steps toward a healthy pregnancy before they even get pregnant. Women can help promote a healthy pregnancy and birth of a healthy baby by taking the following steps before they become pregnant:

- Develop a plan for their reproductive life.
- Increase their daily intake of folic acid (one of the B vitamins) to at least 400 mcg.
- Make sure their immunizations are up-to-date.
- Control diabetes and other medical conditions.
- Avoid smoking, drinking alcohol, and using drugs.
- Attain a healthy weight.
- Learn about their family health history and that of their partner.
- Seek help for depression, anxiety, or other mental health issues.

PRENATAL CARE

Women who suspect they may be pregnant should schedule a visit to their health-care provider to begin prenatal care. Prenatal visits to a health-care provider usually include a physical exam, weight checks, and providing a urine sample. Depending on the stage of the pregnancy, health-care providers may also do blood tests and imaging tests, such as ultrasound exams. These visits also include discussions about the mother's health, the fetus's health, and any questions about the pregnancy.

Prepregnancy and prenatal care can help prevent complications and inform women about important steps they can take to protect their infant and ensure a healthy pregnancy. With regular prenatal care, women can do the following:

- **Reduce the risk of pregnancy complications**. Following a healthy, safe diet, getting regular exercise as advised by a health-care provider, and avoiding exposure to potentially harmful substances such as lead and radiation can help reduce the risk of problems during pregnancy and promote fetal health and development. Controlling existing conditions, such as high blood pressure and diabetes, is important to prevent serious complications and their effects.

- **Reduce the fetus's and infant's risk of complications**. Tobacco smoke and alcohol use during pregnancy have been shown to increase the risk of sudden infant death syndrome (SIDS). Alcohol use also increases the risk of fetal alcohol spectrum disorders (FASDs), which can cause a variety of problems such as abnormal facial features, having a small head, poor coordination, poor memory, intellectual disability, and problems with the heart, kidneys, or bones. According to one recent study supported by the National Institutes of Health (NIH), these and other long-term problems can occur even with low levels of prenatal alcohol exposure.

  In addition, taking 400 mcg of folic acid daily reduces the risk of neural tube defects by 70 percent. Most prenatal vitamins contain the recommended 400 mcg of folic acid as well as other vitamins that pregnant women and their developing fetus need. Folic acid has been added to foods such as cereals, breads, pasta, and other grain-based foods. Although a related form (called "folate") is present in orange juice and leafy, green vegetables (such as kale and spinach), folate is not absorbed as well as folic acid.

- **Help ensure the medications women take are safe**. Women should not take certain medications, including some acne treatments and dietary and herbal supplements, during pregnancy because they can harm the fetus.[1]

PRENATAL CHECKUPS

During pregnancy, regular checkups are very important. This consistent care can help keep you and your baby healthy, spot problems if they occur, and prevent problems during delivery. Typically, routine checkups occur:

- once each month for weeks 4–28
- twice a month for weeks 28–36
- weekly for weeks 36 to birth

Women with high-risk pregnancies need to see their doctors more often.

At your first visit, your doctor will perform a full physical exam, take your blood for lab tests, and calculate your due date. Your doctor might also do a breast exam, a pelvic exam to check your uterus (womb), and a cervical exam, including a Pap test. During this first visit, your doctor will ask you lots of questions about your lifestyle, relationships, and health habits. It is important to be honest with your doctor.

After the first visit, most prenatal visits will include:

- checking your blood pressure and weight
- checking the baby's heart rate
- measuring your abdomen to check your baby's growth

---

[1] "What Is Prenatal Care and Why Is It Important?" *Eunice Kennedy Shriver* National Institute of Child Health and Human Development (NICHD), January 31, 2017. Available online. URL: www.nichd.nih.gov/health/topics/pregnancy/conditioninfo/prenatal-care. Accessed May 19, 2023.

You will also have some routine tests throughout your pregnancy, such as tests to look for anemia, tests to measure the risk of gestational diabetes, and tests to look for harmful infections.

Become a partner with your doctor to manage your care. Keep all of your appointments—every one is important! Ask questions and read to educate yourself about this exciting time.

MONITOR YOUR BABY'S ACTIVITY

After 28 weeks, keep track of your baby's movement. This will help you notice if your baby is moving less than normal, which could be a sign that your baby is in distress and needs a doctor's care. An easy way to do this is the "count-to-10" approach. Count your baby's movements in the evening—the time of day when the fetus tends to be most active. Lie down if you have trouble feeling your baby move. Most women count 10 movements within about 20 minutes. But it is rare for a woman to count less than 10 movements within two hours at times when the baby is active. Count your baby's movements every day, so you know what is normal for you. Call your doctor if you count less than 10 movements within two hours or if you notice your baby is moving less than normal. If your baby is not moving at all, call your doctor right away.

PRENATAL TESTS

Tests are used during pregnancy to check your and your baby's health (refer to Table 16.1). At your first prenatal visit, your doctor will use tests to check for a number of things, such as:

- your blood type and Rh factor
- anemia
- infections, such as toxoplasmosis and sexually transmitted infections (STIs), including hepatitis B, syphilis, chlamydia, and human immunodeficiency virus (HIV)
- signs that you are immune to rubella (German measles) and chickenpox

Throughout your pregnancy, your doctor or midwife may suggest a number of other tests, too. Some tests are suggested for all women, such as screenings for gestational diabetes, Down syndrome, and HIV. Other tests might be offered based on your:

- age
- personal or family health history
- ethnic background
- results of routine tests

Some tests are screening tests. They detect risks for or signs of possible health problems in you or your baby. Based on screening test results, your doctor might suggest diagnostic tests. Diagnostic tests confirm or rule out health problems in you or your baby.

Table 16.1. Common Prenatal Tests

Test	What It Is	How It Is Done
Amniocentesis	This test can diagnose certain birth defects, including: • Down syndrome • cystic fibrosis • spina bifida It is performed at 14–20 weeks. It may be suggested for couples at higher risk of genetic disorders. It also provides DNA for paternity testing.	A thin needle is used to draw out a small amount of amniotic fluid and cells from the sac surrounding the fetus. The sample is sent to a lab for testing.
Biophysical profile (BPP)	This test is used in the third trimester to monitor the overall health of the baby and to help decide if the baby should be delivered early.	BPP involves an ultrasound exam along with a nonstress test. The BPP looks at the baby's breathing, movement, muscle tone, heart rate, and the amount of amniotic fluid.
Chorionic villus sampling (CVS)	This test is done at 10–13 weeks to diagnose certain birth defects, including: • chromosomal disorders, including Down syndrome • genetic disorders, such as cystic fibrosis CVS may be suggested for couples at higher risk of genetic disorders. It also provides DNA for paternity testing.	A needle removes a small sample of cells from the placenta to be tested.

Table 16.1. Continued

Test	What It Is	How It Is Done
First trimester screen	This is a screening test done at 11–14 weeks to detect higher risk of: • chromosomal disorders, including Down syndrome and trisomy 18 • other problems, such as heart defects It can also reveal multiple births. Based on test results, your doctor may suggest other tests to diagnose a disorder.	This test involves both a blood test and an ultrasound exam called "nuchal translucency screening." The blood test measures the levels of certain substances in the mother's blood. The ultrasound exam measures the thickness at the back of the baby's neck. This information, combined with the mother's age, helps doctors determine the risk to the fetus.
Glucose challenge screening	This is a screening test done at 26–28 weeks to determine the mother's risk of gestational diabetes. Based on test results, your doctor may suggest a glucose tolerance test.	First, you consume a special sugary drink from your doctor. A blood sample is taken one hour later to look for high blood sugar levels.
Glucose tolerance test	This test is done at 26–28 weeks to diagnose gestational diabetes.	Your doctor will tell you what to eat a few days before the test. Then, you cannot eat or drink anything but sips of water for 14 hours before the test. Your blood is drawn to test your "fasting blood glucose level." Then you will consume a sugary drink. Your blood will be tested every hour for three hours to see how well your body processes sugar.
Group B *Streptococcus* infection	This test is done at 36–37 weeks to look for bacteria that can cause pneumonia or serious infection in newborns.	A swab is used to take cells from your vagina and rectum to be tested.

Prenatal Medical Tests and Care during Pregnancy

Table 16.1. Continued

Test	What It Is	How It Is Done
Maternal serum screen (also called "quad screen," "triple test," "triple screen," "multiple marker screen," or "AFP")	This is a screening test done at 15–20 weeks to detect higher risk of: • chromosomal disorders, including Down syndrome and trisomy 18 • neural tube defects, such as spina bifida Based on test results, your doctor may suggest other tests to diagnose a disorder.	Blood is drawn to measure the levels of certain substances in the mother's blood.
Nonstress test (NST)	This test is performed after 28 weeks to monitor your baby's health. It can show signs of fetal distress, such as your baby not getting enough oxygen.	A belt is placed around the mother's belly to measure the baby's heart rate in response to its own movements.
Ultrasound exam	An ultrasound exam can be performed at any point during the pregnancy. Ultrasound exams are not routine. But it is not uncommon for women to have a standard ultrasound exam between 18 and 20 weeks to look for signs of problems with the baby's organs and body systems and confirm the age of the fetus and proper growth. It might also be able to tell the sex of your baby. Ultrasound exam is also used as part of the first trimester screen and BPP. Based on exam results, your doctor may suggest other tests or other types of ultrasound to help detect a problem.	Ultrasound uses sound waves to create a "picture" of your baby on a monitor. With a standard ultrasound, a gel is spread on your abdomen. A special tool is moved over your abdomen, which allows your doctor and you to view the baby on a monitor.
Urine test	A urine sample can look for signs of health problems, such as: • urinary tract infection (UTI) • diabetes • preeclampsia If your doctor suspects a problem, the sample might be sent to a lab for more in-depth testing.	You will collect a small sample of clean, midstream urine in a sterile plastic cup. Testing strips that look for certain substances in your urine are dipped in the sample. The sample can also be looked at under a microscope.

UNDERSTANDING PRENATAL TESTS AND TEST RESULTS

If your doctor suggests certain prenatal tests, do not be afraid to ask lots of questions. Learning about the test, why your doctor is suggesting it for you, and what the test results could mean can help you cope with any worries or fears you might have. Keep in mind that screening tests do not diagnose problems. They evaluate risk. Therefore, if a screening test comes back abnormal, this does not mean there is a problem with your baby. More information is needed. Your doctor can explain what test results mean and possible next steps.

AVOID KEEPSAKE ULTRASOUNDS

You might think a keepsake ultrasound is a must-have for your scrapbook. But doctors advise against ultrasound when there is no medical need to do so. Some companies sell "keepsake" ultrasound videos and images. Although ultrasound is considered safe for medical purposes, exposure to ultrasound energy for a keepsake video or image may put a mother and her unborn baby at risk. Do not take that chance.[2]

---

[2] Office on Women's Health (OWH), "Prenatal Care and Tests," U.S. Department of Health and Human Services (HHS), February 22, 2021. Available online. URL: www.womenshealth.gov/pregnancy/youre-pregnant-now-what/prenatal-care-and-tests. Accessed May 19, 2023.

Chapter 17 | **Birthing, Breastfeeding, and Parenting Classes**

First-time mothers-to-be often have lots of questions and even some worries: How will I know I am in labor? Will it hurt? Will my baby know how to breastfeed? How do I care for a newborn? Classes to prepare you for childbirth, breastfeeding, infant care, and parenting are great ways to lessen anxiety and build confidence. In some cities, classes might be offered in different languages.

BIRTHING CLASSES

Birthing classes are often offered through local hospitals and birthing centers. Some classes follow a specific method, such as Lamaze or the Bradley method. Others review labor techniques from a variety of methods. You might want to read about the different methods beforehand to see if one appeals more to you than the others. That way, you will know what to sign up for if more than one type of birthing class is offered. Try to sign up for a class several months before your due date. Classes sometimes fill up quickly. Also, make sure the instructor is qualified.

Most women attend the class with the person who will provide support during labor, such as a spouse, sister, or good friend. This person is sometimes called the "labor coach." During class, the instructor will go over the signs of labor and review the stages of labor. She will talk about positioning for labor and birth and ways to control pain. She will also give you strategies to work through labor pains and to help you stay relaxed and in control. You will practice many of these strategies in class so that you are ready when the big day arrives. Many classes also provide a tour of the birthing facility.

BREASTFEEDING CLASSES

Like any new skill, breastfeeding takes knowledge and practice to be successful. Pregnant women who learn about how to breastfeed are more likely to be successful than those who do not. Breastfeeding classes offer pregnant women and their partners the chance to prepare and ask questions before the baby's arrival. Classes may be offered through hospitals, breastfeeding support programs, La Leche League, or local lactation consultants. Ask your doctor for help finding a breastfeeding class in your area.

PARENTING CLASSES

Many first-time parents have never cared for a newborn. Hospitals, community education centers, and places of worship sometimes offer baby care classes. These classes cover the basics, such as diapering, feeding, and bathing your newborn. You will also learn these basic skills in the hospital before you are discharged.

In some communities, parenting classes are available. Children do not come with how-to manuals. So some parents appreciate learning about the different stages of child development, as well as practical skills for dealing with common issues, such as discipline or parent–child power struggles. Counselors and social workers often teach this type of class. If you are interested in parenting programs, ask your child's doctor for help finding a class in your area.[1]

---

[1] Office on Women's Health (OWH), "Birthing, Breastfeeding, and Parenting Classes," U.S. Department of Health and Human Services (HHS), February 22, 2021. Available online. URL: www.womenshealth.gov/pregnancy/getting-ready-baby/birthing-breastfeeding-and-parenting-classes. Accessed May 17, 2023.

Chapter 18 | **Immunization for Pregnant Women**

Vaccines can help protect both you and your baby from vaccine-preventable diseases. During pregnancy, vaccinated mothers pass on infection-fighting proteins called "antibodies" to their babies. Antibodies provide some immunity (protection) against certain diseases during their first few months of life when your baby is still too young to get vaccinated. It also helps provide important protection for you throughout your pregnancy. To protect yourself and your baby, it is important to understand which vaccines you may need before, during, and after your pregnancy.

WHICH VACCINES DO YOU NEED BEFORE YOU GET PREGNANT?

If you are planning to get pregnant, it is important to make sure you are up-to-date on all of your adult vaccines.

Before your pregnancy, talk with your doctor about your vaccine history. You may need vaccines that protect against the following:

- **Rubella**. Rubella during pregnancy can cause serious birth defects that can lead to death before birth or life-long illness for your child. To find out if you are protected from rubella, you can check with your doctor or have a prepregnancy blood test. It is important to wait a month after getting the vaccine before you try to get pregnant.
- **Hepatitis B**. If you have hepatitis B infection during pregnancy, it can pass to your baby during birth. Hepatitis B can lead to serious, ongoing health problems for your child. Talk with your doctor about

183

getting tested for hepatitis B and whether or not you need to get vaccinated.

WHICH VACCINES DO YOU NEED DURING PREGNANCY?

All pregnant women need to get vaccinated against the flu and whooping cough during each pregnancy.

The Flu Shot

Getting vaccinated against the flu is important because pregnant women are at increased risk of serious complications from the flu. The flu can also cause serious problems, such as early labor and delivery, which can affect your baby's health.

In addition, getting the flu shot during pregnancy makes it less likely that newborns will get the flu for several months after they are born—and that lowers their risk of serious complications such as pneumonia (lung infection). You can get the flu shot during any trimester of your pregnancy.

The Whooping Cough Vaccine

Getting vaccinated against whooping cough helps protect young babies from whooping cough before they are old enough to get vaccinated themselves. About half of babies who get whooping cough end up in the hospital—and the disease can be life-threatening.

The vaccine can be given at any time during pregnancy, but experts recommend getting the vaccine as early as possible in the third trimester (between 27 and 36 weeks of pregnancy). The whooping cough vaccine is also recommended for other adults who spend time with your baby.

Is It Safe to Get Vaccines during Pregnancy?

Yes. It is safe to get the vaccines recommended during pregnancy. Research shows that whooping cough and flu vaccines help provide important disease protection for pregnant women. And experts closely monitor the safety of vaccines.

Like any medicine, vaccines can have side effects. But these side effects are usually mild and go away on their own. The side effects of vaccines that protect against the flu and whooping cough include the following:
- pain, redness, or swelling where the shot was given
- muscle aches
- feeling tired
- fever

Many people experience these side effects—not just pregnant women.

WHICH VACCINES DO YOU NEED AFTER YOUR BABY IS BORN?

After your baby is born, you may need to get vaccines to protect against the following:
- **Whooping cough.** If you did not get the whooping cough vaccine when you were pregnant, you will need to get vaccinated right after delivery. Other people who spend time with the baby may also need to get the whooping cough vaccine.
- **Measles, mumps, rubella, and chickenpox.** If you are not already protected from measles, mumps, rubella, or chickenpox, you will need to get vaccinated before you leave the hospital.

All routinely recommended vaccines are safe for breastfeeding women.

ARE YOU PLANNING TO TRAVEL? MAKE SURE YOU AND YOUR BABY ARE PROTECTED

Many vaccine-preventable diseases that are rare in the United States are still common in other parts of the world. If you are pregnant and planning to travel outside the United States, talk with your doctor about vaccines that may be recommended for you.[1]

---

[1] "Vaccines for Pregnant Women," U.S. Department of Health and Human Services (HHS), May 7, 2021. Available online. URL: www.hhs.gov/immunization/who-and-when/pregnant/index.html. Accessed May 19, 2023.

CAN A VACCINE HARM YOUR DEVELOPING BABY?

Some vaccines, especially live vaccines, should not be given to pregnant women because they may be harmful to the baby. Keep in mind that vaccine recommendations for pregnant women are developed with the highest safety concerns for both mothers and babies.

ARE VACCINES SAFE IF YOU ARE BREASTFEEDING?

Yes. It is safe to receive routine vaccines right after giving birth, even while you are breastfeeding. However, the yellow fever vaccine is not recommended for breastfeeding women unless travel to certain countries is unavoidable and a health-care provider determines that the benefits of vaccination outweigh the risks. Talk with your provider if you are considering the yellow fever vaccine.[2]

---

[2] "Vaccines during Pregnancy FAQs," Centers for Disease Control and Prevention (CDC), August 24, 2020. Available online. URL: www.cdc.gov/vaccinesafety/concerns/vaccines-during-pregnancy.html. Accessed May 19, 2023.

Chapter 19 | Taking Medicines during Pregnancy

Chapter Contents

Section 19.1 | Is It Safe to Use Medicines during Pregnancy?

When deciding whether or not to use a medicine in pregnancy, you and your doctor need to talk about the medicine's benefits and risks. Before you start or stop any medicine while you are pregnant, it is always best to speak with your doctor.

IS IT SAFE TO USE MEDICINE WHILE YOU ARE PREGNANT?
There is no clear-cut answer to this question. Before you start or stop any medicine, it is always best to speak with the doctor who is caring for you while you are pregnant.

HOW SHOULD YOU DECIDE WHETHER TO USE A MEDICINE WHILE YOU ARE PREGNANT?
When deciding whether or not to use a medicine in pregnancy, you and your doctor need to talk about the medicine's benefits and risks.
- **Benefits**. What are the good things the medicine can do for me and my growing baby (fetus)?
- **Risks**. What are the ways the medicine might harm me or my growing baby (fetus)?

There may be times during pregnancy when using medicine is a choice. Some of the medicine choices you and your doctor make while you are pregnant may differ from the choices you make when you are not pregnant. For example, if you get a cold, you may decide to "live with" your stuffy nose instead of using the "stuffy nose" medicine you use when you are not pregnant.

Other times, using medicine is not a choice—it is needed. Some women need to use medicines while they are pregnant. Sometimes, women need medicine for a few days or a couple of weeks to treat a problem such as a bladder infection or strep throat. Other women need to use medicine every day to control long-term health problems such as asthma, diabetes, depression, or seizures. Also, some women have a pregnancy problem that needs treatment with medicine. These problems might include severe nausea and vomiting, earlier pregnancy losses, or preterm labor.

WHERE DO DOCTORS AND NURSES LEARN ABOUT USING MEDICINES DURING PREGNANCY?

Doctors and nurses get information from medicine labels and packages, textbooks, and research journals. They also share knowledge with other doctors and nurses and talk to the people who make and sell medicines.

The U.S. Food and Drug Administration (FDA) is the part of the country's government that controls the medicines that can and cannot be sold in the United States. The FDA lets a company sell a medicine in the United States if it is safe to use and works for a certain health problem. Companies that make medicines usually have to show the FDA doctors and scientists whether birth defects or other problems occur in baby animals when the medicine is given to pregnant animals. Most of the time, drugs are not studied in pregnant women.

The FDA works with drug companies to make clear and complete medicine labels. However, in most cases, there is not much information about how a medicine affects pregnant women and their growing babies. Many prescription medicine labels include the results of studies done on pregnant animals. But medicine does not always affect growing humans and animals in the same way. Here is an example:

- A medicine is given to pregnant rats. If the medicine causes problems in some of the rat babies, it may or may not cause problems in human babies. If there are no problems in the rat babies, it does not prove that the medicine will not cause problems in human babies.
  The FDA asks for studies in two different kinds of animals. This improves the chance that the studies can predict what may happen in pregnant women and their babies.

There is a lot that FDA doctors and scientists do not know about using medicine during pregnancy. In a perfect world, every medicine label would include helpful information about the medicine's effects on pregnant women and their growing babies. Unfortunately, this is not the case.

HOW DO PRESCRIPTION AND OVER-THE-COUNTER MEDICINE LABELS HELP YOUR DOCTOR CHOOSE THE RIGHT MEDICINE FOR YOU WHEN YOU ARE PREGNANT?

Doctors use information from many sources when they choose medicine for a patient, including medicine labels. To help doctors, the FDA created pregnancy letter categories to help explain what is known about using medicine during pregnancy. This system assigns letter categories to all prescription medicines. The letter category is listed on the label of a prescription medicine. The label states whether studies were done in pregnant women or pregnant animals and, if so, what happened. Over-the-counter (OTC) medicines do not have a pregnancy letter category. Some OTC medicines were prescription medicines first and used to have a letter category (refer to Table 19.1). Talk to your doctor and follow the instructions on the label before taking OTC medicines.

Prescription Medicines

The FDA chooses a medicine's letter category based on what is known about the medicine when used in pregnant women and animals.

The FDA is working hard to gather more knowledge about using medicine during pregnancy. The FDA is also trying to make medicine labels more helpful to doctors. Medicine label information for prescription medicines is now changing, and the pregnancy part of the label will change over the next few years. As this prescription information is updated, it is added to an online information clearinghouse called "DailyMed" that gives up-to-date, free information to consumers and health-care providers.

Table 19.1. Definition of Medicine Categories

Pregnancy Category	Definition	Examples of Drugs
A	In human studies, pregnant women used the medicine, and their babies did not have any problems related to using the medicine.	• Folic acid • Levothyroxine (thyroid hormone medicine)
B	In humans, there are no good studies. But, in animal studies, pregnant animals received the medicine, and the babies did not show any problems related to the medicine. Or In animal studies, pregnant animals received the medicine, and some babies had problems. But, in human studies, pregnant women used the medicine, and their babies did not have any problems related to using the medicine.	• Some antibiotics such as amoxicillin • Zofran (ondansetron) for nausea • Glucophage (metformin) for diabetes • Some insulins used to treat diabetes such as regular and NPH insulin
C	In humans, there are no good studies. In animals, pregnant animals treated with the medicine had some babies with problems. However, sometimes, the medicine may still help human mothers and babies more than it might harm. Or No animal studies have been done, and there are no good studies in pregnant women.	• Diflucan (fluconazole) for yeast infections • Ventolin (albuterol) for asthma • Zoloft (sertraline) and Prozac (fluoxetine) for depression
D	Studies in humans and other reports show that when pregnant women use the medicine, some babies are born with problems related to the medicine. However, in some serious situations, the medicine may still help the mother and the baby more than it might harm.	• Paxil (paroxetine) for depression • Lithium for bipolar disorder • Dilantin (phenytoin) for epileptic seizures • Some cancer chemotherapy
X	Studies or reports in humans or animals show that mothers using the medicine during pregnancy may have babies with problems related to the medicine. There are no situations where the medicine can help the mother or baby enough to make the risk of problems worth it. These medicines should never be used by pregnant women.	• Accutane (isotretinoin) for cysticacne • Thalomid (thalidomide) for a type of skin disease

Over-the-Counter Medicines

All OTC medicines have a Drug Facts label. The Drug Facts label is arranged the same way on all OTC medicines. This makes information about using the medicine easier to find. One section of the Drug Facts label is for pregnant women. With OTC medicines, the label usually tells a pregnant woman to speak with her doctor before using the medicine. Some OTC medicines are known to cause certain problems in pregnancy. The labels for these medicines give pregnant women facts about why and when they should not use the medicine. Here are some examples:

- Nonsteroidal anti-inflammatory drugs (NSAIDs), such as ibuprofen (Advil, Motrin), naproxen (Aleve), and aspirin (acetylsalicylate), can cause serious blood flow problems in the baby if used during the last three months of pregnancy (after 28 weeks). Also, aspirin may increase the chance of bleeding problems in the mother and the baby during pregnancy or at delivery.
- The labels for nicotine therapy drugs, such as the nicotine patch and lozenge, remind women that smoking can harm an unborn child. While the medicine is thought to be safer than smoking, the risks of the medicine are not fully known. Pregnant smokers are told to try quitting without the medicine first.

WHAT IF YOU ARE THINKING ABOUT GETTING PREGNANT?

If you are not pregnant yet, you can help your chances of having a healthy baby by planning ahead. Schedule a prepregnancy checkup. At this visit, you can talk to your doctor about the medicines, vitamins, and herbs you use. It is very important that you keep treating your health problems while you are pregnant. Your doctor can tell you if you need to switch your medicine. Ask about vitamins for women who are trying to get pregnant. All women who can get pregnant should take a daily vitamin with folic acid (a B vitamin) to prevent birth defects of the brain and spinal cord. You should begin taking these vitamins before you become pregnant or if you could become pregnant. It is also a good idea to discuss caffeine, alcohol, and smoking with your doctor at this time.

IS IT SAFE TO USE MEDICINE WHILE YOU ARE TRYING TO BECOME PREGNANT?

It is hard to know exactly when you will get pregnant. Once you do get pregnant, you may not know you are pregnant for 10 –14 days or longer. Before you start trying to get pregnant, it is wise to schedule a meeting with your doctor to discuss medicines that you use daily or every now and then. Sometimes, medicines should be changed, and sometimes, they can be stopped before a woman gets pregnant. Each woman is different. So you should discuss your medicines with your doctor rather than making medicine changes on your own.

If you are pregnant or thinking about getting pregnant:

- do not stop any prescribed medicines without first talking to your doctor
- talk to your doctor before using any OTC medicine

WHAT IF YOU GET SICK AND NEED TO USE MEDICINE WHILE YOU ARE PREGNANT?

Whether or not you should use medicine during pregnancy is a serious question to discuss with your doctor. Some health problems need treatment. Not using a medicine that you need could harm you and your baby. For example, a urinary tract infection (UTI) that is not treated may become a kidney infection. Kidney infections can cause preterm labor and low birth weight. You need an antibiotic to cure a UTI. Ask your doctor whether the benefits of taking a certain medicine outweigh the risks for you and your baby.

YOU HAVE A HEALTH PROBLEM. SHOULD YOU STOP USING YOUR MEDICINE WHILE YOU ARE PREGNANT?

If you are pregnant or thinking about becoming pregnant, you should talk to your doctor about your medicines. Do not stop or change them on your own. This includes medicines for depression, asthma, diabetes, seizures (epilepsy), and other health problems. Not using medicine that you need may be more harmful to you and your baby than using the medicine.

For women living with human immunodeficiency virus (HIV), the Centers for Disease Control and Prevention (CDC) recommends using zidovudine (AZT) during pregnancy. Studies show that HIV-positive women who use AZT during pregnancy greatly lower the risk of passing HIV to their babies. If a diabetic woman does not use her medicine during pregnancy, she raises her risk of miscarriage, stillbirth, and some birth defects. If asthma and high blood pressure are not controlled during pregnancy, problems with the fetus may result.

ARE VITAMINS SAFE FOR YOU WHILE YOU ARE PREGNANT?

Women who are pregnant should not take regular vitamins. They can contain doses that are too high. Ask about special vitamins for pregnant women that can help keep you and your baby healthy. These prenatal vitamins should contain at least 400–800 micrograms (μg) of folic acid. It is best to start taking these vitamins before you become pregnant or if you could become pregnant. Folic acid reduces the chance of a baby having a neural tube defect, such as spina bifida, where the spine or brain does not form the right way. Iron can help prevent a low red blood cell (RBC) count (anemia). It is important to take the vitamin dose prescribed by your doctor. Too many vitamins can harm your baby. For example, very high levels of vitamin A have been linked with severe birth defects.

ARE HERBS, MINERALS, OR AMINO ACIDS SAFE FOR YOU WHILE YOU ARE PREGNANT?

No one is sure if these are safe for pregnant women, so it is best not to use them. Even some "natural" products may not be good for women who are pregnant or breastfeeding. Except for some vitamins, little is known about using dietary supplements while pregnant. Some herbal remedy labels claim that they will help with pregnancy. But most often there are no good studies to show if these claims are true or if the herb can cause harm to you or your baby. Talk with your doctor before using any herbal product or dietary supplement. These products may contain things that could harm you or your growing baby during your pregnancy.

In the United States, there are different laws for medicines and for dietary supplements. The part of the FDA that controls dietary supplements is the same part that controls foods sold in the United States. Only dietary supplements containing new dietary ingredients that were not marketed before October 15, 1994, submit safety information for review by the FDA. However, unlike medicines, the FDA does not approve herbal remedies and "natural products" for safety or for what they say they will do. Most have not even been evaluated for their potential to cause harm to you or the growing fetus, let alone shown to be safe for use in pregnancy. Before a company can sell a medicine, the company must complete many studies and send the results to the FDA. Many scientists and doctors at the FDA check the study results. The FDA allows the medicine to be sold only if the studies show that the medicine works and is safe to use.

IN THE FUTURE, WILL THERE BE BETTER WAYS TO KNOW IF MEDICINES ARE SAFE TO USE DURING PREGNANCY?

At this time, drugs are rarely tested for safety in pregnant women for fear of harming the unborn baby. Until this changes, pregnancy exposure registries help doctors and researchers learn how medicines affect pregnant mothers and their growing babies. A pregnancy exposure registry is a study that enrolls pregnant women who are using a certain medicine. The women sign up for the study while pregnant and are followed for a certain length of time after the baby is born. Researchers compare babies of mothers who used the medicine while pregnant to babies of mothers who did not use the medicine. This type of study compares large groups of pregnant mothers and babies to look for medicine effects. A woman and her doctor can use registry results to make more informed choices about using medicine while pregnant.

If you are pregnant and are using a medicine or were using one when you got pregnant, check to see if there is a pregnancy exposure registry for that medicine. The FDA has a list of pregnancy exposure registries that pregnant women can join.[1]

---

[1] Office on Women's Health (OWH), "Pregnancy and Medicines," U.S. Department of Health and Human Services (HHS), February 22, 2021. Available online. URL: www.womenshealth.gov/a-z-topics/pregnancy-and-medicines. Accessed May 19, 2023.

Section 19.2 | Aspirin and Pregnancy

Aspirin is generally not recommended during pregnancy, as it can lead to bleeding problems for both the mother and baby. But, for some women, the benefits of daily low-dose aspirin after the first trimester may outweigh the risk.

Results from multiple clinical trials showed that using low-dose aspirin lowered the risk of preeclampsia in pregnant women at high risk of the condition. Preeclampsia happens when a woman's blood pressure suddenly gets too high during pregnancy. If preeclampsia occurs during pregnancy, the only current cure is delivery of the fetus, often prematurely. In fact, preeclampsia is responsible for 15 percent of preterm births in the United States.

The clinical trials also found that low-dose aspirin reduced the risk of premature delivery and low birth weight of infants. Based on these findings, the U.S. Preventive Services Task Force (USPSTF) issued a recommendation that women at high risk of preeclampsia take a daily low-dose aspirin after 12 weeks of pregnancy to help prevent the condition from developing. The USPSTF recommendation mirrored the 2013 guidelines from the American College of Obstetricians and Gynecologists (ACOG).

DETERMINING A PREGNANT WOMAN'S RISK OF PREECLAMPSIA

Preeclampsia affects 3–5 percent of pregnancies in the United States each year and is a leading cause of maternal and neonatal morbidity/mortality. Women may be at higher risk of preeclampsia if they:

- had preeclampsia in a previous pregnancy, especially if they delivered prematurely
- are obese
- are younger than the age of 20 or older than 35
- are carrying twins or multiples
- had high blood pressure or kidney disease before getting pregnant
- are African American
- have a family history of preeclampsia

- have certain health conditions, such as diabetes, lupus, or polycystic ovary syndrome (PCOS)

However, it can be difficult to predict if a woman will develop preeclampsia. Pregnant women with normal blood pressure at 20 weeks of pregnancy can suddenly develop the symptoms, which include high blood pressure, increased swelling, and protein in the urine. Much of the time, preeclampsia has no visible symptoms.

For this reason, it is important for all pregnant women to get regular prenatal care. This will allow their health-care provider to monitor their health closely and determine if a daily aspirin is needed.[2]

ASPIRIN MAY HELP INCREASE PREGNANCY CHANCES IN WOMEN WITH HIGH INFLAMMATION

A daily low dose of aspirin may help a subgroup of women who have previously lost a pregnancy to successfully conceive and carry a pregnancy to term according to an analysis by researchers at the National Institutes of Health (NIH). The women who benefited from the aspirin treatment had high levels of C-reactive protein (CRP), a substance in the blood indicating system-wide inflammation, which aspirin is thought to counteract. The study appears in the *Journal of Clinical Endocrinology and Metabolism*.

Researchers at the NIH NICHD analyzed data originally obtained from the Effects of Aspirin in Gestation and Reproduction (EAGeR) trial. The trial sought to determine if daily low-dose aspirin could prevent subsequent pregnancy loss among women who had one or two prior losses.

For the current study, researchers classified the women into three groups: low CRP (below 0.70 mg per liter of blood), mid-CRP (from 0.70 to 1.95), and high CRP (at or above 1.95). Women

---

[2] "An Aspirin Day for Preeclampsia Prevention," *Eunice Kennedy Shriver* National Institute of Child Health and Human Development (NICHD), August 25, 2014. Available online. URL: www.nichd.nih.gov/newsroom/resources/spotlight/082514-preeclampsia-prevention. Accessed May 19, 2023.

within each group received either daily low-dose aspirin or a placebo. In their analysis, researchers found no significant differences in birth rates between those receiving aspirin and those receiving placebo in both the low-CRP and mid-CRP groups. For the high-CRP group, those taking the placebo had the lowest rate of live birth at 44 percent, while those taking daily aspirin had a live birth rate of 59 percent—a 35 percent increase. Aspirin also appeared to reduce CRP levels in the high-CRP group when measured during weeks 8, 20, and 36 of pregnancy.[3]

WHAT ARE NONSTEROIDAL ANTI-INFLAMMATORY DRUGS, AND HOW CAN THEY HELP YOU?

Nonsteroidal anti-inflammatory drugs (NSAIDs) have been widely used for decades to treat pain and fever from many different long- and short-term medical conditions such as arthritis, menstrual cramps, headaches, colds, and the flu. NSAIDs work by blocking the production of certain chemicals in the body that cause inflammation.

NSAIDs are available alone and combined with other medicines to treat a wide variety of conditions, including pain, colds, coughs, flu, and insomnia. Examples of NSAIDs include aspirin, ibuprofen, naproxen, diclofenac, and celecoxib.[4]

---

[3] "Aspirin May Help Increase Pregnancy Chances in Women with High Inflammation, NIH Study Finds," *Eunice Kennedy Shriver* National Institute of Child Health and Human Development (NICHD), February 7, 2017. Available online. URL: www.nichd.nih.gov/newsroom/releases/020717_aspirin. Accessed May 19, 2023.
[4] "FDA Recommends Avoiding Use of NSAIDs in Pregnancy at 20 Weeks or Later Because They Can Result in Low Amniotic Fluid," U.S. Food and Drug Administration (FDA), January 27, 2023. Available online. URL: www.fda.gov/drugs/drug-safety-and-availability/fda-recommends-avoiding-use-nsaids-pregnancy-20-weeks-or-later-because-they-can-result-low-amniotic. Accessed May 19, 2023.

Chapter 20 | Nutrition and Pregnancy

Chapter Contents

EATING FOR TWO

Eating healthy foods is more important now than ever! You need more protein, iron, calcium, and folic acid than you did before pregnancy. You also need more calories. But "eating for two" does not mean eating twice as much. Rather, it means that the foods you eat are the main source of nutrients for your baby. A sensible, balanced meal combined with regular physical fitness is still the best recipe for good health during your pregnancy.

CALORIE NEEDS

Your calorie needs will depend on your weight gain goals. Most women need 300 calories a day more during at least the last six months of pregnancy than they do during prepregnancy. Keep in mind that not all calories are equal. Your baby needs healthy foods that are packed with nutrients—not "empty calories" such as those found in soft drinks, candies, and desserts.

Although you want to be careful not to eat more than you need for a healthy pregnancy, make sure not to restrict your diet during pregnancy either. If you do not get the calories you need, your baby might not get the right amounts of proteins, vitamins, and minerals. Low-calorie diets can break down a pregnant woman's stored fat. This can cause your body to make substances called "ketones." Ketones can be found in the mother's blood and urine and are a sign of starvation. Constant production of ketones can result in a child with mental deficiencies.

FOODS GOOD FOR THE MOM AND BABY

A pregnant woman needs more of many important vitamins, minerals, and nutrients than she did before pregnancy. Making healthy food choices every day will help you give your baby what he or she needs to develop. ChooseMyPlate.gov for Moms/Moms-to-Be can show you what to eat as well as how much you need to eat from each food group based on your height, weight, and activity level.

Talk to your doctor if you have special diet needs for these reasons:

- **Diabetes**. Make sure you review your meal plan and insulin needs with your doctor. High blood glucose levels can be harmful to your baby.
- **Lactose intolerance**. Find out about low- or reduced-lactose products and calcium supplements to ensure you are getting the calcium you need.
- **Vegetarian**. Ensure that you are eating enough protein, iron, vitamin B_{12}, and vitamin D.
- **Phenylketonuria (PKU)**. Keep good control of phenylalanine levels in your diet.

FOOD SAFETY

Most foods are safe for pregnant women and their babies. But you will need to use caution or avoid eating certain foods. Follow these guidelines:

- Clean, handle, cook, and chill food properly to prevent foodborne illness, including listeria and toxoplasmosis:
  - Wash hands with soap after touching soil or raw meat.
  - Keep raw meats, poultry, and seafood from touching other foods or surfaces.
  - Cook meat completely.
  - Wash produce before eating.
  - Wash cooking utensils with hot, soapy water.
- Do not eat:
  - refrigerated smoked seafood, such as whitefish, salmon, and mackerel
  - hot dogs or deli meats unless steaming hot
  - refrigerated meat spreads
  - unpasteurized milk or juices
  - store-made salads, such as chicken, egg, or tuna salad
  - unpasteurized soft cheeses, such as unpasteurized feta, Brie, queso blanco, queso fresco, and blue cheeses
  - shark, swordfish, king mackerel, or tilefish (also called "golden" or "white snapper," which have high levels of mercury)

- more than six ounces per week of white (albacore) tuna
- herbs and plants used as medicines without your doctor's approval (The safety of herbal and plant therapies is not always known. Some herbs and plants might be harmful during pregnancy, such as bitter melon (karela), noni juice, and unripe papaya.)
- raw sprouts of any kind (including alfalfa, clover, radish, and mung bean)

DO NOT FORGET FLUIDS

All of your body's systems need water. When you are pregnant, your body needs even more water to stay hydrated and support the life inside you. Water also helps prevent constipation, hemorrhoids, excessive swelling, and urinary tract or bladder infections. Not getting enough water can lead to premature or early labor.

Your body gets the water it needs through the fluids you drink and the foods you eat. How much fluid you need to drink each day depends on many factors, such as your activity level, the weather, and your size. Your body needs more fluids when it is hot and when you are physically active. It also needs more water if you have a fever or if you are vomiting or have diarrhea.

The Institute of Medicine (IOM) recommends that pregnant women drink about 10 cups of fluids daily. Water, juices, coffee, tea, and soft drinks all count toward your fluid needs. But keep in mind that some beverages are high in sugar and "empty" calories. A good way to tell if your fluid intake is okay is if your urine is pale yellow or colorless and you rarely feel thirsty. Thirst is a sign that your body is on its way to dehydration. Do not wait until you feel thirsty to drink.[1]

---

[1] Office on Women's Health (OWH), "Staying Healthy and Safe," U.S. Department of Health and Human Services (HHS), February 22, 2021. Available online. URL: www.womenshealth.gov/pregnancy/youre-pregnant-now-what/staying-healthy-and-safe. Accessed May 22, 2023.

HEALTHY EATING
How Much Should You Eat and Drink?

Consuming healthy foods and low-calorie beverages, particularly water, and the appropriate number of calories may help you and your baby gain the proper amount of weight.

How much food and how many calories you need depends on things such as your weight before pregnancy, your age, and how quickly you gain weight. If you are at a healthy weight, the Centers for Disease Control and Prevention (CDC) says you need no extra calories in your first trimester, about 340 extra calories a day in your second trimester, and about 450 extra calories a day in your third trimester. You may also not need extra calories during the final weeks of pregnancy.

Check with your health-care professional about your weight gain. If you are not gaining the weight you need, he or she may advise you to take in more calories. If you are gaining too much weight, you may need to cut down on calories. Each woman's needs are different. Your needs also depend on whether you were underweight, were overweight, or had obesity before you became pregnant or if you are having more than one baby.

What Kinds of Foods and Beverages Should You Consume?

A healthy eating plan for pregnancy includes nutrient-rich foods and beverages. The *Dietary Guidelines for Americans, 2020–2025* recommend these foods and beverages each day:

- fruits and vegetables (provide vitamins and fiber)
- whole grains, such as oatmeal, whole-grain bread, and brown rice (provide fiber, B vitamins, and other needed nutrients)
- fat-free or low-fat milk and milk products or nondairy soy, almond, rice, or other drinks with added calcium and vitamin D
- protein from healthy sources, such as beans and peas, eggs, lean meats, seafood that is low in mercury (up to 12 ounces per week), and unsalted nuts and seeds, if you can tolerate them and are not allergic to them

A healthy eating plan also limits salt, solid fats (such as butter, lard, and shortening), and sugar-sweetened drinks and foods.

Does your eating plan measure up? How can you improve your habits? Try consuming fruit such as berries or a banana with hot or cold cereal for breakfast, a salad with beans or tofu or other nonmeat protein for lunch, and a lean serving of meat, chicken, turkey, or fish and steamed vegetables for dinner. Think about new, healthful foods and beverages you can try. Write down your ideas and share them with your health-care professional.

Do You Have Any Special Nutrition Needs Now That You Are Pregnant?

Yes. During pregnancy, you need more vitamins and minerals such as folate, iron, and calcium.

Getting the appropriate amount of folate is very important. Folate, a B vitamin also known as "folic acid," may help prevent birth defects. Before pregnancy, you need 400 mcg per day from supplements or fortified foods, in addition to the folate you get naturally from foods and beverages. During pregnancy, you need 600 mcg. While breastfeeding, you need 500 mcg of folate per day. Foods high in folate include orange juice, strawberries, spinach, broccoli, beans, fortified breads, and fortified low-sugar breakfast cereals. These foods may even provide 100 percent of the daily value of folic acid per serving.

Most health-care professionals tell women who are pregnant to take a prenatal vitamin every day and consume healthy foods, snacks, and beverages. Ask your doctor about what you should take.

What Other New Habits May Help You Gain Weight?

Pregnancy can create some new food, beverage, and eating concerns. Meet the needs of your body and be more comfortable with these tips. Check with your health-care professional for any concerns.

- **Eat breakfast every day**. If you feel sick to your stomach in the morning, try dry whole wheat toast or whole grain crackers when you first wake up. Eat them even before you get out of bed. Eat the rest of your breakfast (fruit, oatmeal, hot or cold cereal, or other foods) later in the morning.

- **Eat high-fiber foods.** Eating high-fiber foods, drinking water, and getting daily physical activity may help prevent constipation. Try to eat whole grain cereals, brown rice, vegetables, fruits, and beans.

- **If you have heartburn, eat small meals spread throughout the day.** Try to eat slowly and avoid spicy and fatty foods (such as hot peppers or fried chicken). Have drinks between meals instead of with meals. Do not lie down soon after eating.

What Foods and Drinks Should You Avoid?

Certain foods and drinks can harm your baby if you have them while you are pregnant. Here is a list of items you should avoid:

- **Alcohol.** Do not drink alcohol, such as wine, beer, or hard liquor.

- **Caffeine.** Enjoy decaf coffee or tea, drinks not sweetened with sugar, or water with a dash of juice. Avoid diet drinks and limit drinks with caffeine to less than 200 mg per day—the amount in about 12 ounces of coffee.

- **Fish that may have high levels of mercury (a substance that can build up in fish and harm an unborn baby).** Limit white (albacore) tuna to 6 ounces per week. Do not eat king mackerel, marlin, orange roughy, shark, swordfish, or tilefish. To get the helpful nutrients in fish and shellfish, you may eat up to 12 ounces of seafood per week, choosing from many safe seafood choices, such as cod, salmon, and shrimp.

- **Foods that may cause illness in you or your baby (from viruses, parasites, or bacteria, such as *Listeria* or *Escherichia coli*).** Avoid soft cheeses made from unpasteurized or raw milk; raw cookie dough;

undercooked meats, eggs, and seafood; and deli salads. Take care in choosing and preparing lunch meats, egg dishes, and meat spreads.

- **Anything that is not food.** Some pregnant women may crave something that is not food, such as laundry starch, clay, ashes, or paint chips. This may mean that you are not getting the right amount of a nutrient. Talk to your health-care professional if you crave something that is not food. He or she can help you get the right amount of nutrients.[2]

Section 20.2 | Vegetarian Diets and Pregnancy

A vegetarian is someone who does not eat meat. Some vegetarians, called "vegans," do not eat any animal products, such as eggs or milk. If you are a vegetarian or vegan, you may need to take a dietary supplement, especially if you are pregnant or breastfeeding.

WHAT IS A HEALTHY EATING PLAN FOR WOMEN WHO ARE VEGETARIAN?

A healthy eating pattern for women who are vegetarian is the same as for any woman. Because vegetarians eat mostly plant-based foods, they usually get more fiber-rich foods and low-cholesterol foods than nonvegetarians. But women who are vegetarians still need to make sure they are eating healthy, which includes foods with calcium and protein.

[2] National Institute of Diabetes and Digestive and Kidney Diseases (NIDDK), "Health Tips for Pregnant Women," October 2019. Available online. URL: www.niddk. nih.gov/health-information/weight-management/healthy-eating-physical-activity-for-life/health-tips-for-pregnant-women#eatingPregnant. Accessed May 29, 2023.

DO WOMEN WHO ARE VEGETARIAN NEED TO TAKE A DIETARY SUPPLEMENT?

Not always. You can get all the nutrients you need from a vegetarian eating plan by eating a variety of foods from all of the food groups. But you may need to take extra steps to get enough protein, iron, calcium, vitamin B_{12}, and zinc.

The extra steps you need to take depend on what type of vegetarian you are. For example, low-fat and fat-free milk and milk products are good sources of calcium, vitamin B_{12}, and complete protein. Eggs are a good source of vitamin B_{12}, choline, and complete protein. Therefore, if you do not drink milk or eat eggs, you need to get these nutrients from other foods.

DO VEGETARIANS NEED MORE NUTRIENTS DURING PREGNANCY?

Yes. Just like all women, your body needs more of some nutrients, such as folic acid, during pregnancy to help your baby grow and develop. In general, though, choosing a variety of healthy foods from each of the food groups will help you get the nutrients you need during pregnancy. Be sure to get enough protein, found in beans, nuts, nut butter, and eggs if you eat them.

Use the MyPlate Plan (www.myplate.gov) tool to find out how many calories you need based on your age, sex, height, weight, and physical activity level.[3]

Section 20.3 | Iron Deficiency Anemia and Pregnancy

WHAT IS IRON DEFICIENCY ANEMIA?

Iron deficiency anemia is the most common type of anemia, a condition that happens when your body does not make enough healthy red blood cells (RBCs) or the blood cells do not work correctly.

---

[3] Office on Women's Health (OWH), "Vegetarian Eating," U.S. Department of Health and Human Services (HHS), February 17, 2021. Available online. URL: www.womenshealth.gov/healthy-eating/how-eat-health/vegetarian-eating. Accessed May 22, 2023.

Iron deficiency anemia happens when you do not have enough iron in your body. Your body needs iron to make hemoglobin, the part of the red blood cell that carries oxygen through your blood to all parts of your body.

WHO GETS IRON DEFICIENCY ANEMIA?

Iron deficiency anemia affects more women than men. The risk of iron deficiency anemia is highest for the following women:

- **Pregnant women.** Iron deficiency anemia affects one in six pregnant women. You need more iron during pregnancy to support your unborn baby's development.
- **Women who have heavy menstrual periods.** Up to 5 percent of women of childbearing age develop iron deficiency anemia because of heavy bleeding during their periods.

Infants, small children, and teens are also at high risk of iron deficiency anemia.

WHAT CAUSES IRON DEFICIENCY ANEMIA?

Women can have low iron levels for several reasons:

- **Iron lost through bleeding.** Bleeding can cause you to lose more blood cells and iron than your body can replace. Women may have low iron levels from bleeding caused by:
  - digestive system problems, such as ulcers, colon polyps, or colon cancer
  - regular, long-term use of aspirin and other over-the-counter pain relievers
  - donating blood too often or without enough time in between donations for your body to recover
  - heavier or longer than normal menstrual periods
  - uterine fibroids, which are noncancerous growths in the uterus that can cause heavy bleeding

- **Increased need for iron during pregnancy.** During pregnancy, your body needs more iron than normal to support your developing baby.
- **Not eating enough food that contains iron.** Your body absorbs the iron in animal-based foods, such as meat, chicken, and fish, two to three times better than the iron in plant-based foods. Vegetarians or vegans, who eat little or no animal-based foods, need to choose other good sources of iron to make sure they get enough. Your body also absorbs iron from plant-based foods better when you eat them with foods that have vitamin C, such as oranges and tomatoes. But most people in the United States get enough iron from food.
- **Problems absorbing iron.** Certain health conditions, such as Crohn's disease or celiac disease, or gastric bypass surgery for weight loss can make it harder for your body to absorb iron from food.

WHAT ARE THE SYMPTOMS OF IRON DEFICIENCY ANEMIA?

Iron deficiency anemia often develops slowly. In the beginning, you may not have any symptoms, or they may be mild. As it gets worse, you may notice one or more of the following symptoms:

- fatigue (very common)
- weakness (very common)
- dizziness
- headaches
- low body temperature
- pale or yellow "sallow" skin
- rapid or irregular heartbeat
- shortness of breath or chest pain, especially with physical activity
- brittle nails
- pica (unusual cravings for ice, very cold drinks, or nonfood items such as dirt or paper)

If you think you may have iron deficiency anemia, talk to your doctor or nurse.

HOW IS IRON DEFICIENCY ANEMIA DIAGNOSED?
Talk to your doctor if you think you might have iron deficiency anemia. Your doctor may do the following:
- Talk to you about the foods you eat, the medicines you take, and your family health history.
- Do blood tests. Your doctor will do a complete blood count (CBC). The CBC measures many parts of your blood. If the CBC test shows that you have anemia, your doctor will likely do another blood test to measure the iron levels in your blood and confirm that you have iron deficiency anemia.

If you have iron deficiency anemia, your doctor may want to do other tests to find out what is causing it.

HOW IS IRON DEFICIENCY ANEMIA TREATED?
Treatment for iron deficiency anemia depends on the cause:
- **Blood loss from a digestive system problem**. If you have an ulcer, your doctor may give you antibiotics or other medicine to treat the ulcer. If your bleeding is caused by a polyp or cancerous tumor, you may need surgery to remove it.
- **Blood loss from heavy menstrual periods**. Your doctor may give you hormonal birth control to help relieve heavy periods. If your heavy bleeding does not get better, your doctor may recommend surgery. Types of surgery to control heavy bleeding include endometrial ablation, which removes or destroys your uterine lining, and hysterectomy, which removes all or parts of your uterus.
- **Increased need for iron**. If you have problems absorbing iron or have lower iron levels but do not have severe anemia, your doctor may recommend the following:
  - **Taking iron pills**. It helps build up your iron levels as quickly as possible. Do not take any iron pills without first talking to your doctor or nurse.

- **Eating more foods that contain iron.** Good sources of iron include meat, fish, eggs, beans, peas, and fortified foods (look for cereals fortified with 100% of the daily value for iron).
- **Eating more foods with vitamin C.** Vitamin C helps your body absorb iron. Good sources of vitamin C include oranges, broccoli, and tomatoes.

If you have severe bleeding or symptoms of chest pain or shortness of breath, your doctor may recommend iron or RBC transfusions. Transfusions are for severe iron deficiencies only and are much less common.

WHAT DO YOU NEED TO KNOW ABOUT IRON PILLS?

Your doctor may recommend iron pills to help build up your iron levels. Do not take these pills without talking to your doctor or nurse first. Taking iron pills can cause side effects, including an upset stomach, constipation, and diarrhea. If taken as a liquid, iron supplements may stain your teeth.

You can reduce side effects from iron pills by taking these steps:

- Start with half of the recommended dose. Gradually increase to the full dose.
- Take iron in divided doses. For example, if you take two pills daily, take one in the morning with breakfast and the other after dinner.
- Take iron with food (especially something with vitamin C, such as a glass of orange juice, to help your body absorb the iron).
- If one type of iron pill causes side effects, ask your doctor for another type.
- If you take iron as a liquid instead of as a pill, aim it toward the back of your mouth. This will prevent the liquid from staining your teeth. You can also brush your teeth after taking the medicine to help prevent staining.

WHAT CAN HAPPEN IF IRON DEFICIENCY ANEMIA IS NOT TREATED?

If left untreated, iron deficiency anemia can cause serious health problems. Having too little oxygen in the body can damage organs. With anemia, the heart must work harder to make up for the lack of RBCs or hemoglobin. This extra work can harm the heart.

Iron deficiency anemia can also cause problems during pregnancy.

HOW CAN YOU PREVENT IRON DEFICIENCY ANEMIA?

You can help prevent iron deficiency anemia with the following steps:

- **Treat the cause of blood loss**. Talk to your doctor if you have heavy menstrual periods or if you have digestive system problems, such as frequent diarrhea or blood in your stool.
- **Eat foods with iron**. Good sources of iron include lean meat and chicken; dark, leafy vegetables; and beans.
- **Eat and drink foods that help your body absorb iron.** These include orange juice, strawberries, broccoli, or other fruits and vegetables with vitamin C.
- **Make healthy food choices**. Most people who make healthy, balanced food choices get the iron and vitamins their bodies need from the foods they eat.
- **Avoid drinking coffee or tea with meals**. These drinks make it harder for your body to absorb iron.
- **Talk to your doctor if you take calcium pills**. Calcium can make it harder for your body to absorb iron. If you have a hard time getting enough iron, talk to your doctor about the best way to also get enough calcium.

HOW MUCH IRON DO YOU NEED EVERY DAY?

Table 20.1 lists how much iron you need every day. The recommended amounts are listed in milligrams (mg).

Table 20.1. How Much Iron Women Need Daily

Age (Years)	Women (mg)	Pregnant Women (mg)	Breastfeeding Women (mg)	Vegetarian Women (mg)*
14–18	15	27	10	27
19–50	18	27	9	32
51+	8	N/A	N/A	14

Source: Adapted from the Institute of Medicine (IOM), Food and Nutrition Board (FNB)
*Vegetarians need more iron from food than people who eat meat. This is because the body can absorb iron from meat better than from plant-based foods.

WHAT FOODS CONTAIN IRON?

Food sources of iron include the following:

- fortified breakfast cereals (18 mg per serving)
- oysters (8 mg per 3-ounce serving)
- canned white beans (8 mg per cup)
- dark chocolate (7 mg per 3-ounce serving)
- beef liver (5 mg per 3-ounce serving)
- spinach (3 mg per ½ cup)
- tofu, firm (3 mg per ½ cup)
- kidney beans (2 mg per ½ cup)
- canned tomatoes (2 mg per ½ cup)
- lean beef (2 mg for a 3-ounce serving)
- baked potato (2 mg for a medium potato)

DO YOU NEED MORE IRON DURING PREGNANCY?

Yes. During pregnancy, your body needs more iron to support your growing baby. In fact, pregnant women need almost twice as much iron as women who are not pregnant. Not getting enough iron during pregnancy raises your risk of premature birth or a low-birth-weight baby (less than 5½ pounds). Premature birth is the most common cause of infant death. Both premature birth and low birth weight raise your baby's risk of health and developmental problems at birth and during childhood.

If you are pregnant, talk to your doctor about the following:
- getting 27 mg of iron every day (Take a prenatal vitamin with iron every day or talk to your doctor about taking an iron supplement (pill).)
- testing for iron deficiency anemia
- testing for iron deficiency anemia four to six weeks after childbirth

DO YOU NEED MORE IRON IF YOU ARE BREASTFEEDING?

No, you do not need more iron during breastfeeding. In fact, you need less iron than before you were pregnant. The amount of iron women need during breastfeeding is 10 mg per day for young mothers 14–18 and 9 mg per day for breastfeeding women older than 18.

You need less iron while breastfeeding because you likely will not lose a lot through your menstrual cycle. Many breastfeeding women do not have a period or may have only a light period. Also, if you have taken enough iron during pregnancy (27 mg a day), your breast milk will supply enough iron for your baby.

YOU ARE A VEGETARIAN. HOW CAN YOU MAKE SURE YOU GET ENOUGH IRON?

You can help make sure you get enough iron by choosing foods that contain iron more often. Vegetarians need more iron from food than people who eat meat. This is because the body can absorb iron from meat better than from plant-based foods.

Vegetarian sources of iron include the following:
- cereals and bread with added iron
- lentils and beans
- dark chocolate
- dark green leafy vegetables, such as spinach and broccoli
- tofu
- chickpeas
- canned tomatoes

Talk to your doctor or nurse about whether you get enough iron. Most people get enough iron from food.

CAN YOU GET MORE IRON THAN YOUR BODY NEEDS?

Yes, your body can get too much iron. Extra iron can damage the liver, heart, and pancreas. Try to get no more than 45 mg of iron a day unless your doctor prescribes more.

Some people get too much iron because of a condition called "hemochromatosis" that runs in families. You can also get too much iron from iron pills (if you also get iron from food) or from repeated blood transfusions.[4]

Section 20.4 | Folic Acid

Folic acid is the human-made form of folate, a B vitamin. Folate is found naturally in certain fruits, vegetables, and nuts. Folic acid is found in vitamins and fortified foods.

Folic acid and folate help the body make healthy new red blood cells (RBCs). RBCs carry oxygen to all the parts of your body. If your body does not make enough RBCs, you can develop anemia. Anemia happens when your blood cannot carry enough oxygen to your body, which makes you pale, tired, or weak. Also, if you do not get enough folic acid, you could develop a type of anemia called "folate deficiency anemia."

WHAT ARE FOLIC ACID AND FOLATE?

Everyone needs folic acid to be healthy. But it is especially important for women:

- **Before and during pregnancy**. Folic acid protects unborn children against serious birth defects called

---

[4] Office on Women's Health (OWH), "Iron-Deficiency Anemia," U.S. Department of Health and Human Services (HHS), February 22, 2021. Available online. URL: www.womenshealth.gov/a-z-topics/iron-deficiency-anemia. Accessed May 22, 2023.

"neural tube defects." These birth defects happen in the first few weeks of pregnancy, often before a woman knows she is pregnant. Folic acid might also help prevent other types of birth defects and early pregnancy loss (miscarriage). Since about half of all pregnancies in the United States are unplanned, experts recommend all women get enough folic acid even if they are not trying to get pregnant.

- **To keep the blood healthy by helping RBCs form and grow.** Not getting enough folic acid can lead to a type of anemia called "folate deficiency anemia." Folate deficiency anemia is more common in women of childbearing age than in men.

HOW DO YOU GET FOLIC ACID?

You can get folic acid in the following two ways:

- **Through the foods you eat.** Folate is found naturally in some foods, including spinach, nuts, and beans. Folic acid is found in fortified foods (called "enriched foods"), such as breads, pastas, and cereals. Look for the term "enriched" on the ingredients list to find out whether the food has added folic acid.
- **As a vitamin.** Most multivitamins sold in the United States contain 400 micrograms (mcg), or 100 percent of the daily value, of folic acid. Check the label to make sure.

HOW MUCH FOLIC ACID DO WOMEN NEED?

All women need 400 mcg of folic acid every day. Women who can get pregnant should get 400–800 mcg of folic acid from a vitamin or from food that has added folic acid, such as breakfast cereal. This is in addition to the folate you get naturally from food. Some women may need more folic acid each day. Table 20.2 shows the chart to determine how much folic acid you need.

Table 20.2. The Daily Recommended Intake of Folic Acid for Women

If You	Amount of Folic Acid You May Need Daily
Could get pregnant or are pregnant	400–800 mcg. Your doctor may prescribe a prenatal vitamin with more.
Had a baby with a neural tube defect (such as spina bifida) and want to get pregnant again	4,000 mcg. Your doctor may prescribe this amount. Research shows taking this amount may lower the risk of having another baby with spina bifida.
Have a family member with spina bifida and could get pregnant	4,000 mcg. Your doctor may prescribe this amount.
Have spina bifida and want to get pregnant	4,000 mcg. Your doctor may prescribe this amount. Women with spina bifida have a higher risk of having children with the condition.
Take medicines to treat epilepsy, type 2 diabetes, rheumatoid arthritis, or lupus	Talk to your doctor or nurse. Folic acid supplements can interact with these medicines.
Are on dialysis for kidney disease	Talk to your doctor or nurse.
Have a health condition, such as inflammatory bowel disease or celiac disease, that affects how your body absorbs folic acid	Talk to your doctor or nurse.

ARE SOME WOMEN AT RISK OF NOT GETTING ENOUGH FOLIC ACID?

Yes, certain groups of women do not get enough folic acid each day:

- Women who can get pregnant need more folic acid (400–800 mcg).
- Nearly one in three African American women does not get enough folic acid each day.
- Spanish-speaking Mexican-American women often do not get enough folic acid. However, Mexican-Americans who speak English usually get enough folic acid.

Not getting enough folic acid can cause health problems, including folate deficiency anemia, and problems during pregnancy for you and your unborn baby.

WHAT CAN HAPPEN IF YOU DO NOT GET ENOUGH FOLIC ACID DURING PREGNANCY?

If you do not get enough folic acid before and during pregnancy, your baby is at a higher risk of neural tube defects.

Neural tube defects are serious birth defects that affect the spine, spinal cord, or brain and may cause death. These include the following:

- **Spina bifida**. This condition happens when an unborn baby's spinal column does not fully close during development in the womb, leaving the spinal cord exposed. As a result, the nerves that control the legs and other organs do not work. Children with spina bifida often have lifelong disabilities. They may also need many surgeries.
- **Anencephaly**. This means that most or all of the brain and skull does not develop in the womb. Almost all babies with this condition die before or soon after birth.

DO YOU NEED TO TAKE FOLIC ACID EVERY DAY EVEN IF YOU ARE NOT PLANNING TO GET PREGNANT?

Yes. All women who can get pregnant need to take 400–800 mcg of folic acid every day, even if they are not planning to get pregnant. The following are a few reasons why:

- Your birth control may not work, or you may not use birth control correctly every time you have sex. In a survey by the Centers for Disease Control and Prevention (CDC), almost 40 percent of women with unplanned pregnancies were using birth control.
- Birth defects of the brain and spine can happen in the first few weeks of pregnancy, often before you know you are pregnant. By the time you find out you are pregnant, it might be too late to prevent the birth defects.
- You need to take folic acid every day because it is a water-soluble B vitamin. Water-soluble means that it does not stay in the body for a long time. Your body

metabolizes (uses) folic acid quickly, so your body needs folic acid each day to work properly.

WHAT FOODS CONTAIN FOLATE?

Folate is found naturally in some foods. Foods that are naturally high in folate include the following:
- spinach and other dark green, leafy vegetables
- oranges and orange juice
- nuts
- beans
- poultry (chicken, turkey, etc.) and meat
- whole grains

WHAT FOODS CONTAIN FOLIC ACID?

Folic acid is added to foods that are refined or processed (not whole grain):
- breakfast cereals (Some have 100% of the recommended daily value—or 400 mcg—of folic acid in each serving.)
- breads and pasta
- flours
- cornmeal
- white rice

Since 1998, the U.S. Food and Drug Administration (FDA) has required food manufacturers to add folic acid to processed breads, cereals, flours, cornmeal, pastas, rice, and other grains. For other foods, check the Nutrition Facts label on the package to see if they have folic acid. The label will also tell you how much folic acid is in each serving. Sometimes, the label will say "folate" instead of folic acid.

HOW CAN YOU BE SURE YOU GET ENOUGH FOLIC ACID?

You can get enough folic acid from food alone. Many breakfast cereals have 100 percent of your recommended daily value (400 mcg) of folic acid.

If you are at risk of not getting enough folic acid, your doctor or nurse may recommend that you take a vitamin with folic acid every day. Most U.S. multivitamins have at least 400 mcg of folic acid. Check the label on the bottle to be sure. You can also take a pill that contains only folic acid.

If swallowing pills is hard for you, try a chewable or liquid product with folic acid.

WHAT SHOULD YOU LOOK FOR WHEN BUYING VITAMINS WITH FOLIC ACID?

Look for "United States Pharmacopeia" (USP) or "National Sanitation Foundation" (NSF) on the label when choosing vitamins. These "seals of approval" mean the pills are made properly and have the amounts of vitamins it says on the label. Also, make sure the pills have not expired. If the bottle has no expiration date, do not buy it.

Ask your pharmacist for help with selecting a vitamin or folic acid-only pill. If you are pregnant and already take a daily prenatal vitamin, you probably get all the folic acid you need.

CAN YOU GET ENOUGH FOLIC ACID FROM FOOD ALONE?

Yes, many people get enough folic acid from food alone. Some foods have high amounts of folic acid. For example, many breakfast cereals have 100 percent of the recommended daily value (400 mcg) of folic acid in each serving. Check the label to be sure.

Some women, especially women who could get pregnant, may not get enough folic acid from food. African American women and Mexican Americans are also at a higher risk of not getting enough folic acid each day. Talk to your doctor or nurse about whether you should take a vitamin to get the 400 mcg of folic acid you need each day.

WHAT IS FOLATE DEFICIENCY ANEMIA?

Folate deficiency anemia is a type of anemia that happens when you do not get enough folate. Folate deficiency anemia is most common during pregnancy. Other causes of folate deficiency anemia include alcoholism and certain medicines to treat seizures, anxiety, or arthritis.

The symptoms of folate deficiency anemia include the following:

- fatigue
- headache
- pale skin
- sore mouth and tongue

If you have folate deficiency anemia, your doctor may recommend taking folic acid vitamins and eating more foods with folate.

CAN YOU GET TOO MUCH FOLIC ACID?

Yes, you can get too much folic acid but only from human-made products such as multivitamins and fortified foods, such as breakfast cereals. You cannot get too much from foods that naturally contain folate. You should not get more than 1,000 mcg of folic acid a day unless your doctor prescribes a higher amount. Too much folic acid can hide signs that you lack vitamin B_{12}, which can cause nerve damage.

ARE FOLIC ACID PILLS COVERED UNDER INSURANCE?

Yes. Under the Affordable Care Act (ACA; the health-care law), all Health Insurance Marketplace plans and most other insurance plans cover folic acid pills for women who could get pregnant at no cost to you. Check with your insurance provider to find out what is included in your plan.[5]

---

[5] Office on Women's Health (OWH), "Folic Acid," U.S. Department of Health and Human Services (HHS), February 12, 2021. Available online. URL: www.womenshealth.gov/a-z-topics/folic-acid. Accessed May 29, 2023.

Section 20.5 | What You Need to Know about Mercury in Fish and Shellfish

For most people, the risk from eating contaminated fish and shellfish is not a health concern. However, some groups of people such as pregnant women, children, and the elderly are at a greater health risk than others. Additionally, some individuals are at a higher risk simply because they eat substantially more fish than others.

If you are pregnant, a young child, an older adult, or someone with a weakened immune system, to avoid foodborne illness from bacteria (often called "food poisoning"), you are advised not to eat:

- raw fish, partially cooked seafood (such as shrimp and crab), or refrigerated smoked seafood
- raw shellfish (including oysters, clams, mussels, and scallops) or their juices

PEOPLE WHO ARE PREGNANT, MAY BECOME PREGNANT, OR ARE BREASTFEEDING

The nutritional value of fish is important during growth and development before birth, in early infancy for breastfed infants, and in childhood. The health risks from mercury in fish and shellfish depend on the amount of fish and shellfish a person eats and the levels of mercury in the specific fish and shellfish. Some fish contain higher levels of mercury that may harm an unborn baby or a young child's developing nervous system.

As a result, people who are pregnant or may become pregnant and people who are nursing risk exposing their children to contamination if they eat these fish.

The U.S. Environmental Protection Agency (EPA) and U.S. Food and Drug Administration (FDA) recommend that people who are pregnant, may become pregnant, or are breastfeeding eat two to three servings (8–12 ounces) of fish each week from choices that are lower in mercury. The advice includes a Please provide link to this chart (www.epa.gov/fish-tech/epa-fda-advice-about-eating-fish-and-shellfish) that shows how often people and children can eat more than 60 types of fish and shellfish. The fish are grouped into "best choices," "good choices," and "choices to avoid" based on the mercury content.[6]

FISH FACTS

Fish and shellfish can be an important part of a healthy diet. They are a great source of protein and heart-healthy omega-3 fatty acids. Some researchers believe low fish intake may be linked to depression in women during and after pregnancy. Research also suggests that omega-3 fatty acids consumed by pregnant women may aid in babies' brain and eye development.

Women who are or may become pregnant and nursing mothers need 12 ounces of fish per week to reap the health benefits. Unfortunately, some pregnant and nursing women do not eat any fish because they worry about mercury in seafood. Mercury is a metal that, at high levels, can harm the brain of your unborn baby—even before it is conceived. Mercury mainly gets into our bodies by eating large, predatory fish. Yet many types of seafood have little or no mercury at all. So the risk of mercury exposure depends on the amount and type of seafood you eat.

Women who are nursing, are pregnant, or may become pregnant can safely eat a variety of cooked seafood but should steer clear of fish with high levels of mercury. Keep in mind that removing all fish from your diet will rob you of important omega-3 fatty acids. To reach 12 ounces while limiting exposure to mercury, follow these tips:

- Do not eat these fish that are high in mercury:
  - swordfish
  - tilefish
  - king mackerel
  - shark
- Eat up to 6 ounces (about one serving) per week:
  - canned albacore or chunk white tuna (also sold as tuna steaks), which has more mercury than canned light tuna

[6] "Should I Be Concerned about Eating Fish and Shellfish?" U.S. Environmental Protection Agency (EPA), September 9, 2022. Available online. URL: https://epa.gov/choose-fish-and-shellfish-wisely/should-i-be-concerned-about-eating-fish-and-shellfish. Accessed May 29, 2023.

- Eat up to 12 ounces (about two servings) per week of cooked* fish and shellfish with little or no mercury, such as:
  - shrimp
  - crab
  - clams
  - oysters
  - scallops
  - canned light tuna
  - salmon
  - pollock
  - catfish
  - cod
  - tilapia

Do not eat uncooked fish or shellfish (such as clams, oysters, or scallops), which includes refrigerated uncooked seafood labeled nova-style, lox, kippered, smoked, or jerky.

- Check before eating fish caught in local waters. State health departments have guidelines on fish from local waters. Or get local fish advisories at the EPA. If you are unsure about the safety of a fish from local waters, eat only 6 ounces per week and do not eat any other fish that week.
- Eat a variety of cooked seafood rather than just a few types.

Foods supplemented with docosahexaenoic acid/eicosapentaenoic acid (DHA/EPA; such as "omega-3 eggs") and prenatal vitamins supplemented with DHA are other sources of the type of omega-3 fatty acids found in seafood.[7]

---

[7] Office on Women's Health (OWH), "Staying Healthy and Safe," U.S. Department of Health and Human Services (HHS), February 22, 2021. Available online. URL: https://womenshealth.gov/pregnancy/youre-pregnant-now-what/staying-healthy-and-safe. Accessed May 29, 2023.

Section 20.6 | Caffeine Use during Pregnancy

CAFFEINE

Moderate amounts of caffeine appear to be safe during pregnancy. Moderate means less than 200 mg of caffeine per day, which is the amount in about 12 ounces of coffee. Most caffeinated teas and soft drinks have much less caffeine. Some studies have shown a link between higher amounts of caffeine and miscarriage and preterm birth. But there is no solid proof that caffeine causes these problems. The effects of too much caffeine are unclear. Ask your doctor whether drinking a limited amount of caffeine is okay for you.[8]

PREPREGNANCY CAFFEINE CONSUMPTION LINKED TO MISCARRIAGE RISK

A woman is more likely to miscarry if she and her partner drink more than two caffeinated beverages a day during the weeks leading up to conception, according to a study from researchers at the National Institutes of Health (NIH) and Ohio State University, Columbus. Similarly, women who drank more than two daily caffeinated beverages during the first seven weeks of pregnancy were also more likely to miscarry.

However, women who took a daily multivitamin before conception and through early pregnancy were less likely to miscarry than women who did not.

"The findings provide useful information for couples who are planning a pregnancy and who would like to minimize their risk for early pregnancy loss," said the study's first author, Germaine Buck Louis, Ph.D., director of the Division of Intramural Population Health Research at the NIH's *Eunice Kennedy Shriver* National Institute of Child Health and Human Development (NICHD).

---

[8] Office on Women's Health (OWH), "Staying Healthy and Safe," U.S. Department of Health and Human Services (HHS), February 22, 2021. Available online. URL: https://womenshealth.gov/pregnancy/youre-pregnant-now-what/staying-healthy-and-safe. Accessed May 29, 2023.

The researchers analyzed data from the Longitudinal Investigation of Fertility and the Environment (LIFE) study, which was established to examine the relationship between fertility, lifestyle, and exposure to environmental chemicals. The LIFE study enrolled 501 couples from four counties in Michigan and 12 counties in Texas, from 2005 to 2009.

For this study, researchers compared lifestyle factors such as cigarette use, caffeinated beverage consumption, and multivitamin use among 344 couples with a singleton pregnancy from the weeks before they conceived through the seventh week of pregnancy.

The researchers reported their results using a statistical concept known as a "hazard ratio," which estimates the chances of a particular health outcome occurring during the study time frame. For example, the researchers evaluated caffeinated beverage consumption in terms of the daily likelihood of pregnancy loss over a given time period. A score greater than one indicates an increased risk of pregnancy loss each day following conception, and a score less than one indicates a reduced daily risk.

Of the 344 pregnancies, 98 (28%) ended in miscarriage. For the prepregnancy period, miscarriage was associated with females aged 35 or above for a hazard ratio of 1.96 (nearly twice the miscarriage risk of younger women). The study was not designed to conclusively prove cause and effect. The study authors cited possible explanations for the higher risk, including advanced age of sperm and egg in older couples or cumulative exposure to substances in the environment, which could be expected to increase as people age.

Both male and female consumption of more than two caffeinated beverages a day was also associated with an increased hazard ratio: 1.74 for females and 1.73 for males. Earlier studies, the authors noted, have documented increased pregnancy loss associated with caffeine consumption in early pregnancy. However, those studies could not rule out whether caffeine consumption contributed to pregnancy loss or was a sign of an unhealthy pregnancy. It is possible, the authors wrote, that these earlier findings could have been the result of a healthy pregnancy, rather than caffeine consumption interfering with pregnancy. For example, the increase in food aversions and vomiting associated with a healthy pregnancy led the women to give up caffeinated beverages.

Because their study found caffeine consumption before pregnancy was associated with a higher risk of miscarriage, it is more likely that caffeinated beverage consumption during this time directly contributes to pregnancy loss.

"Our findings also indicate that the male partner matters, too," Dr. Buck Louis said. "Male preconception consumption of caffeinated beverages was just as strongly associated with pregnancy loss as females."

Finally, the researchers saw a reduction in miscarriage risk of women who took a daily multivitamin. During the prepregnancy period, researchers found a hazard ratio of 0.45—a 55 percent reduction in risk of pregnancy loss. Women who continued to take the vitamins through early pregnancy had a hazard ratio of 0.21 or a risk reduction of 79 percent. The authors cited other studies that found that vitamin B_6 and folic acid—included in prepregnancy and pregnancy vitamin formulations—can reduce miscarriage risk. Folic acid supplements are recommended for women of childbearing age as their use in the weeks leading up to and following conception reduces the risk of having a child with a neural tube defect.[9]

[9] "Couples' Pre-pregnancy Caffeine Consumption Linked to Miscarriage Risk," *Eunice Kennedy Shriver* National Institute of Child Health and Human Development (NICHD), March 24, 2016. Available online. URL: https://nichd.nih.gov/newsroom/releases/032416-miscarriage-caffeine. Accessed May 29, 2023.

Chapter 21 | Exercise during Pregnancy

EXPECTING? KEEP ACTIVE!

Pregnancy should not keep women from a healthy dose of activity. Both during pregnancy and after delivery, exercise can help the mother through improved cardiovascular fitness and in many other ways. Postpartum benefits also include mood improvement and weight management. Some evidence points toward shortened labor and reduced risk of certain complications. The 2008 *Physical Activity Guidelines for Americans* spell it out based on solid evidence and in lay terms.

The following are the key recommendations:

- Healthy women who are not already highly active or doing vigorous-intensity activity should get at least 150 minutes (2 hours and 30 minutes) of moderate-intensity aerobic activity per week during pregnancy and the postpartum period. Preferably, this activity should be spread throughout the week.

- Pregnant women who habitually engage in vigorous-intensity aerobic activity or are highly active can continue physical activity during pregnancy and the postpartum period, provided that they remain healthy and discuss with their health-care provider how and when activity should be adjusted over time.

Pregnant women should review the recommendations in full, including activities to avoid and the wisdom of seeking a health-care professional who can provide knowledgeable guidance. Armed with solid information and motivated by the desire to achieve the best health for themselves and their babies, pregnant women can remain active through pregnancy and beyond.[1]

STAY ACTIVE DURING PREGNANCY: QUICK TIPS

Physical activity is important for everyone, including people who are pregnant. Staying active during pregnancy can help you feel better right away—and it can even make your labor shorter and recovery faster.

Getting active during pregnancy may also make it less likely you will have complications such as:

- gestational diabetes (a type of diabetes that happens during pregnancy)
- preeclampsia (a condition that causes high blood pressure and other problems)
- postpartum depression

If you were already physically active before your pregnancy, it is healthy to keep it up. Even if you are doing more vigorous activities—such as running—it is safe to keep doing them while you are pregnant. And, if you were not active before your pregnancy, it is not too late to start!

LISTEN TO YOUR BODY

Remember that lots of things count as physical activity—so listen to your body and find what works for you at each stage of your pregnancy. And keep in mind that physical activity may feel different when you are pregnant. If an activity does not feel right, try something else instead.

---

[1] Office of Disease Prevention and Health Promotion (ODPHP), "Exercise during Pregnancy: You'll Both Benefit," U.S. Department of Health and Human Services (HHS), April 7, 2010. Available online. URL: https://health.gov/news-archive/blog/2010/04/exercise-during-pregnancy-youll-both-benefit. Accessed May 25, 2023.

AIM FOR 150 MINUTES A WEEK OF MODERATE-INTENSITY AEROBIC ACTIVITY

- If you were not physically active before, start slowly—even five minutes of physical activity has real health benefits, and you can build up to more over time.
- Choose activities that make your heart beat faster—such as walking fast, dancing, swimming, or raking leaves.

DO MUSCLE-STRENGTHENING ACTIVITIES AT LEAST TWO DAYS A WEEK

- If you are used to lifting weights or doing other muscle-strengthening activities, it is safe and healthy to continue while you are pregnant.
- Remember that lifting weights is not the only way to strengthen your muscles; for example, you can use resistance bands or do body weight activities, such as squats and lunges.
- Make sure you are not holding your breath while you do muscle-strengthening activities.

AVOID HIGH-RISK ACTIVITIES

- Avoid doing any activities while lying flat on your back after the first trimester (12 weeks) because it can cause problems with blood flow—try propping yourself up with a pillow instead.
- Stay away from activities that increase your risk of falling, such as downhill skiing or horseback riding.
- Avoid playing sports where you could get hit in the belly, such as basketball or soccer.

TALK WITH YOUR DOCTOR OR MIDWIFE

Prenatal checkups are a great time to talk about physical activity. Ask your doctor or midwife the following questions:

- How can being active help me have a healthier pregnancy?

- What activities would you recommend for me?
- Are there any activities I need to avoid?[2]

SHOULD YOU EXERCISE DURING YOUR PREGNANCY?

Almost all women can and should be physically active during pregnancy. First, talk to your health-care provider, particularly if you have high blood pressure, diabetes, anemia, bleeding, or other disorders or if you are obese or underweight. Whether or not you were active before you were pregnant, ask about a safe level of exercise for you. Aim for at least 30 minutes of moderate-intensity physical activity (one in which you breathe harder but do not overwork or overheat) on most, if not every day of the week.

SEVEN BENEFITS OF REGULAR, MODERATE PHYSICAL ACTIVITY DURING PREGNANCY

- Helps you and your baby gain the proper amounts of weight.
- Reduces the discomforts of pregnancy, such as backaches, leg cramps, constipation, bloating, and swelling.
- Lowers the risk of gestational diabetes (diabetes found for the first time when a woman is pregnant).
- Boosts mood and energy level.
- Improves sleep.
- Helps with an easier, shorter labor.
- Assists faster recovery from delivery and return to a healthy weight.

FIVE TIPS FOR GETTING GOING!

- Go for a walk around the block or through a shopping mall with your spouse or a friend.
- Join a prenatal yoga, water aerobics, or fitness class, letting the instructor know you are pregnant before beginning.

---

[2] Office of Disease Prevention and Health Promotion (ODPHP), "Stay Active during Pregnancy: Quick Tips," U.S. Department of Health and Human Services (HHS), May 24, 2023. Available online. URL: https://health.gov/myhealthfinder/pregnancy/nutrition-and-physical-activity/stay-active-during-pregnancy-quick-tips. Accessed May 25, 2023.

- Follow an exercise video for pregnant women.
- At your gym, community center, Young Men's Christian Association (YMCA), or Young Women's Christian Association (YWCA), sign up for a fitness session for the pregnant.
- Stand up, stretch, and move at least once an hour if you sit most of the day, as well as during commercials when watching TV.

FIVE STEPS FOR SAFE EXERCISE DURING PREGNANCY

- Choose moderate activities unlikely to injure, such as walking, water aerobics, swimming, yoga, or using a stationary bike.
- Stop exercising when you start to feel tired and never exercise until you are exhausted or overheated.
- Drink plenty of water.
- Wear comfortable clothing that fits well and supports and protects your breasts.
- Stop exercising if you feel dizzy, become short of breath, feel pain in your back, experience swelling or numbness, feel sick to your stomach, or your heart beats too fast or at an uneven rate.

WHAT SHOULD YOU NOT DO?

For you and your baby's health and safety, it is best to avoid:

- being active outside during hot weather
- steam rooms, hot tubs, and saunas
- certain yoga poses or other activities that call for lying flat on your back after the twentieth week of pregnancy
- contact sports such as football and boxing that might injure you
- sports such as tennis or basketball that make you jump or change directions quickly

- horseback riding, in-line skating, downhill skiing, and other activities that can result in falls[3]

TIPS FOR SAFE AND HEALTHY PHYSICAL ACTIVITY

Follow these tips for safe and healthy fitness:
- When you exercise, start slowly, progress gradually, and cool down slowly.
- You should be able to talk while exercising. If not, you may be overdoing it.
- Take frequent breaks.
- Do not exercise on your back after the first trimester. This can put too much pressure on an important vein and limit blood flow to the baby.
- Avoid jerky, bouncing, and high-impact movements. Connective tissues stretch much more easily during pregnancy. So these types of movements put you at risk of joint injury.
- Be careful not to lose your balance. As your baby grows, your center of gravity shifts making you more prone to falls. For this reason, activities such as jogging, using a bicycle, or playing racquet sports might be riskier as you near the third trimester.
- Do not exercise at high altitudes (more than 6,000 feet). It can prevent your baby from getting enough oxygen.
- Make sure you drink lots of fluids before, during, and after exercising.
- Do not work out in extreme heat or humidity.
- If you feel uncomfortable, short of breath, or tired, take a break and take it easier when you exercise again.

Stop exercising and call your doctor as soon as possible if you have any of the following:
- dizziness
- headache

---

[3] MedlinePlus, "Winter 2008," National Institutes of Health (NIH), February 10, 2009. Available online. URL: https://magazine.medlineplus.gov/pdf/winter2008.pdf. Accessed May 25, 2023.

- chest pain
- calf pain or swelling
- abdominal pain
- blurred vision
- fluid leaking from the vagina
- vaginal bleeding
- less fetal movement
- contractions

WORK OUT YOUR PELVIC FLOOR

Your pelvic floor (Kegel exercises) muscles support the rectum, vagina, and urethra in the pelvis. Toning these muscles with Kegel exercises will help you push during delivery and recover from birth. It will also help control bladder leakage and lower your chance of getting hemorrhoids.

Pelvic muscles are the same ones used to stop the flow of urine. Still, it can be hard to find the right muscles to squeeze. You can be sure you are exercising the right muscles if when you squeeze them, you stop urinating. Or you can put a finger into the vagina and squeeze. If you feel pressure around the finger, you have found the pelvic floor muscles. Try not to tighten your stomach, legs, or other muscles.

Kegel Exercises

- Tighten the pelvic floor muscles for a count of three and then relax for a count of three.
- Repeat 10–15 times, three times a day.
- Start Kegel exercises lying down. This is the easiest position. When your muscles get stronger, you can do Kegel exercises sitting or standing, as you like.[4]

---

[4] Office on Women's Health (OWH), "Staying Healthy and Safe," U.S. Department of Health and Human Services (HHS), February 22, 2021. Available online. URL: https://womenshealth.gov/pregnancy/youre-pregnant-now-what/staying-healthy-and-safe#b. Accessed May 25, 2023.

BENEFITS OF PHYSICAL ACTIVITY DURING PREGNANCY

- Reduces the risk of excessive weight gain during pregnancy.
- Reduces the risk of gestational diabetes during pregnancy.
- Reduces symptoms of postpartum depression.

EXAMPLES OF MODERATE-INTENSITY PHYSICAL ACTIVITY*

- brisk walking
- some forms of yoga
- water aerobics
- bike riding

After the first trimester, try to avoid activities that require lying flat on your back. [5]

---

[5] "Physical Activity Recommendations for Pregnant and Postpartum Women," Centers for Disease Control and Prevention (CDC), September 30, 2021. Available online: https://cdc.gov/physicalactivity/basics/pdfs/pa-pregnant-and-postpartum-women-508.pdf. Accessed May 25, 2023.

Chapter 22 | Weight Gain during Pregnancy

WHY IS GAINING A HEALTHY AMOUNT OF WEIGHT DURING PREGNANCY IMPORTANT?

Gaining an appropriate amount of weight during pregnancy helps your baby grow to a healthy size. But gaining too much or too little weight may lead to serious health problems for you and your baby.

Too much weight gain during pregnancy raises your chances for developing gestational diabetes (diabetes during pregnancy) and high blood pressure during pregnancy. It also increases your risk of type 2 diabetes and high blood pressure later in life. If you are overweight or obese when you get pregnant, your chances for health problems may be even higher. You could also be more likely to have a cesarean section (C-section).

Gaining a healthy amount of weight helps you have an easier pregnancy and delivery. It may also help make it easier for you to get back to a healthy weight after delivery. Research shows that recommended amounts of weight gain during pregnancy can also lower the chances that you or your child will have obesity and weight-related problems later in life.

HOW MUCH WEIGHT SHOULD YOU GAIN DURING YOUR PREGNANCY?

How much weight you should gain depends on your body mass index (BMI) before pregnancy. The BMI is a measure of your weight in relation to your height. You can use a formula to calculate your BMI (www.nhlbi.nih.gov/health/educational/lose_wt/BMI/bmicalc.htm).

It is important to gain weight very slowly. The old myth that you are "eating for two" is not true. During the first three months, your baby is only the size of a walnut and does not need many extra calories. The following rate of weight gain is advised:

- 1–4 pounds total in the first three months
- 2–4 pounds each month from four months until delivery

Talk to your health-care professional about how much weight gain is appropriate for you. Work with him or her to set goals for your weight gain. Take into account your age, weight, and health. Track your weight at home or when you visit your health-care professional.

Do not try to lose weight if you are pregnant. Your baby needs to be exposed to healthy foods and low-calorie beverages (particularly water) to grow properly. Some women may lose a small amount of weight at the start of pregnancy. Speak to your health-care professional if this happens to you.[1]

WHY IS IT IMPORTANT TO GAIN THE RECOMMENDED AMOUNT OF WEIGHT DURING PREGNANCY?

Gaining less than the recommended amount of weight in pregnancy is associated with delivering a baby who is too small. Some babies born too small may have difficulty starting breastfeeding, may be at increased risk of illness, and may experience developmental delays (not meeting the milestones for his or her age).

Gaining more than the recommended amount of weight in pregnancy is associated with having a baby who is born too large, which can lead to delivery complications, cesarean delivery, and obesity during childhood. Gaining more than the recommended amount of weight can also increase the amount of weight you hold on to after pregnancy, which can lead to obesity.

---

[1] "Health Tips for Pregnant Women," National Institute of Diabetes and Digestive and Kidney Diseases (NIDDK), October 1, 2019. Available online. URL: www.niddk.nih.gov/health-information/weight-management/healthy-eating-physical-activity-for-life/health-tips-for-pregnant-women?dkrd=/health-information/weight-management/health-tips-pregnant-women. Accessed May 25, 2023.

Weight Gain during Pregnancy

Tables 22.1 and 22.2 show the general weight gain recommendations for women with one baby or with twins.

Table 22.1. Weight Gain Recommendations for Women Pregnant with One Baby

If before Pregnancy, You Were	You Should Gain (pounds)
Underweight (BMI less than 18.5)	28–40
Normal weight (BMI of 18.5–24.9)	25–35
Overweight (BMI of 25.0–29.9)	15–25
Obese (BMI ≥30.0)	11–20

Table 22.2. Weight Gain Recommendations for Women Pregnant with Twins

If before Pregnancy, You Were	You Should Gain (pounds)
Underweight (BMI less than 18.5)	50–62*
Normal weight (BMI of 18.5–24.9)	37–54
Overweight (BMI of 25.0–29.9)	31–50
Obese (BMI ≥30.0)	25–42

All recommendations are from the Institute of Medicine (IOM), with the exception of underweight women with twins.

WHAT STEPS CAN YOU TAKE TO MEET PREGNANCY WEIGHT GAIN RECOMMENDATIONS?

- **Know your caloric needs.** In general, the first trimester (or first three months) does not require any extra calories. Typically, women need about 340 additional calories per day during the second trimester (second three months) and about 450 additional calories per day during the third trimester (last three months).
- **Work with your health-care provider.** Work with your health-care provider on your weight gain goals at the beginning of and regularly throughout your pregnancy.

- **Track your pregnancy weight gain.** Track your pregnancy weight gain at the beginning and regularly throughout pregnancy and compare your progress to recommended ranges of healthy weight gain.
- **Eat a balanced diet.** Eat a diet high in whole grains, vegetables, fruits, low-fat dairy, and lean protein. Most foods are safe to eat during pregnancy, but you will need to use caution with or avoid certain foods.
- **Know foods to avoid in pregnancy.** Talk with your health-care provider or visit the checklist of foods to avoid during pregnancy (www.foodsafety.gov/people-at-risk/pregnant-women) for more information about food safety in pregnancy.
- **Limit added sugars and solid fats.** These are found in foods such as soft drinks, desserts, fried foods, whole milk, and fatty meats.
- **Do moderate-intensity aerobic activity.** Work up to or maintain at least 150 minutes (two and a half hours) of moderate-intensity aerobic activity (such as brisk walking) per week. A duration of 150 minutes may sound overwhelming, but you can achieve your goal by breaking up your physical activity into 10 minutes at a time. Physical activity is healthy and safe for most pregnant women. Talk to your health-care provider to determine if you have any physical activity restrictions.[2]

---

[2] "Weight Gain during Pregnancy," Centers for Disease Control and Prevention (CDC), June 13, 2022. Available online. URL: www.cdc.gov/reproductivehealth/maternalinfanthealth/pregnancy-weight-gain.htm#trackers. Accessed May 25, 2023.

Chapter 23 | Risk Factors for Sleep Apnea during Pregnancy

Snoring, older age, and obesity may increase a pregnant woman's risk of sleep apnea—or interrupted breathing during sleep—according to researchers funded by the National Institutes of Health (NIH). The study, which appears in the *American Journal of Obstetrics and Gynecology* (AJOG), was supported by the NIH's *Eunice Kennedy Shriver* National Institute of Child Health and Human Development (NICHD) and the National Heart, Lung, and Blood Institute (NHLBI).

"The NIH study found an easy, inexpensive way to screen large numbers of women at higher risk of sleep apnea during pregnancy," said study coauthor Uma Reddy, M.D., of the NICHD's Pregnancy and Perinatology Branch. "Right now, this means we will be able to rapidly identify women who may benefit from further testing. Depending on what we learn from future studies, our findings could also lead to improvements in pregnancy outcomes."

In an earlier study of first-time pregnancies, the researchers found that sleep apnea increases a woman's risk of hypertensive disorders and gestational diabetes. Currently, there are no medical guidelines or treatment recommendations for sleep apnea during pregnancy. The NIH supports a study of potential treatments for pregnancy-related sleep apnea and is planning a larger one to be conducted by the NICHD-funded Maternal-Fetal Medicine Units (MFMU) Network.

In the study, participants responded to questionnaires about their sleep habits, snoring, and daytime sleepiness in early pregnancy (6–15 weeks) and midpregnancy (22–29 weeks). The women also underwent sleep apnea testing using an at-home monitoring device.

The researchers found that 3.6 percent of 3,264 women in early pregnancy and 8.3 percent of 2,512 women in midpregnancy had sleep apnea. Risk factors for having the condition included frequent snoring (three or more nights per week), older maternal age, and being overweight or obese as determined by the body mass index (BMI).

Because each woman's risk varies according to individual characteristics, the authors developed a calculator using maternal age, BMI, and frequency of snoring to arrive at her probability of sleep apnea in early pregnancy and midpregnancy. This tool may be used by obstetric providers to identify women at risk of the condition, so they can be referred for definitive testing.

A common treatment for sleep apnea is continuous positive airway pressure (CPAP) therapy, which involves wearing a mask that fits over the nose or the nose and mouth. Air is pumped through a tube attached to the mask, increasing pressure into the airways to keep them from collapsing. Dr. Reddy explained, however, that it is not currently known if using CPAP therapy during pregnancy will prevent hypertension, diabetes, or other complications of sleep apnea. She added that pregnant women who have or think they have sleep apnea should discuss their concerns with a physician.[1]

[1] "NIH-Funded Researchers Identify Risk Factors for Sleep Apnea during Pregnancy," National Institutes of Health (NIH), February 13, 2018. Available online. URL: www.nih.gov/news-events/news-releases/nih-funded-researchers-identify-risk-factors-sleep-apnea-during-pregnancy. Accessed May 25, 2023.

Chapter 24 | Sex during Pregnancy

Many parents-to-be find it difficult to discuss sex during pregnancy, perhaps because the subject feels culturally taboo to them, but they can count on experiencing changes in their sex life during pregnancy. Because of this reality, it is important to find a balanced way to feel happy as a couple in the midst of these changes. Some of the common questions about sex during pregnancy are addressed below.

IS SEX SAFE DURING PREGNANCY?

Yes, sexual activity is considered safe during all stages of a healthy pregnancy. During a healthy, normal pregnancy, the risk of complications, such as preterm labor or miscarriage, is low for couples who enjoy sex during pregnancy. In fact, unless your health-care provider advises you not to, it is absolutely safe for you to have sex up until your water breaks.

IS PREGNANT SEX DIFFERENT FROM REGULAR SEX?

Some women may feel discomfort during pregnant sex because of tender heavy breasts, hormonal fluctuations, exhaustion, increased self-consciousness about weight gain, increased influx of blood in the lower parts of the body (which causes heightened sensitivity and engorgement of the genitals), vaginal fluid changes, and so on, while others experience little discomfort.

WILL SEX HARM THE FETUS?

Penetration during intercourse will not harm the developing fetus, as it is cushioned by the amniotic fluid (watery yellow fluid within the amniotic sac) and encircled by the muscles of the uterus. The mucus plug seal in the cervix guards against infection.

CAN INTERCOURSE OR ORGASM CAUSE A MISCARRIAGE OR CONTRACTIONS?

In a healthy pregnancy, the answer is no. It will not provoke a miscarriage. The contractions during and after orgasm are totally different from labor. As a safety precaution, some providers may advise not to have sex during the final week of pregnancy as it is suspected that prostaglandins (hormones in semen) may stimulate labor contractions in past-due or full-term pregnancies.

WHICH SEX POSITIONS ARE MOST COMFORTABLE DURING PREGNANCY?

As the pregnancy progresses, the missionary position (the man on top) may not be comfortable for some couples. Alternative sex positions to try during pregnancy, which keep the weight off of the stomach, are:

- straddling while the partner sits in a chair, table, or on a counter to control pace and penetration
- women on top or doggy position in order to balance the weight between hands and knees
- lying side-by-side (spooning position) to avoid deep penetration

Open communication is the secret to determining what works best for the individual and the couple for pregnancy sex.

ARE CONDOMS NECESSARY?

If the relationship is not mutually monogamous or if one partner chooses to have sex with a new partner, then condom use is the safest way to avoid sexually transmitted infections (STIs).

WHEN SHOULD YOU NOT HAVE SEX DURING PREGNANCY?

Health-care providers will say "no sex" if they determine the pregnancy to be high risk with:

- a history or threat of preterm labor (premature uterine contractions/birth/delivery before 37 weeks of pregnancy)
- a history or threat of miscarriage
- vaginal bleeding or cramps with no known cause
- incompetent cervix—a condition in which the cervix becomes weak, which could lead to a premature/early opening of the cervix (This would raise the risk of a premature birth/delivery.)
- placenta previa—a condition in which the placenta (a blood-rich structure that nourishes the fetus) lies too low
- leakage of the amniotic fluid (the fluid that surrounds the fetus; this is also called "ruptured membrane" or "waters broken.")
- multiple fetuses—if the couple is expecting twins, triplets, or multiples
- either parent found to have a sexually transmitted disease (STD)

WHAT SHOULD YOU NOT DO DURING PREGNANCY SEX?

- Avoid deep penetration.
- Avoid holding your breath during penetration.
- Avoid direct nipple stimulation.
- Avoid lying flat on your back after the first trimester—always use a pillow under one side.
- Avoid anal sex (as suggested by some of the health-care providers).
- Avoid blowing air into the partner's vagina during oral sex, as this can cause an air embolism (blockage of a blood vessel by an air bubble), which can be fatal to both the mother and fetus.
- Avoid new sexual partners whose sexual history is unknown.

- Avoid all forms of sex (oral, anal, or vaginal) if the partner has an active STI since having an STI during pregnancy is potentially dangerous for both the parents-to-be and the unborn baby.

WHEN DO YOU HAVE TO CALL THE DOCTOR?

Orgasm in late pregnancy may cause mild contractions (called "Braxton Hicks contractions"), which are common near the end of the third trimester but will resolve after a few minutes of rest. If the contractions continue or you experience unusual symptoms such as developing pain, bleeding, or leaking fluid, then contact your doctor right away. Always remember that "normal" is a relative term when discussing "sex during pregnancy" and make sure to discuss what feels right for both you and your partner.

References

Hirsch, Larissa. MD. "Sex during Pregnancy," KidsHealth from Nemours, October 2016. Available online. URL: https://kidshealth.org/en/parents/sex-pregnancy.html. Accessed June 25, 2023.

Johnson, Traci C. MD. "Sex during and after Pregnancy," WebMD, January 21, 2017. Available online. URL: www.webmd.com/baby/guide/sex-and-pregnancy#2. Accessed June 25, 2023.

"Sex during Pregnancy: What's Ok, What's Not," Mayoclinic, July 10, 2018. Available online. URL: www.mayoclinic.org/healthy-lifestyle/pregnancy-week-by-week/in-depth/sex-during-pregnancy/art-20045318. Accessed June 25, 2023.

Chapter 25 | Working and Traveling during Pregnancy

Chapter Contents

Section 25.1 | Pregnancy and Your Job

Pregnancy can affect your safety as a worker. If you are pregnant, you are encouraged to discuss possible job hazards with your employer, health and safety office at work (if there is one), and doctor, as soon as possible. Many pregnant women are able to adjust their job duties temporarily or take extra steps to protect themselves.

Current occupational exposure limits were set based on studies of nonpregnant adults. What is considered safe for you may not be safe for your fetus. Although most employees are able to safely do their job throughout pregnancy, pregnancy can sometimes affect worker safety.

If you are pregnant and working, you may have to consider the following:

- Changes in your metabolism increase how quickly you absorb some chemicals (e.g., some metals).
- Because of physical changes, the personal protective equipment that you could wear correctly before pregnancy may not fit properly, such as lab coats or respirators.
- When pregnant, changes in your immune system, lung capacity, and even ligaments can alter your risk of injury or illness due to some workplace hazards.
- A fetus might be more vulnerable to some chemicals because of its rapid growth and development, particularly early in pregnancy when its organs are developing.[1]

KNOW YOUR PREGNANCY RIGHTS

When sharing your good news with coworkers, discrimination might be the last thing on your mind. But the truth is that many women are treated unfairly—or even fired—after revealing the

[1] National Institute for Occupational Safety and Health (NIOSH), "Pregnancy and Your Job–Reproductive Health," Centers for Disease Control and Prevention (CDC), May 1, 2023. Available online. URL: https://cdc.gov/niosh/index. htm. Accessed May 25, 2023.

news of their pregnancy. As long as a pregnant woman is able to perform the major functions of her job, not hiring or firing her because she is pregnant is against the law. It is against the law to dock her pay or demote her to a lesser position because of pregnancy. It is also against the law to hold back benefits for pregnancy because a woman is not married. All are forms of pregnancy discrimination, and all are illegal.

Women are protected under the Pregnancy Discrimination Act (PDA; www.eeoc.gov/fact-sheet/facts-about-pregnancy-discrimination). It says that businesses with at least 15 employees must treat women who are pregnant in the same manner as other job applicants or employees with similar abilities or limitations.

The Family and Medical Leave Act (FMLA) also protects the jobs of workers who are employed by companies with 50 employees or more and who have worked for the company for at least 12 months. These companies must allow employees to take 12 weeks of unpaid leave for medical reasons, including pregnancy and childbirth. Your job cannot be given away during this 12-week period.

Many state laws also protect pregnant women's rights. These laws appear clear-cut. But issues that arise on the job seldom are. Go to the U.S. Equal Employment Opportunity Commission (EEOC) website (www.eeoc.gov) to learn more about your rights during pregnancy and what to do if you think your rights have been violated.[2]

---

[2] Office on Women's Health (OWH), "Know Your Pregnancy Rights," U.S. Department of Health and Human Services (HHS), February 22, 2021. Available online. URL: https://womenshealth.gov/pregnancy/youre-pregnant-now-what/know-your-pregnancy-rights. Accessed May 25, 2023.

Section 25.2 | Travel and Pregnancy

TRAVEL DURING PREGNANCY

Everyday life does not stop once you are pregnant. Most healthy pregnant women are able to continue with their usual routine and activity level. That means going to work, running errands, and, for some, traveling away from home. To take care of yourself and help keep your baby safe, consider these points before taking a long trip or traveling far from home:

- Talk to your doctor before making any travel decisions that will take you far from home. Ask if any health conditions you might have can make travel during pregnancy unsafe. Also, consider the destination. Is the food and water safe? Will you need immunizations before you go? Is there good medical care available in the event of an emergency? Will your health insurance cover medical care at your destination?
- Avoid sitting for long periods during car or air travel. Prolonged sitting can affect blood flow in your legs. Try to limit driving to no more than five or six hours each day. Take frequent breaks to stretch your legs. Stand up and move your legs often during air travel. Wearing support pantyhose can also help blood flow.
- Occasional air travel is safe for most pregnant women, and most airlines will allow women to fly up to 36 weeks of pregnancy. Make sure to wear your seat belt during the flight and take steps to ease the discomfort of prolonged travel and sitting. Frequent air travel during pregnancy increases the risk of fetal exposure to cosmic radiation. If you are a pregnant pilot, aircrew member, or other frequent flier, check with your employer about flying restrictions.
- Bring a copy of your medical record and find out about medical care at your destination, so you will be prepared in the event of an emergency.

- If you suspect a problem with your pregnancy during your trip, do not wait until you come home to see your doctor. Seek medical care right away.

BUCKLE UP!

Wearing a seat belt during car and air travel is safe while pregnant. The lap strap should go under your belly, across your hips. The shoulder strap should go between your breasts and to the side of your belly. Make sure it fits snugly.[3]

Section 25.3 | International Travel during Pregnancy

Pregnant travelers can generally travel safely with appropriate preparation. But they should avoid some destinations, including those with the risk of Zika and malaria. Learn more about traveling during pregnancy and steps you can take to keep you and your baby healthy.

ZIKA AND MALARIA

Zika can cause severe birth defects. The Zika virus is spread through mosquito bites and sex. If you are pregnant, do not travel to areas with the risk of Zika. If you must travel to an area with Zika, use insect repellent and take other steps to avoid bug bites. If you have a sex partner who lives in or has traveled to an area with Zika, you should use condoms for the rest of your pregnancy.

Pregnant travelers should avoid travel to areas with malaria, as it can be more severe in pregnant women. Malaria increases the risk of serious pregnancy problems, including premature birth, miscarriage, and stillbirth. If you must travel to an area with malaria, talk

[3] Office on Women's Health (OWH), "Staying Healthy and Safe," U.S. Department of Health and Human Services (HHS), February 22, 2021. Available online. URL: https://womenshealth.gov/pregnancy/youre-pregnant-now-what/staying-healthy-and-safe. Accessed May 25, 2023.

to your doctor about taking malaria prevention medicine. Malaria is spread by mosquitoes, so use insect repellent and take other steps to avoid bug bites.

BEFORE TRAVEL

Before you book a cruise or air travel, check the airlines or cruise operator policies for pregnant women. Some airlines will let you fly until 36 weeks, but others may have an earlier cutoff. Cruises may not allow you to travel after 24–28 weeks of pregnancy, and you may need to have a note from your doctor stating you are fit to travel.

Make an Appointment

Before travel, make an appointment with your health-care provider or a travel health specialist that takes place at least one month before you leave. They can help you get destination-specific vaccines, medicines, and information. Discussing your health concerns, itinerary, and planned activities with your provider allows them to give more specific advice and recommendations.

Plan for the Unexpected

It is important to plan for unexpected events as much as possible. Doing so can help you get quality health care or avoid being stranded at a destination. A few steps you can take to plan for unexpected events are to get travel insurance, learn where to get health care during travel, pack a travel health kit, and enroll in the Department of State's STEP (https://step.state.gov/step).

Be sure your health-care policy covers pregnancy and neonatal complications while overseas. If it does not, get travel health insurance that covers those items. Consider getting medical evacuation insurance, too.

Recognize signs and symptoms that require immediate medical attention, including pelvic or abdominal pain, bleeding, contractions, symptoms of preeclampsia (unusual swelling, severe headaches, nausea and vomiting, and vision changes), and dehydration.

Prepare a Travel Health Kit

Pregnant travelers may want to include in your kit prescription medications, hemorrhoid cream, antiemetic drugs, antacids, prenatal vitamins, medication for vaginitis or yeast infection, and support hose, in addition to the items recommended for all travelers.

DURING TRAVEL

Your feet may become swollen on a long flight, so wear comfortable shoes and loose clothing and try to walk around every hour or so. Sitting for a long time, like on a long flight, increases your chances of getting blood clots, or deep vein thrombosis. Pregnant women are also more likely to get blood clots. To reduce your risk of a blood clot, your doctor may recommend compression stockings or leg exercises you can do in your seat.

Prepare a Travel Health Kit

Contaminated food or drinks can cause traveler's diarrhea and other diseases and disrupt your travel. Travelers to low- or middle-income destinations are especially at risk. Generally, foods served hot are usually safe to eat as well as dry and packaged foods. Bottled, canned, and hot drinks are usually safe to drink.

Pregnant women should not use bismuth subsalicylate, which is in Pepto-Bismol and Kaopectate. Travelers to low- or middle-income destinations are more likely to get sick from food or drinks. Iodine tablets for water purification should not be used since they can harm thyroid development of the fetus.

AFTER TRAVEL

If you traveled and feel sick, particularly if you have a fever, talk to a health-care provider immediately and tell them about your travel. Avoid contact with other people while you are sick.[4]

---

[4] "Pregnant Travelers," Centers for Disease Control and Prevention (CDC), June 28, 2022. Available online. URL: wwwnc.cdc.gov/travel/page/pregnant-travelers. Accessed May 25, 2023.

Chapter 26 | Nicotine, Alcohol, and Substance Use during Pregnancy

Chapter Contents

Section 26.1 | Smoking and Pregnancy

Most people know that smoking causes cancer and other major health problems. And smoking while you are pregnant can cause serious problems, too. Your baby could be born too early, have a birth defect, or die from sudden infant death syndrome (SIDS). Even being around cigarette smoke can cause health problems for you and your baby.

It is best to quit smoking before you get pregnant. But, if you are already pregnant, quitting can still help protect you and your baby from health problems. It is never too late to quit smoking. If you smoked and had a healthy pregnancy in the past, there is no guarantee that your next pregnancy will be healthy. When you smoke during pregnancy, you put your health and your baby's health at risk.

HOW DOES SMOKING AFFECT FERTILITY?

Smoking can cause fertility problems for you or your partner. Women who smoke have more trouble getting pregnant than women who do not smoke. In men, smoking can damage sperm and contribute to impotence (erectile dysfunction (ED)). Both problems can make it harder for a man to father a baby when he and his partner are ready.

HOW CAN SMOKING HARM YOU AND YOUR BABY?

- Your baby may be born too small, even after a full-term pregnancy. Smoking slows your baby's growth before birth.
- Your baby may be born too early (premature birth). Premature babies often have health problems.
- Smoking can damage your baby's developing lungs and brain. The damage can last through childhood and into the teen years.
- Smoking doubles your risk of abnormal bleeding during pregnancy and delivery. This can put both you and your baby in danger.

- Smoking raises your baby's risk of birth defects, including cleft lip, cleft palate, or both. A cleft is an opening in your baby's lip or in the roof of his or her mouth (palate). He or she can have trouble eating properly and is likely to need surgery.
- Babies of moms who smoke during pregnancy—and babies exposed to cigarette smoke after birth—have a higher risk of SIDS.

HOW CAN A PREMATURE BIRTH HARM YOUR BABY?

If you smoke during pregnancy, you are more likely to give birth too early. A baby born three weeks or more before your due date is premature. Babies born too early miss important growth that happens in the womb during the final weeks and months of pregnancy.

The earlier a baby is born, the greater the chances for serious health problems or death. Premature babies can have:

- low birth weight
- feeding difficulties
- breathing problems right away
- breathing problems that last into childhood
- cerebral palsy (brain damage that causes trouble with movement and muscle tone)
- developmental delays (when a baby or child is behind in language, thinking, or movement skills)
- problems with hearing or eyesight

Premature babies may need to stay at the hospital for days, weeks, or even months.[1]

HEALTH EFFECTS OF SMOKING AND SECONDHAND SMOKE ON PREGNANCIES

- Women who smoke have more difficulty becoming pregnant and have a higher risk of never becoming pregnant.

---

[1] "Smoking, Pregnancy, and Babies," Centers for Disease Control and Prevention (CDC), May 5, 2022. Available online. URL: www.cdc.gov/tobacco/campaign/tips/diseases/pregnancy.html. Accessed May 25, 2023.

- Smoking during pregnancy can cause tissue damage in the unborn baby, particularly in the lungs and brain, and some studies suggest a link between maternal smoking and cleft lip.
- Studies also suggest a relationship between tobacco and miscarriage. Carbon monoxide in tobacco smoke can keep the developing baby from getting enough oxygen. Tobacco smoke also contains other chemicals that can harm unborn babies.

HEALTH EFFECTS OF SMOKING AND SECONDHAND SMOKE ON BABIES

- Mothers who smoke are more likely to deliver their babies early. Preterm delivery is a leading cause of death, disability, and disease among newborns.
- One in every five babies born to mothers who smoke during pregnancy has a low birth weight. Mothers who are exposed to secondhand smoke while pregnant are more likely to have lower birth weight babies. Babies born too small or too early are not as healthy.
- Both babies whose mothers smoke while pregnant and babies who are exposed to secondhand smoke after birth are more likely to die from SIDS than babies who are not exposed to cigarette smoke. Babies whose mothers smoke are about three times more likely to die from SIDS.
- Babies whose mothers smoke while pregnant or who are exposed to secondhand smoke after birth have weaker lungs than other babies, which increases the risk of many health problems.[2]

HOW CAN QUITTING SMOKING HELP YOU AND YOUR BABY?

The best time to quit smoking is before you get pregnant, but quitting at any time during pregnancy can help your baby get a better

---

[2] "Smoking during Pregnancy," Centers for Disease Control and Prevention (CDC), April 28, 2020. Available online. URL: www.cdc.gov/tobacco/basic_information/health_effects/pregnancy/index.htm. Accessed May 25, 2023.

start on life. Talk to your doctor about the best ways to quit while you are pregnant or trying to get pregnant.

When you stop smoking:

- your baby gets more oxygen, even after just one day
- your baby will grow better
- your baby is less likely to be born too early
- you will have more energy and breathe more easily
- you will be less likely to develop heart disease, stroke, lung cancer, lung disease, and other smoking-related diseases

SUPPORT FOR QUITTING SMOKING DURING PREGNANCY

Most pregnant women who smoke want to quit, but quitting is not always easy during pregnancy. What is more, if you are pregnant and still smoking, you may feel ashamed and alone. The right kind of support can help a pregnant woman get through the unique challenges of quitting during this phase of life.

STAY SMOKE-FREE FOR A HEALTHY CHILD

Staying smoke-free is important. Tobacco smoke contains a deadly mix of more than 7,000 chemicals. When your child is not exposed to smoke, you can expect him or her to have the following:

- fewer coughs and chest colds
- a lower risk of bronchitis or pneumonia (lung problems)
- fewer ear infections
- fewer asthma attacks and wheezing problems[3]

---

[3] See footnote [1].

Section 26.2 | Alcohol Use and Pregnancy

There is no known safe amount of alcohol use during pregnancy or while trying to get pregnant. There is also no safe time for alcohol use during pregnancy. All types of alcohol are equally harmful, including all wines and beer. Fetal alcohol spectrum disorders (FASDs) are preventable if a baby is not exposed to alcohol before birth.

WHY ALCOHOL IS DANGEROUS

Alcohol in the mother's blood passes to the baby through the umbilical cord. Alcohol use during pregnancy can cause miscarriage, stillbirth, and a range of lifelong physical, behavioral, and intellectual disabilities. These disabilities are known as "FASDs." Children with FASDs might have the following characteristics and behaviors:

- abnormal facial features, such as a smooth ridge between the nose and upper lip (this ridge is called the "philtrum")
- small head size
- shorter-than-average height
- low body weight
- poor coordination
- hyperactive behavior
- difficulty with attention
- poor memory
- difficulty in school (especially with math)
- learning disabilities
- speech and language delays
- intellectual disability or low intelligence quotient (IQ)
- poor reasoning and judgment skills
- sleep and sucking problems as a baby
- vision or hearing problems
- problems with the heart, kidney, or bones

HOW MUCH ALCOHOL IS DANGEROUS?

There is no known safe amount of alcohol use during pregnancy.

WHEN ALCOHOL IS DANGEROUS

There is no safe time for alcohol use during pregnancy. Alcohol can cause problems for the baby throughout pregnancy, including before a woman knows she is pregnant. Alcohol use in the first three months of pregnancy can cause the baby to have abnormal facial features. Growth and central nervous system problems (e.g., low birth weight, behavioral problems) can occur from alcohol use anytime during pregnancy. The baby's brain is developing throughout pregnancy and can be affected by exposure to alcohol at any time. It is never too late to stop alcohol use during pregnancy. Stopping alcohol use will improve the baby's health and well-being.[4]

Section 26.3 | Fetal Alcohol Spectrum Disorders

Fetal alcohol spectrum disorders (FASDs) are a group of conditions that can occur in a person who was exposed to alcohol before birth. These effects can include physical problems and problems with behavior and learning. Often, a person with an FASD has a mix of these problems.

CAUSE AND PREVENTION OF FETAL ALCOHOL SPECTRUM DISORDERS

Fetal alcohol spectrum disorders can occur when a person is exposed to alcohol before birth. Alcohol in the mother's blood passes to the baby through the umbilical cord. There is no known safe amount of alcohol during pregnancy or when trying to get pregnant. There is also no safe time to drink during pregnancy.

---

[4] National Center on Birth Defects and Developmental Disabilities (NCBDDD), "Alcohol Use during Pregnancy," Centersfor Disease Control and Prevention (CDC), November 4, 2022. Available online. URL: www.cdc.gov/ncbddd/fasd/alcohol-use.html. Accessed May 25, 2023.

Alcohol can cause problems for a developing baby throughout pregnancy, including before a woman knows she is pregnant. All types of alcohol are equally harmful, including all wines and beer.

To prevent FASDs, a woman should avoid alcohol if she is pregnant or might be pregnant. This is because a woman could get pregnant and not know for up to four to six weeks. It is never too late to stop alcohol use during pregnancy. Because brain growth takes place throughout pregnancy, stopping alcohol use will improve the baby's health and well-being.

SIGNS AND SYMPTOMS OF FETAL ALCOHOL SPECTRUM DISORDERS

Fetal alcohol spectrum disorders refer to a collection of diagnoses that represent the range of effects that can happen to a person who was exposed to alcohol before birth. These conditions can affect each person in different ways and can range from mild to severe.

A person with an FASD might have:

- low body weight
- poor coordination
- hyperactive behavior
- difficulty with attention
- poor memory
- difficulty in school (especially with math)
- learning disabilities
- speech and language delays
- intellectual disability or low intelligence quotient (IQ)
- poor reasoning and judgment skills
- sleep and sucking problems as a baby
- vision or hearing problems
- problems with the heart, kidneys, or bones
- shorter-than-average height
- small head size
- abnormal facial features, such as a smooth ridge between the nose and upper lip (this ridge is called the "philtrum")

DIAGNOSIS OF FETAL ALCOHOL SPECTRUM DISORDERS

Different FASD diagnoses are based on particular symptoms and include the following:

- **Fetal alcohol syndrome (FAS).** FAS represents the most involved end of the FASD spectrum. People with FAS have central nervous system (CNS) problems, minor facial features, and growth problems. People with FAS can have problems with learning, memory, attention span, communication, vision, or hearing. They might have a mix of these problems. People with FAS often have a hard time in school and trouble getting along with others.

- **Alcohol-related neurodevelopmental disorder (ARND).** People with ARND might have intellectual disabilities and problems with behavior and learning. They might do poorly in school and have difficulties with math, memory, attention, judgment, and poor impulse control.

- **Alcohol-related birth defects (ARBDs).** People with ARBDs might have problems with the heart, kidneys, or bones or with hearing. They might have a mix of these.

- **Neurobehavioral disorder associated with prenatal alcohol exposure (ND-PAE).** ND-PAE was first included as a recognized condition in the *Diagnostic and Statistical Manual 5* (*DSM 5*) of the American Psychiatric Association (APA) in 2013. A child or youth with ND-PAE will have problems in three areas:
  - thinking and memory, where the child may have trouble planning or may forget material he or she has already learned
  - behavior problems, such as severe tantrums, mood issues (e.g., irritability), and difficulty shifting attention from one task to another
  - trouble with day-to-day living, which can include problems with bathing, dressing for the weather, and playing with other children

In addition, to be diagnosed with ND-PAE, the mother of the child must have consumed more than minimal levels of alcohol before the child's birth, which the APA defines as more than 13 alcoholic drinks per month of pregnancy (i.e., any 30-day period of pregnancy) or more than two alcoholic drinks in one sitting.

Areas Evaluated for Fetal Alcohol Spectrum Disorders Diagnoses

The term FASDs is not meant for use as a clinical diagnosis. Diagnosing FASDs can be hard because there is no medical test, such as a blood test, for these conditions. And other disorders, such as attention deficit hyperactivity disorder (ADHD) and Williams syndrome, have some symptoms such as FASDs.

To diagnose FASDs, doctors look for:

- prenatal alcohol exposure although confirmation is not required to make a diagnosis
- CNS problems (e.g., small head size, problems with attention and hyperactivity, poor coordination)
- lower-than-average height, weight, or both
- abnormal facial features (e.g., a smooth ridge between the nose and upper lip)

TREATMENT FOR FETAL ALCOHOL SPECTRUM DISORDERS

Fetal alcohol spectrum disorders last a lifetime. There is no cure for FASDs, but research shows that early intervention treatment services can improve a child's development.

There are many types of treatment options, including medication to help with some symptoms, behavior and education therapy, parent training, and other alternative approaches. No one treatment is right for every child. Good treatment plans will include close monitoring, follow-ups, and changes as needed along the way.

Also, "protective factors" can help reduce the effects of FASDs and help people with these conditions reach their full potential.

Protective factors include:

- diagnosis before six years of age
- loving, nurturing, and stable home environment during the school years

- absence of violence
- involvement in special education and social services[5]

Section 26.4 | Substance Use during Pregnancy

Research shows that use of tobacco, alcohol, or illicit drugs or misuse of prescription drugs by pregnant women can have severe health consequences for infants. This is because many substances pass easily through the placenta, so substances that a pregnant woman takes also reach the fetus. Research shows that smoking tobacco or marijuana, taking prescription pain relievers, or using illegal drugs during pregnancy is associated with double or even triple the risk of stillbirth. Estimates suggest that about 5 percent of pregnant women use one or more addictive substances.

Regular use of some drugs can cause neonatal abstinence syndrome (NAS), in which the baby goes through withdrawal upon birth. Most research in this area has focused on the effects of opioids (prescription pain relievers or heroin). However, data have shown that use of alcohol, barbiturates, benzodiazepines, and caffeine during pregnancy may also cause the infant to show withdrawal symptoms at birth. The type and severity of an infant's withdrawal symptoms depend on the drug(s) used, how long and how often the mother used, how her body breaks the drug down, and whether the infant was born full term or prematurely.

Symptoms of drug withdrawal in a newborn can develop immediately or up to 14 days after birth and can include:
- blotchy skin coloring
- diarrhea
- excessive or high-pitched crying
- abnormal sucking reflex
- fever

[5] National Center on Birth Defects and Developmental Disabilities (NCBDDD), "Basics about FASDs," Centers for Disease Control and Prevention (CDC), November 4, 2022. Available online. URL: https://cdc.gov/ncbddd/fasd/facts.html. Accessed May 26, 2023.

- hyperactive reflexes
- increased muscle tone
- irritability
- poor feeding
- rapid breathing
- seizures
- sleep problems
- slow weight gain
- stuffy nose and sneezing
- sweating
- trembling
- vomiting

Effects of using some drugs could be long-term and possibly fatal to the baby. They are as follows:

- birth defects
- low birth weight
- premature birth
- small head circumference
- sudden infant death syndrome (SIDS)

ILLEGAL DRUGS
Marijuana (Cannabis)

A 2017 opinion posted by the American College of Obstetrics and Gynecology (ACOG) suggests that cannabis effects on fetal growth (e.g., low birth weight and length) may be more pronounced in women who consume marijuana frequently, especially in the first and second trimesters. The ACOG recommends that pregnant women or women contemplating pregnancy should be encouraged to discontinue the use of marijuana.

There is no human research connecting marijuana use to the chance of miscarriage; however, animal studies indicate that the risk of miscarriage increases if marijuana is used early in pregnancy. Some associations have been found between marijuana use during pregnancy and future developmental and hyperactivity disorders in children. There is substantial evidence of a statistical association between marijuana smoking among pregnant women and low birth weight. Researchers theorize that elevated levels of carbon dioxide might restrict fetal growth in women who use marijuana during pregnancy. Some women report using marijuana to treat severe nausea associated with their pregnancy; however, there is no research confirming that this is a safe practice, and it is generally not recommended.

Human research has shown that some babies born to women who used marijuana during their pregnancies display altered responses to visual stimuli, increased trembling, and a high-pitched cry, which could indicate problems with neurological development.

Stimulants (Cocaine and Methamphetamine)

Research shows that pregnant women who use cocaine are at a higher risk of maternal migraines and seizures, premature membrane rupture, and placental abruption (separation of the placental lining from the uterus). Pregnancy is accompanied by normal cardiovascular changes, and cocaine use exacerbates these changes—sometimes leading to serious problems with high blood pressure (hypertensive crisis), spontaneous miscarriage, preterm labor, and difficult delivery. Babies born to mothers who use cocaine during pregnancy may also have low birth weight and smaller head circumferences and are shorter in length than babies born to mothers who do not use cocaine. They also show symptoms of irritability, hyperactivity, tremors, high-pitched cry, and excessive sucking at birth. These symptoms may be due to the effects of cocaine itself, rather than withdrawal, since cocaine and its metabolites are still present in the baby's body up to five to seven days after delivery.

Methylenedioxymethamphetamine (Ecstasy, Molly)

Research suggests that prenatal methylenedioxymethamphetamine (MDMA) exposure may cause learning, memory, and motor problems in the baby.

Heroin

Heroin use during pregnancy can result in NAS specifically associated with opioid use. NAS occurs when heroin passes through the placenta to the fetus during pregnancy, causing the baby to become dependent on opioids. Symptoms include excessive crying, high-pitched cry, irritability, seizures, and gastrointestinal problems, among others.

MEDICATIONS
Prescription and Over-the-Counter Drugs

Pregnancy can be a confusing time for women facing many choices about legal drugs, such as tobacco and alcohol, as well as prescription and over-the-counter (OTC) drugs that may affect the developing fetus. These are difficult issues for researchers to study because scientists cannot give potentially dangerous drugs to pregnant women. Here are some of the known facts about popular medications and pregnancy.

There are more than 6 million pregnancies in the United States every year, and about 9 out of 10 pregnant women take medication. The U.S. Food and Drug Administration (FDA) issued rules on drug labeling to provide clearer instructions for pregnant and nursing women, including a summary of the risks of use during pregnancy and breastfeeding, a discussion of the data supporting the summary, and other information to help prescribers make safe decisions.

Even so, we know little about the effects of taking most medications during pregnancy. Fewer than 10 percent of prescriptions have enough information to determine fetal risks. This is because pregnant women are often not included in studies to determine safety of new medications before they come on the market. One study shows that use of short-acting prescription opioids such as oxycodone during pregnancy, especially when combined with tobacco and/or certain antidepressant medications, is associated with an increased likelihood of NAS in the infant.

Although some prescription and OTC medications are safe to take during pregnancy, a pregnant woman should tell her doctor about all prescription and OTC medications and herbal or dietary supplements she is taking or planning to take. This will allow her doctor to weigh the risks and benefits of a medication during pregnancy. In some cases, the doctor may recommend the continued use of specific medications even though they could have some impact on the fetus. Suddenly stopping the use of a medication may be more risky for both the mother and fetus than continuing to use the medication while under a doctor's care.

Some prescription and OTC medications are generally compatible with breastfeeding. Others, such as some antianxiety and antidepressant medications, have unknown effects, so mothers who are using these medications should consult with their doctor before breastfeeding. Nursing mothers should contact their infant's health-care provider if their infants show any of these reactions to the breast milk: diarrhea, excessive crying, vomiting, skin rashes, loss of appetite, or sleepiness.[6]

[6] "Substance Use While Pregnant and Breastfeeding," National Institute on Drug Abuse (NIDA), April 1, 2020. Available online. URL: https://nida.nih.gov/publications/research-reports/substance-use-in-women/substance-use-while-pregnant-breastfeeding. Accessed May 26, 2023.

Chapter 27 | Prenatal Radiation Exposures and Home Monitoring

Chapter Contents

Section 27.1 | X-rays, Pregnancy, and You

Pregnancy is a time to take good care of yourself and your unborn child. Many things are especially important during pregnancy, such as eating right, cutting out cigarettes and alcohol, and being careful about the prescription and over-the-counter (OTC) drugs you take. Diagnostic x-rays and other medical radiation procedures of the abdominal area also deserve extra attention during pregnancy.

Diagnostic x-rays can give the doctor important and even life-saving information about a person's medical condition. But, like many things, diagnostic x-rays have risks as well as benefits. They should be used only when they will give the doctor information needed to treat you.

You will probably never need an abdominal x-ray during pregnancy. But, sometimes, because of a particular medical condition, your physician may feel that a diagnostic x-ray of your abdomen or lower torso is needed. If this should happen, do not be upset. The risk to you and your unborn child is very small, and the benefit of finding out about your medical condition is far greater. In fact, the risk of not having a needed x-ray could be much greater than the risk from the radiation. But even small risks should not be taken if they are unnecessary.

You can reduce those risks by telling your doctor if you are, or think you might be, pregnant whenever an abdominal x-ray is prescribed. If you are pregnant, the doctor may decide that it would be best to cancel the x-ray examination, to postpone it, or to modify it to reduce the amount of radiation. Or, depending on your medical needs and realizing that the risk is very small, the doctor may feel that it is best to proceed with the x-ray as planned. In any case, you should feel free to discuss the decision with your doctor.

WHAT KIND OF X-RAYS CAN AFFECT THE UNBORN CHILD?

During most x-ray examinations—such as those of the arms, legs, head, teeth, or chest—your reproductive organs are not exposed to the direct x-ray beam. So these kinds of procedures, when properly done, do not involve any risk to the unborn child. However, x-rays of the mother's lower torso—abdomen, stomach, pelvis, lower back, or kidneys—may expose the unborn child to the direct x-ray beam. They are of more concern.

WHAT ARE THE POSSIBLE EFFECTS OF X-RAYS?

There is scientific disagreement about whether the small amounts of radiation used in diagnostic radiology can actually harm the unborn child, but it is known that the unborn child is very sensitive to the effects of things such as radiation, certain drugs, excess alcohol, and infection. This is true, in part, because the cells are rapidly dividing and growing into specialized cells and tissues. If radiation or other agents were to cause changes in these cells, there could be a slightly increased chance of birth defects or certain illnesses, such as leukemia, later in life.

It should be pointed out, however, that the majority of birth defects and childhood diseases occur even if the mother is not exposed to any known harmful agent during pregnancy. Scientists believe that heredity and random errors in the developmental process are responsible for most of these problems.

WHAT IF YOU ARE X-RAYED BEFORE YOU KNOW YOU ARE PREGNANT?

Do not be alarmed. Remember that the possibility of any harm to you and your unborn child from an x-ray is very small. There are, however, rare situations in which a woman who is unaware of her pregnancy may receive a very large number of abdominal x-rays over a short period, or she may receive radiation treatment of the lower torso. Under these circumstances, the woman should discuss the possible risks with her doctor.

HOW CAN YOU HELP MINIMIZE THE RISKS?

- Most important, tell your physician if you are pregnant or think you might be. This is important for many medical decisions, such as drug prescriptions and nuclear medicine procedures, as well as x-rays. And, remember, this is true even in the very early weeks of pregnancy.

- Occasionally, a woman may mistake the symptoms of pregnancy for the symptoms of a disease. If you have any of the symptoms of pregnancy—consider whether you might be pregnant and tell your doctor or x-ray technologist (the person doing the examination) before having an x-ray of the lower torso. A pregnancy test may be called for.
- If you are pregnant or think you might be, do not hold a child who is being x-rayed. If you are not pregnant and you are asked to hold a child during an x-ray, be sure to ask for a lead apron to protect your reproductive organs. This is to prevent damage to your genes that could be passed on and cause harmful effects in your future descendants.
- Whenever an x-ray is requested, tell your doctor about any similar x-rays you have had recently. It may not be necessary to do another. It is a good idea to keep a record of the x-ray examinations you and your family have had taken so that you can provide this kind of information accurately.
- Feel free to talk with your doctor about the need for an x-ray examination. You should understand the reason x-rays are requested in your particular case.[1]

[1] "X-rays, Pregnancy and You," U.S. Food and Drug Administration (FDA), December 9, 2017. Available online. URL: https://fda.gov/radiation-emitting-products/medical-x-ray-imaging/x-rays-pregnancy-and-you. Accessed May 29, 2023.

Section 27.2 | Ultrasound Imaging and Pregnancy

Ultrasound imaging (sonography) uses high-frequency sound waves to view inside the body. Because ultrasound images are captured in real time, they can also show movement of the body's internal organs as well as blood flowing through the blood vessels. Unlike x-ray imaging, there is no ionizing radiation exposure associated with ultrasound imaging.

In an ultrasound exam, a transducer (probe) is placed directly on the skin or inside a body opening. A thin layer of gel is applied to the skin so that the ultrasound waves are transmitted from the transducer through the gel into the body. The ultrasound image is produced based on the reflection of the waves off of the body structures. The strength (amplitude) of the sound signal and the time it takes for the wave to travel through the body provide the information necessary to produce an image.

USES OF ULTRASOUND IMAGING

Ultrasound imaging is a medical tool that can help a physician evaluate, diagnose, and treat medical conditions. Common ultrasound imaging procedures include:

- abdominal ultrasound (to visualize abdominal tissues and organs)
- bone sonometry (to assess bone fragility)
- breast ultrasound (to visualize breast tissue)
- doppler fetal heart rate monitors (to listen to the fetal heart beat)
- doppler ultrasound (to visualize blood flow through a blood vessel, organs, or other structures)
- echocardiogram (to view the heart)
- fetal ultrasound (to view the fetus in pregnancy)
- ultrasound-guided biopsies (to collect a sample of tissue)
- ophthalmic ultrasound (to visualize ocular structures)
- ultrasound-guided needle placement (in blood vessels or other tissues of interest)

BENEFITS/RISKS OF ULTRASOUND IMAGING

Ultrasound imaging has been used for over 20 years and has an excellent safety record. It is based on nonionizing radiation, so it does not have the same risks as x-rays or other types of imaging systems that use ionizing radiation.

Although ultrasound imaging is generally considered safe when used prudently by appropriately trained health-care providers, ultrasound energy has the potential to produce biological effects on the body. Ultrasound waves can heat the tissues slightly. In some cases, it can also produce small pockets of gas in body fluids or tissues (cavitation). The long-term consequences of these effects are still unknown. Because of the particular concern for effects on the fetus, organizations, such as the American Institute of Ultrasound in Medicine (AIUM), have advocated prudent use of ultrasound imaging in pregnancy. Furthermore, the use of ultrasound solely for nonmedical purposes, such as obtaining fetal keepsake videos, has been discouraged. Keepsake images or videos are reasonable if they are produced during a medically indicated exam and if no additional exposure is required.

INFORMATION FOR PATIENTS INCLUDING EXPECTANT MOTHERS

For all medical imaging procedures, the U.S. Food and Drug Administration (FDA) recommends that patients talk to their health-care provider to understand the reason for the examination, the medical information that will be obtained, the potential risks, and how the results will be used to manage the medical condition or pregnancy. Because ultrasound is not based on ionizing radiation, it is particularly useful for women of childbearing age when computed tomography (CT) or other imaging methods would otherwise result in exposure to radiation.

Expectant Mothers

Ultrasound is the most widely used medical imaging method for viewing the fetus during pregnancy. Routine examinations are performed to assess and monitor the health status of the fetus and mother. Ultrasound examinations provide parents with a valuable opportunity to view and hear the heartbeat of the fetus, bond with the unborn baby, and capture images to share with family and friends.

In fetal ultrasound, three-dimensional (3D) ultrasound allows the visualization of some facial features and possibly other parts, such as fingers and toes of the fetus. Four-dimensional (4D) ultrasound is 3D ultrasound in motion. While ultrasound is generally considered to be safe with very low risks, the risks may increase with unnecessary prolonged exposure to ultrasound energy or when untrained users operate the device.

Expectant mothers should also be aware of concerns with purchasing over-the-counter (OTC) fetal heartbeat monitoring systems (also called "doptones"). These devices should only be used by trained health-care providers when medically necessary. The use of these devices by untrained persons could expose the fetus to prolonged and unsafe energy levels or could provide information that is interpreted incorrectly by the user.[2]

Section 27.3 | Home Uterine Monitors Are Not Useful for Predicting Premature Birth

Two methods thought to hold promise in predicting preterm delivery in first-time pregnancies identified only a small proportion of cases and do not appear suitable for widespread screening, according to a large study by a National Institutes of Health (NIH) research network.

The study focused on spontaneous preterm delivery—labor that occurs naturally—rather than delivery initiated for medical need, such as cesarean surgery or induced labor.

The study authors evaluated routine ultrasound examination of the uterine cervix, the lower part of the uterus that shortens

---

[2] "Ultrasound Imaging," U.S. Food and Drug Administration (FDA), September 28, 2020. Available online. URL: https://fda.gov/radiation-emitting-products/medical-imaging/ultrasound-imaging. Accessed May 29, 2023.

and opens during labor. Previous studies have indicated that a short cervix early in pregnancy could be a warning sign of impending preterm birth. The researchers also evaluated testing for fetal fibronectin, a glue-like protein that secures the amniotic sac to the inside of the uterus. Some studies have suggested that the presence of fetal fibronectin in the vagina early in pregnancy could signal early labor.

However, after screening more than 9,000 women throughout pregnancy, each test identified only a small proportion of the women who would eventually deliver preterm.

"These methods of assessing women in their first pregnancy do not identify most of those who will later go on to have a spontaneous preterm delivery," said the study's senior author, Uma Reddy, M.D., Professor of Obstetrics, Gynecology, and Reproductive Sciences; Section Chief, Maternal-Fetal Medicine, Yale School of Medicine. "There is a need to develop better screening tests that can be performed early in pregnancy."

The study included 9,410 women pregnant with a single fetus at eight research centers in the United States. It was conducted as part of the Nulliparous Pregnancy Outcomes Study: Monitoring Mothers-to-Be (nuMoM2b), which aims to improve the care of women during their first pregnancy and to find new ways to identify impending preterm birth and other adverse pregnancy conditions.

The women underwent ultrasound testing to measure cervical length at 16–22 weeks of pregnancy and again from 22 to 31 weeks of pregnancy. Fetal fibronectin tests were conducted at 6–14 weeks, 16–22 weeks, and 22–30 weeks. A short cervix was defined as less than 25 mm.

Of the women tested at 16–22 weeks, 35–439 women (8%) who delivered spontaneously before the 37th week of pregnancy had a short cervix. At 22–31 weeks, 94–403 women (23.3%) who delivered prematurely had a short cervix.

For the fibronectin test at 16–22 weeks, 30 of 410 women (7.3%) who delivered spontaneously before the 37th week had high fibronectin levels. At 22–30 weeks, 31 of 384 women

(8.1%) who delivered prematurely had high fibronectin levels. The authors defined a high fibronectin level as 50 ng/mL or greater.

The researchers found no benefit to combining the results of the two tests. They concluded that alone and together, the methods did not identify enough preterm births to support routine screening of first-time pregnancies.[3]

[3] News and Events, "Common Tests for Preterm Birth Not Useful for Routine Screening of First-Time Pregnancies," National Institutes of Health (NIH), March 14, 2017. Available online. URL: https://www.nih.gov/news-events/news-releases/common-tests-preterm-birth-not-useful-routine-screening-first-time-pregnancies. Accessed May 29, 2023.

Chapter 28 | Common Safety Concerns during Pregnancy

Chapter Contents

Section 28.1 | Hot Tubs, High Temperatures, and Pregnancy Risks

Low water volumes combined with high temperatures and heavy bather loads make public hot tub operation challenging. The result can be low disinfectant levels that allow the growth and spread of a variety of germs (e.g., *Pseudomonas* and *Legionella*) that can cause skin and respiratory recreational water illnesses (RWIs). Operators who focus on hot tub maintenance and operation to ensure continuous, high water quality are the first line of defense in preventing the spread of RWIs.

- Obtain state- or local authority-recommended operator and chemical handling training.
- Ensure availability of trained operation staff during weekends when hot tubs are used most.
- Maintain free chlorine (3–10 parts per million (ppm)) or bromine (4–8 ppm) levels continuously.
- Maintain the pH level of the water at 7.2–7.8.
- Test pH and disinfectant levels at least twice per day (hourly when in heavy use).
- Maintain accurate records of disinfectant/pH measurements and maintenance activities.
- Maintain filtration and recirculation systems according to manufacturer recommendations.
- Inspect accessible recirculation system components for a slime layer and clean as needed.
- Scrub hot tub surfaces to remove any slime layer.
- Enforce bather load limits.
- Drain and replace all or portions of the water on a weekly to monthly basis, depending on usage and water quality. Depending on the filter type, clean the filter or replace the filter media before refilling the hot tub.
- Treat the hot tub with a biocidal shock treatment on a daily to weekly basis, depending on water quality and frequency of water replacement.

- Institute a preventive maintenance program to replace equipment or parts before they fail (e.g., feed pump tubing, sensor probes).
- Provide disinfection guidelines for fecal accidents and body fluid spills.
- Develop a clear communication chain for reporting operation problems.
- Cover hot tubs, if possible, to minimize loss of disinfectant and reduce the levels of environmental contamination (e.g., debris and dirt).
- Educate hot tub users about appropriate hot tub use.

ADDITIONAL HOT TUB SAFETY MEASURES

- Prevent the water temperature from exceeding 104 °F (40 °C).
- Exclude children less than five years old from using hot tubs.
- Maintain a locked safety cover for the hot tub when possible.
- Recommend that all pregnant women consult a physician before hot tub use, particularly in the first trimester.
- Prevent entrapment injuries with appropriate drain design and configuration.[1]

Section 28.2 | Cosmetics and Pregnancy

WHAT DOES THE LAW SAY ABOUT COSMETIC SAFETY?

It is important to know that the law does not require cosmetic products or ingredients to have U.S. Food and Drug Administration (FDA) approval before they go on the market. However, cosmetics must be safe when consumers use them according to product labeling, or as the products are customarily used.

---

[1] "Operating Public Hot Tubs," Centers for Disease Control and Prevention (CDC), May 25, 2016. Available online. URL: https://cdc.gov/healthywater/pdf/swimming/resources/operating-public-hot-tubs-factsheet.pdf. Accessed May 29, 2023.

Companies and individuals who manufacture or market cosmetics are legally responsible for making sure their products are safe. The FDA can take action against an unsafe cosmetic that does not comply with the law, but first, health-care providers need reliable information showing that it is unsafe when people use it as intended.

The law treats color additives differently. Color additives must be approved by the FDA before they are used in cosmetics or other FDA-regulated products. Some must even be from batches certified in the FDA's own labs. The law also makes a special exception for coal tar hair dyes, which include most permanent, semipermanent, and temporary hair dyes on the market. The FDA cannot take action against a coal tar hair dye if it has the following statement on the label—along with instructions for doing a skin test:

- Caution—This product contains ingredients which may cause skin irritation on certain individuals, and a preliminary test according to accompanying directions should first be made. This product must not be used for dyeing the eyelashes or eyebrows; to do so may cause blindness.

HOW DOES THE FDA MONITOR COSMETIC SAFETY?

The FDA monitors the safety of cosmetics in several ways. For example, the FDA periodically buys cosmetics and analyzes them, especially if health-care providers are aware of a potential problem. The FDA scientists keep up with the latest research, and the FDA conducts its own research as well. Health-care providers also evaluate reports of problems that are sent to us by consumers who have had bad reactions to watch for trends that will tell us if a particular product may require action on the FDA's part.

When health-care providers look into the safety of a cosmetic product or ingredient on the market, health-care providers consider factors such as how it is used and who is likely to use it. This includes whether there are likely to be safety concerns when women use the product during pregnancy. When health-care providers identify a safety problem, health-care providers let the public know and take action against the product.

SAFETY INFORMATION IN COSMETIC LABELING

Cosmetics must be labeled properly. For example, they must have any directions for use and any warnings needed to make sure consumers use the product safely.

Also, cosmetics marketed on a retail basis to consumers, such as in stores or person-to-person, must have a list of ingredients on the label. For cosmetics sold by mail order, including online, this list must be on the label, in a catalog, on a website, enclosed with the shipment, or sent separately when the consumer asks for it. This list lets consumers know if a product contains ingredients they want to avoid.

SOME "PERSONAL CARE PRODUCTS" THAT ARE NOT COSMETICS

Not all "personal care products," including those you might use during and after pregnancy, are cosmetics. For example, a product that is intended to affect the structure or function of your body or to treat or prevent disease is regulated as a drug or sometimes both a cosmetic and a drug. This is true even if it affects how you look. Stretch mark treatments, creams for treating irritated or cracked nipples, sunscreens, antiperspirants, and treatments for dandruff and acne are some common examples.

Generally, nonprescription drugs must conform to special regulations, called "monographs," for their product category or be approved by the FDA before they go on the market.[2]

---

[2] "Cosmetics & Pregnancy," U.S. Food and Drug Administration (FDA), March 4, 2022. Available online. URL: https://fda.gov/cosmetics/resources-consumers-cosmetics/cosmetics-pregnancy. Accessed May 29, 2023.

Part 4 | High-Risk Pregnancies

Chapter 29 | What Is a High-Risk Pregnancy?

WHAT IS A HIGH-RISK PREGNANCY?

A high-risk pregnancy is one that threatens the health or life of the mother or her fetus. It often requires specialized care from specially trained providers. Some pregnancies become high risk as they progress, while some women are at increased risk for complications even before they get pregnant for a variety of reasons. Early and regular prenatal care helps many women have healthy pregnancies and deliveries without complications. Risk factors for a high-risk pregnancy can include the following:

- **Existing health conditions.** These conditions include high blood pressure, diabetes, and being human immunodeficiency virus (HIV) positive.
- **Overweight and obesity.** Obesity increases the risk of high blood pressure, preeclampsia, gestational diabetes, stillbirth, neural tube defects, and cesarean delivery. The *Eunice Kennedy Shriver* National Institute of Child Health and Human Development (NICHD) researchers have found that obesity can raise infants' risk of heart problems at birth by 15 percent.
- **Multiple births.** The risk of complications is higher in women carrying more than one fetus (twins and higher-order multiples). Common complications include preeclampsia, premature labor, and preterm birth. More than one-half of all twins and as many as 93 percent of triplets are born at less than 37 weeks of gestation.

- **Young or old maternal age.** Pregnancy in teens and women aged 35 or older increases the risk for preeclampsia and gestational high blood pressure.

Women with high-risk pregnancies should receive care from a special team of health-care providers to ensure the best possible outcomes.[1]

WHAT ARE SOME FACTORS THAT MAKE A PREGNANCY HIGH RISK?

Several factors can make a pregnancy high risk, including existing health conditions, the mother's age, lifestyle, and health issues that happen before or during pregnancy.

This chapter provides some possible factors that could create a high-risk pregnancy situation. This list is not meant to be all-inclusive, and each pregnancy is different, so the specific risks for one pregnancy may not be risks for another. Women who have any questions about their pregnancy should talk to a health-care provider.

Existing Health Conditions

- **High blood pressure.** Even though high blood pressure can be risky for the mother and fetus, most women with slightly high blood pressure and no other diseases have healthy pregnancies and healthy deliveries because they get their blood pressure under control before pregnancy. Uncontrolled high blood pressure, however, can damage the mother's kidneys and increase the risk for low birth weight or preeclampsia. It is very important for women to have their blood pressure checked at every prenatal visit so that health-care providers can detect any changes and make decisions about treatment.
- **Polycystic ovary syndrome (PCOS).** Women with PCOS have higher rates of pregnancy loss before 20 weeks

[1] "What Is a High-Risk Pregnancy?" *Eunice Kennedy Shriver* National Institute of Child Health and Human Development (NICHD), January 31, 2017. Available online. URL: www.nichd.nih.gov/health/topics/pregnancy/conditioninfo/high-risk. Accessed May 17, 2023.

of pregnancy, diabetes during pregnancy (gestational diabetes), preeclampsia, and cesarean section.

- **Diabetes**. It is important for women with diabetes to manage their blood sugar levels both before getting pregnant and throughout pregnancy. During the first few weeks of pregnancy, often before a woman even knows she is pregnant, high blood sugar levels can cause birth defects. Even women whose diabetes is well under control may have changes in their metabolism during pregnancy that require extra care or treatment to promote a healthy birth. Babies of mothers with diabetes tend to be large and are likely to have low blood sugar soon after birth. That is another reason for women with diabetes to keep tight control of their blood sugar.

- **Kidney disease**. Women with mild kidney disease often have healthy pregnancies. But kidney disease can cause difficulties getting and staying pregnant as well as problems during pregnancy, including preterm delivery, low birth weight, and preeclampsia. Nearly one-fifth of women who develop preeclampsia early in pregnancy are found to have undiagnosed kidney disease. Pregnant women with kidney disease require additional treatments, changes in diet and medication, and frequent visits to their health-care provider.

- **Autoimmune disease**. Conditions such as lupus and multiple sclerosis can increase a woman's risk for problems during pregnancy and delivery. For example, women with lupus are at increased risk for preterm birth and stillbirth. Some women may find that their symptoms improve during pregnancy, while others have flare-ups and other challenges. Certain medicines to treat autoimmune diseases may be harmful to the fetus, meaning a woman with an autoimmune disease will need to work closely with a health-care provider throughout pregnancy.

- **Thyroid disease**. The thyroid is a small gland in the neck that makes hormones that help control heart rate and blood pressure. Uncontrolled thyroid disease, such as an overactive or underactive thyroid, can cause problems for the fetus, such as heart failure, poor weight gain, and brain development problems. Thyroid problems are usually treatable with medicine or surgery. However, the NICHD-supported study found that treating mildly low thyroid function during pregnancy did not improve outcomes for mothers or their babies.

- **Obesity.** Being obese before pregnancy is associated with a number of risks for poor pregnancy outcomes. For example, obesity increases a woman's chance of developing diabetes during pregnancy, which can contribute to difficult births. Obesity can also cause a fetus to be larger than normal, making the birth process more difficult. The NICHD research also found that obesity increases the risk for sleep apnea and disordered sleep breathing during pregnancy. Obesity before pregnancy is associated with an increased risk of structural problems with the baby's heart. There can also be problems if overweight or obese women gain too much weight during pregnancy. The NICHD research has shown that an integrated approach can help obese women limit their weight gain during pregnancy, leading to better pregnancy outcomes. The Institute of Medicine (IOM) recommends that overweight women gain no more than 15–25 pounds during pregnancy and that women with obesity gain no more than 11–20 pounds.

- **HIV/Acquired immunodeficiency syndrome (AIDS).** HIV can pass to a fetus during pregnancy, labor and delivery, and breastfeeding. Fortunately, there are effective treatments that can reduce and prevent the spread of HIV from the mother to the fetus or child. Medications for the mother and for the infant, as well as surgical delivery of the baby before the "water breaks" and feeding formula instead of breastfeeding, can prevent mother-to-child transmission and have led to a dramatic decrease in transmission—to less than 1 percent in the United States and other developed countries.

- **Zika infection.** Although scientists and health-care providers have known about Zika for decades, the link between Zika infection during pregnancy and pregnancy risks and birth defects has only recently come to light. The NICHD-supported research has shown that infants born to mothers who were infected with Zika just before and during pregnancy were at higher risk for different problems with the brain and nervous system. The most noticeable condition is microcephaly, a condition in which the head is smaller than normal. Zika infection during pregnancy can also increase the woman's risk for pregnancy loss and stillbirth. Researchers are still just learning the possible mechanisms of Zika's effects on pregnancy.

Age

- **Young age.** Pregnant teens are more likely to develop pregnancy-related high blood pressure and anemia (lack of healthy red blood cells) and to go through preterm (early) labor and delivery than women who are older. Teens are also more likely to not know they have a sexually transmitted infection (STI). Some STIs can cause problems with the pregnancy or for the baby. Teens may be less likely to get prenatal care or to keep prenatal appointments. Prenatal care is important because it allows a health-care provider to evaluate, identify, and treat risks, such as counseling teens not to take certain medications during pregnancy, sometimes before these risks become problems.
- **First-time pregnancy after age 35.** Most older first-time mothers have normal pregnancies, but research shows that older women are at higher risk for certain problems than younger women, including the following:
  - pregnancy-related high blood pressure (called "gestational hypertension") and diabetes (called "gestational diabetes")
  - pregnancy loss

- ectopic pregnancy (when the embryo attaches itself outside the uterus), a condition that can be life-threatening
- cesarean (surgical) delivery
- delivery complications, such as excessive bleeding
- prolonged labor (lasting more than 20 hours)
- labor that does not advance
- genetic disorders, such as Down syndrome, in the baby

Lifestyle Factors

- **Alcohol use.** Drinking alcohol during pregnancy can increase the baby's risk for fetal alcohol spectrum disorders (FASDs), sudden infant death syndrome (SIDS), and other problems. The FASDs are a variety of effects on the fetus that result from the mother's use of alcohol during pregnancy. The effects range from mild to severe, and they include intellectual and developmental disabilities, behavior problems, abnormal facial features, and disorders of the heart, kidneys, bones, and hearing. The FASDs are completely preventable: If a woman does not drink alcohol while she is pregnant, her child will not have an FASD.

  Women who drink are also more likely to have a miscarriage or stillbirth. The research shows that there is no safe amount of alcohol to drink while pregnant. According to one study supported by the National Institutes of Health (NIH), infants can suffer long-term developmental problems even with low levels of prenatal alcohol exposure.

- **Tobacco use.** Smoking during pregnancy puts the fetus at risk for preterm birth, certain birth defects, and SIDS. One study showed that smoking doubled or even tripled the risk of stillbirth or fetal death after 20 weeks of pregnancy. Research has also found that smoking during pregnancy leads to changes in an infant's immune system. Secondhand smoke also puts a woman and her developing fetus at increased risk for health problems.

- **Drug use**. Research shows that smoking marijuana and taking drugs during pregnancy can also harm the fetus and affect infant health. One study showed that smoking marijuana and using illegal drugs doubled the risk of stillbirth. Research also shows that smoking marijuana during pregnancy can interfere with normal brain development in the fetus, possibly causing long-term problems.

Conditions of Pregnancy

- **Multiple gestation**. Pregnancy with twins, triplets, or more fetuses, called "multiple gestation," increases the risk of infants being born prematurely (before 37 weeks of pregnancy). Both giving birth after age 30 and taking fertility drugs have been linked with multiple births. Having three or more infants increases the chance that a woman will need to have the infants delivered by cesarean section. Twins and triplets are more likely to be smaller for their size than single infants. If infants are born prematurely, they are more likely to have difficulty breathing.
- **Gestational diabetes**. Gestational diabetes occurs when a woman who did not have diabetes before develops diabetes when she is pregnant. Gestational diabetes can cause problems for both the mother and the fetus, including preterm labor and delivery and high blood pressure. It also increases the risk that a woman and her baby will develop type 2 diabetes later in life. Many women with gestational diabetes have healthy pregnancies because they work with a health-care provider to manage their condition.
- **Preeclampsia and eclampsia**. Preeclampsia is a sudden increase in a pregnant woman's blood pressure after the 20th week of pregnancy. It can affect the mother's kidneys, liver, and brain. The condition can be fatal for both the mother and the fetus or cause long-term health problems. Eclampsia is a more severe form of preeclampsia that includes seizures and possibly coma.

- **Previous preterm birth.** Women who went into labor or who had their baby early (before 37 weeks of pregnancy) with a previous pregnancy are at higher risk for preterm labor and birth with their current pregnancy. Health-care providers will want to monitor women at high risk for preterm labor and birth in case treatment is needed. The NICHD research has shown that among women at high risk for preterm labor and birth because of a previous preterm birth, giving progesterone can help delay birth. In addition, women who become pregnant within 12 months after their latest delivery may be at increased risk for preterm birth. Women who have recently given birth may want to talk with a health-care provider about contraception to help delay the next pregnancy.

- **Birth defects or genetic conditions in the fetus.** In some cases, health-care providers can detect health problems in the fetus during pregnancy. Depending on the nature of the problems, the pregnancy may be considered high risk because treatments are needed while the fetus is still in the womb or immediately after birth. For example, if certain forms of spina bifida are detected in the fetus, the problems can be repaired before birth. Certain heart problems that are common among infants with Down syndrome need to be corrected with surgery immediately after birth. Knowing a fetus has Down syndrome before birth can help health-care providers and parents be prepared to give treatment right away.[2]

[2] "What Are Some Factors That Make a Pregnancy High Risk?" *Eunice Kennedy Shriver* National Institute of Child Health and Human Development (NICHD), November 6, 2018. Available online. URL: www.nichd.nih.gov/health/topics/high-risk/conditioninfo/factors. Accessed May 17, 2023.

Chapter 30 | Common Risky Pregnancies

Section 30.1 | Teen Pregnancy

Most teenage girls do not plan to get pregnant, but many do. Teen pregnancies carry extra health risks to both the mother and the baby. Often, teens do not get prenatal care soon enough, which can lead to problems later on. They have a higher risk for pregnancy-related high blood pressure and its complications. Risks for the baby include premature birth and low birth weight.

If you are a pregnant teen, you can help yourself and your baby by:

- getting regular prenatal care
- taking your prenatal vitamins for your health and to prevent some birth defects
- avoiding smoking, alcohol, and drugs
- using a condom, if you are having sex, to prevent sexually transmitted diseases (STDs) that could hurt your baby (If your or your partner is allergic to latex, you can use polyurethane condoms.)[1]

THE ADVERSE EFFECTS OF TEEN PREGNANCY

The high social and economic costs of teen pregnancy and child-bearing can have short- and long-term negative consequences for teen parents, their children, and their community. Through recent research, it has been recognized that pregnancy and childbirth have a significant impact on the educational outcomes of teen parents.

- By age 22, only around 50 percent of teen mothers have received a high school diploma, and only 30 percent have earned a General Education Development (GED) certificate, whereas 90 percent of women who did not give birth during adolescence receive a high school diploma.
- Only about 10 percent of teen mothers complete a two- or four-year college program.

---

[1] MedlinePlus, "Teenage Pregnancy," National Institutes of Health (NIH), April 30, 2018. Available online. URL: https://medlineplus.gov/teenagepregnancy.html. Accessed May 17, 2023.

- Teen fathers have a 25–30 percent lower probability of graduating from high school than teenage boys who are not fathers.

Children who are born to teen mothers also experience a wide range of problems. For example, they are more likely to:
- have a higher risk for low birth weight and infant mortality
- have lower levels of emotional support and cognitive stimulation
- have fewer skills and be less prepared to learn when they enter kindergarten
- have behavioral problems and chronic medical conditions
- rely more heavily on publicly funded health care
- have higher rates of foster care placement
- be incarcerated at some time during adolescence
- have lower school achievement and drop out of high school
- give birth as a teen
- be unemployed or underemployed as a young adult

These immediate and long-lasting effects continue for teen parents and their children even after adjusting for the factors that increased the teen's risk for pregnancy—for example, growing up in poverty, having parents with low levels of education, growing up in a single-parent family, and having low attachment to and performance in school.

Teen pregnancy costs U.S. taxpayers about $11 billion per year due to increased health care and foster care, increased incarceration rates among children of teen parents, and lost tax revenue because of lower educational attainment and income among teen mothers. Some recent cost studies estimate that the cost may be as high as $28 billion per year or an average of $5,500 for each teen parent. The majority of this cost is associated with teens who give birth before the age of 18.[2]

---

[2] "The Adverse Effects of Teen Pregnancy," Youth.gov, October 17, 2012. Available online. URL: https://youth.gov/youth-topics/pregnancy-prevention/adverse-effects-teen-pregnancy. Accessed May 17, 2023.

Section 30.2 | Multiple Pregnancy: Twins, Triplets, and Beyond

If you are pregnant with more than one baby, you are far from alone. In the past two decades, the number of multiple births has climbed way up in the United States.

INFORMATION ABOUT MULTIPLES

In 2005, 133,122 twin babies and 6,208 triplet babies were born in the United States. In 1980, there were only 69,339 twin and 1,337 triplet births.

What is the reason for this increase? For one, more women are having babies after the age of 30. Women in their 30s are more likely than younger women to conceive more than one baby naturally. Another reason is that more women are using fertility treatments to help them conceive.

HOW TWINS ARE FORMED?

Twins form (refer to Figure 30.1) in one of the following two ways:

- **Identical twins**. These twins occur when a single fertilized egg splits into two. Identical twins look almost exactly alike and share the exact same genes. Most identical twins happen by chance.
- **Fraternal twins**. These twins form when two separate eggs are fertilized by two separate sperm. Fraternal twins do not share the exact same genes—they are no more alike than they are to their siblings from different pregnancies. Fraternal twins tend to run in some families.

Multiple births can be fraternal, identical, or a combination. Multiples associated with fertility treatments are mainly fraternal.

PREGNANCY WITH MULTIPLES

Years ago, most twins came as a surprise. Now, thanks to advances in prenatal care, most women learn about a multiple pregnancy

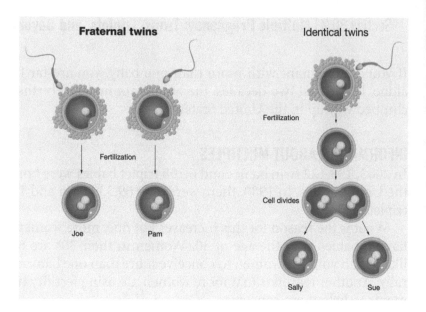

Figure 30.1. Identical Twins and Fraternal Twins

National Human Genome Research Institute (NHGRI)

early. You might suspect you are pregnant with multiples if you have more severe body changes, including the following:

- rapid weight gain in the first trimester
- intense nausea and vomiting
- extreme breast tenderness

Your doctor can confirm whether you are carrying more than one baby through ultrasound. If you are pregnant with twins or other multiples, you will need to see your doctor more often than women who are carrying only one baby because your risk of complications is greater. Women carrying more than one baby are at higher risk of:

- preterm birth
- low birth weight
- preeclampsia
- gestational diabetes
- cesarean birth

Common Risky Pregnancies

More frequent prenatal visits help your doctor monitor the health of you and your babies. Your doctor will also tell you how much weight to gain, if you need to take extra vitamins, and how much activity is safe. With close monitoring, your babies will have the best chance of being born near term and at a healthy weight.

After delivery and once your babies come home, you may feel overwhelmed and exhausted. Ask for help from your partner, family, and friends. Volunteer help and support groups for parents of multiples can also ease the transition.[3]

---

[3] Office on Women's Health (OWH), "Twins, Triplets, and Other Multiples," U.S. Department of Health and Human Services (HHS), February 22, 2021. Available online. URL: www.womenshealth.gov/pregnancy/youre-pregnant-now-what/twins-triplets-and-other-multiples. Accessed May 17, 2023.

Chapter 31 | Asthma and Pregnancy

WHAT IS ASTHMA?

Asthma is a chronic lung disease that affects the bronchial tubes. Your bronchial tubes carry air into and out of your lungs. When you breathe, your lungs take in oxygen. The oxygen travels through your bloodstream to all parts of your body.

In people who have asthma, the lungs and walls of the bronchial tubes become inflamed and oversensitive. When people with asthma breathe in "asthma triggers," such as smoke, air pollution, cold air, mold, or chemicals, the bronchial tubes tighten in response. This limits airflow and makes it difficult to breathe. Asthma triggers may be different for each person and may change over time.

WHO GETS ASTHMA?

Before age 15, asthma affects more boys than girls. After age 15, asthma is more common among girls and women than among boys and men.

Researchers believe the hormones estrogen and progesterone might affect women's airways. Changing hormone levels throughout the menstrual cycle and during pregnancy and menopause may affect airways in women with asthma.

Some women are more at risk for asthma:

- **African American and Puerto Rican women**. Asthma is more likely to affect African American and Puerto Rican women than women of other racial and ethnic groups.

- **Women who live in cities, especially in low-income areas**. Air pollution, indoor allergens (such as cockroaches), and tobacco smoke are more common in urban, low-income areas.

WHAT ARE THE SYMPTOMS OF ASTHMA?

Asthma symptoms include the following:
- wheezing
- coughing
- shortness of breath
- chest tightness

You may have only one or two of these symptoms, or you may get all of them. You may also get asthma symptoms only at night or in cold weather. Or you may get asthma symptoms after exposure to an allergen or other trigger or when you have a cold or are exercising.

HOW IS ASTHMA DIAGNOSED?

Many people develop asthma during childhood, but asthma can happen at any age. Asthma can be difficult to diagnose. Asthma symptoms can be similar to those of other conditions, such as chronic obstructive pulmonary disease (COPD), pneumonia, bronchitis, anxiety disorders, and heart disease.

To diagnose asthma, your doctor or nurse may:
- ask about your symptoms and what seems to trigger them
- ask about your health history
- do a physical exam
- ask about your daily habits
- ask what types of allergens or irritants might be in your workplace or home that could trigger your asthma symptoms

Your doctor or nurse may also do tests, including the following:
- **Spirometry**. A machine called a "spirometer" measures how much air you can breathe. It also

measures how fast you can blow air out. Your doctor or nurse may give you medicines and then retest you to see if the results are better after you take the medicines.

- **Bronchoprovocation**. Your doctor or nurse tests your lung function using spirometry. During the test, you will put stress on your lungs by exercising or breathing in increasing doses of a special chemical or cold air.

Your doctor or nurse may want to test for other problems that might be causing your symptoms. These include sleep apnea, vocal cord problems, or stomach acid backing up into the throat.

HOW IS ASTHMA TREATED?

Asthma is a chronic disease. This means that it can be treated but not cured. However, some people are able to manage asthma so that symptoms do not happen again or rarely happen.

You can control asthma and prevent problems by:

- working with your doctor or nurse to set up and follow a personal asthma action plan
- taking medicines as your doctor or nurse prescribes them for you
- staying away from your asthma triggers
- getting a flu shot (The flu can be very dangerous for women with asthma. Find a clinic near you where you can get the flu shot.)

WHAT IS AN ASTHMA ACTION PLAN?

Your doctor or nurse will work with you to come up with an action plan for treating your asthma. The action plan includes the following:

- what medicines to take
- when to take your medicines
- how to monitor your asthma, such as with a special tool called a "peak flow meter," which measures how well air is flowing out of your lungs

309

- ways to stay away from asthma triggers
- when to call your doctor or nurse or go to the emergency room

WHAT TYPES OF MEDICINES TREAT ASTHMA?

Asthma medicines work by opening the lung airways or by reducing the inflammation in the lungs. Some asthma medicines are pills, but most come from an inhaler (you breathe the medicine in). Asthma medicines fall into the following two groups:

- **Long-term control medicines.** These medicines help you have fewer and less severe asthma attacks. But they do not work to stop an asthma attack that has already started. You take long-term control medicines every day to relieve inflammation and help open the airways. Common types of long-term control medicines include inhaled corticosteroids and long-acting beta agonists. Inhaled corticosteroids help reduce inflammation in the lungs so that you are less likely to have an asthma attack. They will probably be the first type of long-term asthma control medicine your doctor will give you. If your asthma is not controlled with an inhaled corticosteroid, the U.S. Food and Drug Administration (FDA) approves adding a long-acting beta agonist to your long-term control treatment. Beta agonists help open your airways, but you should only use long-acting beta agonists alongside an inhaled corticosteroid.
- **Quick-relief or "rescue" medicines.** These medicines help stop attacks once they start. Quick-relief medicines include short-acting inhaled beta agonists such as albuterol. Quick-relief medicines usually make your symptoms go away within minutes. They do this by quickly relaxing tightened muscles around the airways.

ARE COMPLEMENTARY OR ALTERNATIVE THERAPIES SAFE TO TREAT ASTHMA?

Research has not shown complementary (add-on) or alternative treatments to stop an asthma attack or prevent asthma symptoms.

More research is needed about whether complementary or alternative therapies work or are safe for asthma treatment.

WHAT ARE COMMON ASTHMA TRIGGERS?

Many different things can trigger an asthma attack. And what triggers one person's asthma may not trigger another person's asthma. Common asthma triggers include the following:

- tobacco smoke
- animal urine, saliva, and dander (dead skin that comes from pets such as cats and dogs)
- dust mites
- cockroaches
- air pollution
- mold
- pollens and other allergens in the air (such as from trees and grass)
- fragrances (including personal care products such as lotions or household products such as candles that have fragrance added)
- physical activity (called "exercise-induced asthma")
- cold air
- wood smoke
- preservatives in alcohol called "sulfites"
- certain chemicals in cleaning products or other types of chemicals you might use at work or at home

HOW CAN YOU PREVENT AN ASTHMA ATTACK?

You can take medicines to help prevent and stop asthma attacks. You can also help prevent attacks by staying away from asthma triggers and following these steps:

- **Monitor the air quality and pollen counts**. If you have asthma, get updates on the air quality index and pollen count in your local area. Air quality tells you how much pollution will be in the air based on the weather. Pollen levels are higher during certain times of the year when different types of plants release pollen into the air.

- Tune in to news media and weather reports on television, the radio, or online for air quality and pollen counts.
- Sign up to get a text message, email, or notification when the air quality is bad in your community.
- Download a free app for your phone that tells you what the pollen count is in your community. Use the keywords such as "pollen" or "asthma" in your app store to find the right app.
- **Stay inside when pollen is high or air quality is bad.** If you have asthma, you are probably more sensitive to bad air quality and high pollen counts. Bad air quality or pollen may trigger asthma symptoms or an asthma attack. Try not to work or play hard outside when pollen or air pollution levels are high.
- **Use air conditioning.** If you have air conditioning, use it when outdoor asthma triggers (pollution or pollen) are high or to keep the humidity lower in your home. If mold triggers your asthma, using a dehumidifier to keep the humidity level low (between 30 and 50% humidity) in your home can help prevent symptoms.
- **Ask your doctor about taking medicine right before you exercise.** This may help you prevent asthma symptoms. Fatigue, wheezing, and coughing brought on by exercise can be signs of asthma that is not controlled. Talk to your doctor or nurse about your symptoms. You may need to adjust your medicine.
- **Do not use household products with chemical irritants.** Some cleaners, paints, pesticides, or air fresheners can trigger asthma symptoms. Try "fragrance-free" products if fragrances trigger your asthma.
- **Keep cockroaches away.** Clean up food spills and clutter right away. Seal cracks that cockroaches and other pests can get through. Keep all food in airtight containers. Use traps or bait, not sprays, to kill cockroaches.
- **Vacuum once a week.** If you can, use a vacuum with a high-efficiency particulate air (HEPA) filter. Leave the

room and have someone without asthma vacuum rugs, upholstered furniture, and curtains. Dust with a damp cloth to trap dust mites.

- **Stay away from pet dander.** If pet dander triggers asthma, keep your pet out of your bedroom and regularly vacuum areas where they spend time.
- **Do not smoke.** Do not allow anyone to smoke inside your home or car.
- **Use the exhaust fan when cooking.** The exhaust fan helps move away dangerous gases created by burning wood, natural gas, and kerosene.
- **Wash off allergens or pollutants.** Shower after going outside so that you wash off any allergens or pollution. Wash bedding in hot water regularly to kill dust mites.

HOW DOES ASTHMA AFFECT WOMEN?

Studies show that asthma may affect women differently compared with men.

- Women may experience more asthma symptoms than men. Women with asthma go to the hospital for asthma treatment more often and use more quick-relief or "rescue" medicines than men with asthma.
- Women with asthma have more trouble sleeping and more anxiety than men with asthma.
- Women's lungs are smaller than men's. This may make women more sensitive to asthma triggers and make it harder for women to breathe during an asthma attack.

HOW DOES ASTHMA AFFECT PREGNANCY?

Many women who have asthma do not have any problems during pregnancy. But asthma can cause problems for you and your baby during pregnancy because of changing hormone levels. Your unborn baby depends on the air you breathe in for oxygen. Asthma attacks during pregnancy can prevent your unborn baby from getting enough oxygen.

Pregnant women with asthma have a higher risk for:

- preeclampsia
- gestational diabetes
- problems with the placenta, including placental abruption
- premature birth (babies born before 37 weeks of pregnancy)
- low birth weight baby (less than 5½ pounds)
- cesarean section (C-section)
- serious bleeding after childbirth (called "postpartum hemorrhage")

Pregnancy may also make asthma symptoms seem worse due to acid reflux or heartburn. If you have asthma and are thinking about becoming pregnant, talk to your doctor or nurse. Having your asthma under control before you get pregnant can help prevent problems during pregnancy.

IS ASTHMA MEDICINE SAFE TO TAKE DURING PREGNANCY?

Some asthma medicines may be safe to take during pregnancy. Talk to your doctor or nurse about whether it is safe to continue taking your medicine during pregnancy.

Your doctor or nurse may suggest a different medicine to take. Do not stop taking your medicine or change your medicine without talking to your doctor or nurse first. Not using the medicine that you need may be more harmful to you and your baby than using the medicine. Untreated asthma can cause serious problems during pregnancy.

Also, talk with your doctor or nurse about getting a flu shot. The flu can be very dangerous for women with asthma, especially during pregnancy when your immune system is different from normal.[1]

---

[1] Office on Women's Health (OWH), "Asthma," U.S. Department of Health and Human Services (HHS), May 31, 2022. Available online. URL: www.womenshealth.gov/a-z-topics/asthma. Accessed May 17, 2023.

Chapter 32 | Cancer and Pregnancy

Chapter Contents

Section 32.1 | Breast Cancer and Pregnancy

WHAT IS BREAST CANCER?

Breast cancer is a disease in which malignant (cancer) cells form in the tissues of the breast. The breast is made up of lobes and ducts. Each breast has 15–20 sections called "lobes." Each lobe has many smaller sections called "lobules." Lobules end in dozens of tiny bulbs that can make milk. The lobes, lobules, and bulbs are linked by thin tubes called "ducts."

Each breast also has blood vessels and lymph vessels. The lymph vessels carry an almost colorless, watery fluid called "lymph." Lymph vessels carry lymph between lymph nodes. Lymph nodes are small, bean-shaped structures found throughout the body. They filter lymph and store white blood cells that help fight infection and disease. Groups of lymph nodes are found near the breast in the axilla (under the arm), above the collarbone, and in the chest.

Sometimes, breast cancer occurs in women who are pregnant or have just given birth. Breast cancer occurs about once in every 3,000 pregnancies. It occurs most often in women aged 32–38 years. Because many women are choosing to delay having children, it is likely that the number of new cases of breast cancer during pregnancy will increase.

SIGNS OF BREAST CANCER

The following are a few signs that may be caused by breast cancer. Check with your doctor if you have any of the following:

- a lump or thickening in or near the breast or in the underarm area
- a change in the size or shape of the breast
- a dimple or puckering in the skin of the breast
- a nipple turned inward into the breast
- fluid, other than breast milk, from the nipple, especially if it is bloody
- scaly, red, or swollen skin on the breast, nipple, or areola (the dark area of skin around the nipple)

317

- dimples in the breast that look like the skin of an orange, called "peau d'orange"

TESTS FOR BREAST CANCER

It may be difficult to detect (find) breast cancer early in pregnant or nursing women. The breasts usually get larger, tender, or lumpy in women who are pregnant, are nursing, or have just given birth. This occurs because of normal hormone changes that take place during pregnancy. These changes can make small lumps difficult to detect. The breasts may also become denser. It is more difficult to detect breast cancer in women with dense breasts using mammography. Because these breast changes can delay diagnosis, breast cancer is often found at a later stage in these women.

Breast exams should be part of prenatal and postnatal care. To detect breast cancer, pregnant and nursing women should examine their breasts themselves. Women should also receive clinical breast exams during their regular prenatal and postnatal checkups. Talk to your doctor if you notice any changes in your breasts that you do not expect or that worry you.

Tests that examine the breasts are used to diagnose breast cancer. The following tests and procedures may be used:

- **Physical exam and health history**. A physical exam of the body is to check general signs of health, including checking for signs of disease, such as lumps or anything else that seems unusual. A history of the patient's health habits and past illnesses and treatments will also be taken.
- **Clinical breast exam (CBE)**. CBE is an exam of the breast by a doctor or other health professional. The doctor will carefully feel the breasts and under the arms for lumps or anything else that seems unusual.
- **Ultrasound exam**. During this procedure, high-energy sound waves (ultrasound) are bounced off internal tissues or organs and make echoes. The echoes form a picture of body tissues called a "sonogram." The picture can be printed to look at later.

- **Mammogram.** This is an x-ray of the breast. A mammogram can be done with little risk to the fetus. Mammograms in pregnant women may appear negative even though cancer is present.
- **Biopsy.** The removal of cells or tissues for analysis is called biopsy, so they can be viewed under a microscope by a pathologist to check for signs of cancer. If a lump in the breast is found, a biopsy may be done.

The following are the three types of breast biopsies:
- **Excisional biopsy.** The removal of an entire lump of tissue.
- **Core biopsy.** The removal of tissue using a wide needle.
- **Fine-needle aspiration (FNA) biopsy.** The removal of tissue or fluid, using a thin needle.

If cancer is found, tests are done to study the cancer cells. Decisions about the best treatment are based on the results of these tests and the trimester of the pregnancy. The tests give information about:
- how quickly the cancer may grow
- how likely it is that the cancer will spread to other parts of the body
- how well certain treatments might work
- how likely the cancer is to recur (come back)

After breast cancer has been diagnosed, tests are done to find out if cancer cells have spread within the breast or to other parts of the body. The process used to find out if the cancer has spread within the breast or to other parts of the body is called "staging." The information gathered from the staging process determines the stage of the disease. It is important to know the stage in order to plan treatment.

Some procedures may expose the fetus to harmful radiation or dyes. These procedures are done only if absolutely necessary. Certain actions, such as using a lead-lined shield to cover the abdomen, are done to help protect the fetus from radiation as much as possible.

319

The following tests and procedures may be used to stage breast cancer during pregnancy:

- **Chest x-ray**. This is an x-ray of the organs and bones inside the chest. An x-ray is a type of energy beam that can go through the body and onto film, making a picture of areas inside the body.
- **Bone scan**. This scan is to check if there are rapidly dividing cells, such as cancer cells, in the bone. A very small amount of radioactive material is injected into a vein and travels through the bloodstream. The radioactive material collects in bones with cancer and is detected by a scanner.
- **Ultrasound exam**. During this procedure, high-energy sound waves (ultrasound) are bounced off internal tissues or organs, such as the liver, and make echoes. The echoes form a picture of body tissues called a "sonogram." The picture can be printed to be looked at later.
- **Magnetic resonance imaging (MRI)**. MRI is a procedure that uses a magnet, radio waves, and a computer to make a series of detailed pictures of areas inside the body, such as the brain. This procedure is also called "nuclear magnetic resonance imaging" (NMRI).

TREATMENT OPTIONS FOR BREAST CANCER

Treatment options for pregnant women depend on the stage of the disease and the trimester of the pregnancy. The following are the three types of standard treatment.

Surgery

Most pregnant women with breast cancer have surgery to remove the breast. Some of the lymph nodes under the arm may be removed, so they can be checked under a microscope by a pathologist for signs of cancer.

Types of surgery to remove the cancer include the following:

- **Modified radical mastectomy**. Surgery to remove the whole breast that has cancer. This may include the removal of the nipple, areola (the dark-colored skin around the nipple), and skin over the breast. Most of the lymph nodes under the arm are also removed.

- **Breast-conserving surgery.** Surgery to remove the cancer and some normal tissue around it, but not the breast itself. Part of the chest wall lining may also be removed if the cancer is near it. This type of surgery may also be called "lumpectomy," "partial mastectomy," "segmental mastectomy," "quadrantectomy," or "breast-sparing surgery."

After the doctor removes all of the cancer that can be seen at the time of surgery, some patients may be given chemotherapy or radiation therapy after surgery to kill any cancer cells that are left. For pregnant women with early-stage breast cancer, radiation therapy and hormone therapy are given after the baby is born. Treatment given after surgery to lower the risk that the cancer will come back is called "adjuvant therapy."

Radiation Therapy

Radiation therapy is a cancer treatment that uses high-energy x-rays or other types of radiation to kill cancer cells or keep them from growing. External radiation therapy uses a machine outside the body to send radiation toward the area of the body with cancer.

External radiation therapy may be given to pregnant women with early-stage (stage I or II) breast cancer after the baby is born. Women with late-stage (stage III or IV) breast cancer may be given external radiation therapy after the first three months of pregnancy, or if possible, radiation therapy is delayed until after the baby is born.

Chemotherapy

Chemotherapy is a cancer treatment that uses drugs to stop the growth of cancer cells, either by killing the cells or by stopping the cells from dividing. When chemotherapy is taken by mouth or injected into a vein or muscle, the drugs enter the bloodstream and can reach cancer cells throughout the body (systemic chemotherapy).

Chemotherapy is usually not given during the first three months of pregnancy. Chemotherapy given after this time does not usually harm the fetus but may cause early labor or low birth weight.

Ending the pregnancy does not seem to improve the mother's chance of survival. Because ending the pregnancy is not likely to improve the mother's chance of survival, it is not usually a treatment option. Treatment for breast cancer may cause side effects.

TREATMENT OPTIONS FOR BREAST CANCER DURING PREGNANCY
Early-Stage Breast Cancer
Pregnant women with early-stage breast cancer (stages I and II) are usually treated in the same way as patients who are not pregnant, with some changes to protect the fetus. Treatment may include the following:

- modified radical mastectomy, if the breast cancer was diagnosed early in pregnancy
- breast-conserving surgery, if the breast cancer is diagnosed later in pregnancy (Radiation therapy may be given after the baby is born.)
- modified radical mastectomy or breast-conserving surgery during pregnancy (After the first three months of pregnancy, certain types of chemotherapy may be given before or after surgery.)

Hormone therapy and trastuzumab should not be given during pregnancy.

Late-Stage Breast Cancer
There is no standard treatment for patients with late-stage breast cancer (stage III or IV) during pregnancy. Treatment may include the following:

- radiation therapy
- chemotherapy

Radiation therapy and chemotherapy should not be given during the first three months of pregnancy.

SPECIAL ISSUES ABOUT BREAST CANCER DURING PREGNANCY

Lactation (breast milk production) and breastfeeding should be stopped if surgery or chemotherapy is planned. If surgery is planned, breastfeeding should be stopped to reduce blood flow in the breasts and make them smaller. Many chemotherapy drugs, especially cyclophosphamide and methotrexate, may occur in high levels in breast milk and may harm the baby. Women receiving chemotherapy should not breastfeed. Stopping lactation does not improve the mother's prognosis. Breast cancer does not appear to harm the fetus. Breast cancer cells do not seem to pass from the mother to the fetus. Pregnancy does not seem to affect the survival of women who have had breast cancer in the past.

For women who have had breast cancer, pregnancy does not seem to affect their survival. However, some doctors recommend that a woman wait two years after treatment for breast cancer before trying to have a baby so that any early return of the cancer would be detected. This may affect a woman's decision to become pregnant.[1]

Section 32.2 | Gestational Trophoblastic Tumors

Gestational trophoblastic disease (GTD) is a group of rare diseases in which abnormal trophoblast cells grow inside the uterus after conception. In GTD, a tumor develops inside the uterus from tissue that forms after conception (the joining of the sperm and the egg). This tissue is made of trophoblast cells and normally surrounds the fertilized egg in the uterus. Trophoblast cells help connect the fertilized egg to the wall of the uterus and form part of the placenta (the organ that passes nutrients from the mother to the fetus).

Sometimes, there is a problem with the fertilized egg and trophoblast cells. Instead of a healthy fetus developing, a tumor forms. Until there are signs or symptoms of the tumor, the pregnancy will seem like a normal pregnancy.

---

[1] "Breast Cancer Treatment during Pregnancy (PDQ®)—Patient Version," National Cancer Institute (NCI), December 14, 2022. Available online. URL: www.cancer.gov/types/breast/patient/pregnancy-breast-treatment-pdq. Accessed May 18, 2023.

Most GTDs are benign (not cancer) and do not spread, but some types become malignant (cancer) and spread to nearby tissues or distant parts of the body. GTD is a general term that includes different types of disease:

- hydatidiform moles (HMs)
  - complete HM
  - partial HM
- gestational trophoblastic neoplasia (GTN)
  - invasive moles
  - choriocarcinomas
  - placental-site trophoblastic tumors (PSTTs; very rare)
  - epithelioid trophoblastic tumors (ETTs; even more rare)

HM is the most common type of GTD. HMs are slow-growing tumors that look like sacs of fluid. An HM is also called a "molar pregnancy." The cause of HMs is not known. HMs may be complete or partial:

- **Complete HMs.** A complete HM forms when sperm fertilizes an egg that does not contain the mother's deoxyribonucleic acid (DNA). The egg has DNA from the father, and the cells that were meant to become the placenta are abnormal.
- **Partial HMs.** A partial HM forms when sperm fertilizes a normal egg and there are two sets of DNA from the father in the fertilized egg. Only part of the fetus forms, and the cells that were meant to become the placenta are abnormal.

Most HMs are benign, but they sometimes become cancer. Having one or more of the following risk factors increases the risk that an HM will become cancer:

- a pregnancy before 20 or after 35 years of age
- a very high level of beta human chorionic gonadotropin (beta-hCG), a hormone made by the body during pregnancy

- a large tumor in the uterus
- an ovarian cyst larger than 6 cm
- high blood pressure during pregnancy
- an overactive thyroid gland (extra thyroid hormone is made)
- severe nausea and vomiting during pregnancy
- trophoblastic cells in the blood, which may block small blood vessels
- serious blood clotting problems caused by the HM

GTN is a type of GTD that is almost always malignant. GTN includes the following:

- **Invasive moles**. Invasive moles are made up of trophoblast cells that grow into the muscle layer of the uterus. Invasive moles are more likely to grow and spread than an HM. Rarely, a complete or partial HM may become an invasive mole. Sometimes, an invasive mole will disappear without treatment.
- **Choriocarcinomas**. A choriocarcinoma is a malignant tumor that forms from trophoblast cells and spreads to the muscle layer of the uterus and nearby blood vessels. It may also spread to other parts of the body, such as the brain, lungs, liver, kidney, spleen, intestines, pelvis, or vagina. A choriocarcinoma is more likely to form in women who have had any of the following:
  - molar pregnancy, especially with a complete HM
  - normal pregnancy
  - tubal pregnancy (the fertilized egg implants in the fallopian tube rather than the uterus)
  - miscarriage
- **Placental-site trophoblastic tumors**. A PSTT is a rare type of GTN that forms where the placenta attaches to the uterus. The tumor forms from trophoblast cells and spreads into the muscle of the uterus and into blood vessels. It may also spread to the lungs, pelvis, or lymph nodes. A PSTT grows very slowly, and signs or symptoms may appear months or years after a normal pregnancy.

- **Epithelioid trophoblastic tumors**. An ETT is a very rare type of GTN that may be benign or malignant. When the tumor is malignant, it may spread to the lungs.

Age and a previous molar pregnancy affect the risk of GTD. Anything that increases your risk of getting a disease is called a "risk factor." Having a risk factor does not mean that you will get cancer; not having risk factors does not mean that you will not get cancer. Talk to your doctor if you think you may be at risk. Risk factors for GTD include the following:
- being pregnant when you are younger than 20 or older than 35 years of age
- having a personal history of HM

SIGNS OF GESTATIONAL TROPHOBLASTIC DISEASE

Signs of GTD include abnormal vaginal bleeding and a uterus that is larger than normal. These and other signs and symptoms may be caused by GTD or by other conditions. Check with your doctor if you have any of the following:
- vaginal bleeding not related to menstruation
- a uterus that is larger than expected during pregnancy
- pain or pressure in the pelvis
- severe nausea and vomiting during pregnancy
- high blood pressure with headache and swelling of feet and hands early in the pregnancy
- vaginal bleeding that continues for longer than normal after delivery
- fatigue, shortness of breath, dizziness, and a fast or irregular heartbeat caused by anemia

GTD sometimes causes an overactive thyroid. Signs and symptoms of an overactive thyroid include the following:
- fast or irregular heartbeat
- shakiness
- sweating
- frequent bowel movements

- trouble sleeping
- feeling anxious or irritable
- weight loss

TESTS FOR GESTATIONAL TROPHOBLASTIC DISEASE

The following tests and procedures may be used:

- **Physical exam and history.** A physical exam of the body is to check general signs of health, including checking for signs of disease, such as lumps or anything else that seems unusual. A history of the patient's health habits and past illnesses and treatments will also be taken.
- **Pelvic exam.** This includes exam of the vagina, cervix, uterus, fallopian tubes, ovaries, and rectum. A speculum is inserted into the vagina, and the doctor or nurse looks at the vagina and cervix for signs of disease. A Pap test of the cervix is usually done. The doctor or nurse also inserts one or two lubricated, gloved fingers of one hand into the vagina and places the other hand over the lower abdomen to feel the size, shape, and position of the uterus and ovaries. The doctor or nurse also inserts a lubricated, gloved finger into the rectum to feel for lumps or abnormal areas.
- **Ultrasound exam of the pelvis.** In this procedure, high-energy sound waves (ultrasound) are bounced off internal tissues or organs in the pelvis and make echoes. The echoes form a picture of body tissues called a "sonogram." Sometimes, a transvaginal ultrasound (TVUS) will be done. For TVUS, an ultrasound transducer (probe) is inserted into the vagina to make the sonogram.
- **Blood chemistry studies.** In this procedure, a blood sample is checked to measure the amounts of certain substances released into the blood by organs and tissues in the body. An unusual (higher or lower than normal) amount of a substance can be a sign of disease. Blood is also tested to check the liver, kidney, and bone marrow.

- **Serum tumor marker test**. In this test, a sample of blood is checked to measure the amounts of certain substances made by organs, tissues, or tumor cells in the body. Certain substances are linked to specific types of cancer when found in increased levels in the body. These are called "tumor markers." For GTD, the blood is checked for the level of beta-hCG, a hormone that is made by the body during pregnancy. Beta-hCG in the blood of a woman who is not pregnant may be a sign of GTD.
- **Urinalysis**. This is a test to check the color of urine and its contents, such as sugar, protein, blood, bacteria, and the level of beta-hCG.

PROGNOSIS AND TREATMENT OPTIONS FOR GESTATIONAL TROPHOBLASTIC DISEASE

Gestational trophoblastic disease can usually be cured. Treatment and prognosis depend on the following:

- the type of GTD
- whether the tumor has spread to the uterus, lymph nodes, or distant parts of the body
- the number of tumors and where they are in the body
- the size of the largest tumor
- the level of beta-hCG in the blood
- how soon the tumor was diagnosed after the pregnancy began
- whether GTD occurred after a molar pregnancy, miscarriage, or normal pregnancy
- previous treatment for GTN

Treatment options also depend on whether the woman wishes to become pregnant in the future. After GTN has been diagnosed, tests are done to find out if the cancer has spread from where it started to other parts of the body.

The process used to find out the extent or spread of cancer is called "staging." The information gathered from the staging process helps determine the stage of the disease. For GTN, its stage is one of the factors used to plan treatment. The following tests and procedures may be done to find out the stage of the disease:

- **Chest x-ray.** This is an x-ray of the organs and bones inside the chest. An x-ray is a type of energy beam that can go through the body onto film, making pictures of areas inside the body.
- **Computerized tomography (CT) scan/computerized axial tomography (CAT) scan.** CT or CAT is a procedure that makes a series of detailed pictures of areas inside the body taken from different angles. The pictures are made by a computer linked to an x-ray machine. A dye may be injected into a vein or swallowed to help the organs or tissues show up more clearly. This procedure is also called "computed tomography."
- **Magnetic resonance imaging (MRI) with gadolinium.** MRI is a procedure that uses a magnet, radio waves, and a computer to make a series of detailed pictures of areas inside the body, such as the brain and spinal cord. A substance called "gadolinium" is injected into a vein. The gadolinium collects around the cancer cells, so they show up brighter in the picture. This procedure is also called "nuclear magnetic resonance imaging" (NMRI).
- **Lumbar puncture.** In this procedure, cerebrospinal fluid (CSF) from the spinal column is collected. This is done by placing a needle between two bones in the spine and into the CSF around the spinal cord and removing a sample of the fluid. The sample of CSF is checked under a microscope for signs that cancer has spread to the brain and spinal cord. This procedure is also called an "LP" or "spinal tap."

TREATMENT FOR GESTATIONAL TROPHOBLASTIC DISEASE
Hydatidiform Moles

Treatment for an HM may include the following:

- surgery (dilatation and curettage with suction evacuation) to remove the tumor

After surgery, beta-hCG blood tests are done every week until the beta-hCG level returns to normal. Patients also have follow-up doctor visits monthly for up to six months. If the level of beta-hCG does not return to normal or increases, it may mean the HM was not completely removed, and it has become cancer. Pregnancy causes beta-hCG levels to increase, so your doctor will ask you not to become pregnant until the follow-up is finished.

For a disease that remains after surgery, treatment is usually chemotherapy.

Gestational Trophoblastic Neoplasia
LOW-RISK GESTATIONAL TROPHOBLASTIC NEOPLASIA

Treatment for low-risk GTN (invasive mole or choriocarcinoma) may include the following:

- chemotherapy with one or more anticancer drugs (Treatment is given until the beta-hCG level is normal for at least three weeks after treatment ends.)

If the level of beta-hCG in the blood does not return to normal or the tumor spreads to distant parts of the body, chemotherapy regimens used for high-risk metastatic GTN are given.

HIGH-RISK METASTATIC GESTATIONAL TROPHOBLASTIC NEOPLASIA

Treatment for high-risk metastatic GTN (invasive mole or choriocarcinoma) may include the following:

- combination chemotherapy
- intrathecal chemotherapy and radiation therapy to the brain (for cancer that has spread to the lung to keep it from spreading to the brain)

- high-dose chemotherapy or intrathecal chemotherapy and/or radiation therapy to the brain (for cancer that has spread to the brain)

PLACENTAL-SITE GESTATIONAL TROPHOBLASTIC TUMORS AND EPITHELIOID TROPHOBLASTIC TUMORS

Treatment for stage I placental-site gestational trophoblastic tumors and ETTs may include the following:
- surgery to remove the uterus

Treatment for stage II placental-site gestational trophoblastic tumors and ETTs may include the following:
- surgery to remove the tumor, which may be followed by combination chemotherapy

Treatment for stage III and IV placental-site gestational trophoblastic tumors and ETTs may include the following:
- combination chemotherapy
- surgery to remove cancer that has spread to other places, such as the lung or abdomen

Recurrent or Resistant Gestational Trophoblastic Neoplasia

Treatment for recurrent or resistant gestational trophoblastic tumors may include the following:
- chemotherapy with one or more anticancer drugs for tumors previously treated with surgery
- combination chemotherapy for tumors previously treated with chemotherapy
- surgery for tumors that do not respond to chemotherapy[2]

---

[2] "Gestational Trophoblastic Disease Treatment (PDQ®)—Patient Version," National Cancer Institute (NCI), February 25, 2022. Available online. URL: www.cancer.gov/types/gestational-trophoblastic/patient/gtd-treatment-pdq. Accessed May 18, 2023.

Chapter 33 | A Guide to Pregnancy for Women with Diabetes

If you have diabetes and plan to have a baby, you should try to get your blood glucose levels close to your target range before you get pregnant. Staying in your target range during pregnancy, which may be different from when you are not pregnant, is also important. High blood glucose, also called "blood sugar," can harm your baby during the first weeks of pregnancy, even before you know you are pregnant. If you have diabetes and are already pregnant, see your doctor as soon as possible to make a plan to manage your diabetes. Working with your health-care team and following your diabetes management plan can help you have a healthy pregnancy and a healthy baby. If you develop diabetes for the first time while you are pregnant, you have gestational diabetes.

HOW CAN DIABETES AFFECT YOUR BABY?
A baby's organs, such as the brain, heart, kidneys, and lungs, start forming during the first eight weeks of pregnancy. High blood glucose levels can be harmful during this early stage and can increase the chance that your baby will have birth defects, such as heart defects or defects of the brain or spine.

High blood glucose levels during pregnancy can also increase the chance that your baby will be born too early, weigh too much, or have breathing problems or low blood glucose right after birth.

High blood glucose can also increase the chance that you will have a miscarriage or a stillborn baby. Stillborn means the baby dies in the womb during the second half of pregnancy.

HOW CAN YOUR DIABETES AFFECT YOU DURING PREGNANCY?

Hormonal and other changes in your body during pregnancy affect your blood glucose levels, so you might need to change how you manage your diabetes. Even if you have had diabetes for years, you may need to change your meal plan, physical activity routine, and medicines. If you have been taking oral diabetes medicine, you may need to switch to insulin. As you get closer to your due date, your management plan might change again.

WHAT HEALTH PROBLEMS COULD YOU DEVELOP DURING PREGNANCY BECAUSE OF YOUR DIABETES?

Pregnancy can worsen certain long-term diabetes problems, such as eye problems and kidney disease, especially if your blood glucose levels are too high.

You also have a greater chance of developing preeclampsia, sometimes called "toxemia," which is when you develop high blood pressure and too much protein in your urine during the second half of pregnancy. Preeclampsia can cause serious or life-threatening problems for you and your baby. The only cure for preeclampsia is to give birth. If you have preeclampsia and have reached 37 weeks of pregnancy, your doctor may want to deliver your baby early. Before 37 weeks, you and your doctor may consider other options to help your baby develop as much as possible before he or she is born.

HOW CAN YOU PREPARE FOR PREGNANCY IF YOU HAVE DIABETES?

If you have diabetes, keeping your blood glucose as close to normal as possible before and during your pregnancy is important to stay healthy and have a healthy baby. Getting checkups before and during pregnancy, following your diabetes meal plan, being physically active as your health-care team advises, and taking diabetes medicines if you need to will help you manage your diabetes. Stopping smoking and taking vitamins, as your doctor advises, can also help you and your baby stay healthy.

Work with Your Health-Care Team

Regular visits with members of a health-care team who are experts in diabetes and pregnancy will ensure that you and your baby get the best care. Your health-care team may include:

- a medical doctor who specializes in diabetes care, such as an endocrinologist or a diabetologist
- an obstetrician with experience treating women with diabetes
- a diabetes educator who can help you manage your diabetes
- a nurse practitioner who provides prenatal care during your pregnancy
- a registered dietitian to help with meal planning
- specialists who diagnose and treat diabetes-related problems, such as vision problems, kidney disease, and heart disease
- a social worker or psychologist to help you cope with stress, worry, and the extra demands of pregnancy

You are the most important member of the team. Your health-care team can give you expert advice, but you are the one who must manage your diabetes every day.

Get a Checkup

Have a complete checkup before you get pregnant or as soon as you know you are pregnant. Your doctor should check for:

- high blood pressure
- eye disease
- heart and blood vessel disease
- nerve damage
- kidney disease
- thyroid disease

Pregnancy can make some diabetes health problems worse. To help prevent this, your health-care team may recommend adjusting your treatment before you get pregnant.

Do Not Smoke

Smoking can increase your chance of having a stillborn baby or a baby born too early. Smoking is especially harmful to people with diabetes. Smoking can increase diabetes-related health problems such as eye disease, heart disease, and kidney disease.

See a Registered Dietitian Nutritionist

If you do not already see a dietitian, you should start seeing one before you get pregnant. Your dietitian can help you learn what to eat, how much to eat, and when to eat to reach or stay at a healthy weight before you get pregnant. Together, you and your dietitian will create a meal plan to fit your needs, schedule, food preferences, medical conditions, medicines, and physical activity routine.

During pregnancy, some women need to make changes in their meal plan, such as adding extra calories, protein, and other nutrients. You will need to see your dietitian every few months during pregnancy as your dietary needs change.

Be Physically Active

Physical activity can help you reach your target blood glucose numbers. Being physically active can also help keep your blood pressure and cholesterol levels in a healthy range, relieve stress, strengthen your heart and bones, improve muscle strength, and keep your joints flexible.

Before getting pregnant, make physical activity a regular part of your life. Aim for 30 minutes of activity five days a week. Talk with your health-care team about what activities are best for you during your pregnancy.

HOW TO EAT BETTER AND BE MORE ACTIVE WHILE YOU ARE PREGNANT

Avoid Alcohol

You should avoid drinking alcoholic beverages while you are trying to get pregnant and throughout pregnancy. When you drink, the alcohol also affects your baby. Alcohol can lead to serious, lifelong health problems for your baby.

Adjust Your Medicines

Some medicines are not safe during pregnancy, and you should stop taking them before you get pregnant. Tell your doctor about all the medicines you take, such as those for high cholesterol and high blood pressure. Your doctor can tell you which medicines to stop taking and may prescribe a different medicine that is safe to use during pregnancy.

Doctors most often prescribe insulin for both type 1 and type 2 diabetes during pregnancy. If you are already taking insulin, you might need to change the kind, the amount, or how and when you take it. You may need less insulin during your first trimester but probably will need more as you go through pregnancy. Your insulin needs may double or even triple as you get closer to your due date. Your health-care team will work with you to create an insulin routine to meet your changing needs.

Take Vitamin and Mineral Supplements

Folic acid is an important vitamin for you to take before and during pregnancy to protect your baby's health. You will need to start taking folic acid at least one month before you get pregnant. You should take a multivitamin or supplement that contains at least 400 micrograms (mcg) of folic acid. Once you become pregnant, you should take 600 mcg daily. Ask your doctor if you should take other vitamins or minerals, such as iron or calcium supplements or a multivitamin.

WHAT DO YOU NEED TO KNOW ABOUT BLOOD GLUCOSE TESTING BEFORE AND DURING PREGNANCY?

How often you check your blood glucose levels may change during pregnancy. You may need to check them more often than you do now. If you did not need to check your blood glucose before pregnancy, you will probably need to start. Ask your health-care team how often and at what times you should check your blood glucose levels. Your blood glucose targets will change during pregnancy. Your health-care team may also want you to check your ketone levels if your blood glucose is too high.

Target Blood Glucose Levels before Pregnancy

When you are planning to become pregnant, your daily blood glucose targets may be different from your previous targets. Ask your health-care team which targets are right for you.

You can keep track of your blood glucose levels using My Daily Blood Glucose Record (www.niddk.nih.gov/-/media/Files/Diabetes/BloodGlucose_508.pdf). You can also use an electronic blood glucose tracking system on your computer or mobile device. Record the results every time you check your blood glucose. Your blood glucose records can help you and your health-care team decide whether your diabetes care plan is working. You can also make notes about your insulin and ketones. Take your tracker with you when you visit your health-care team.

Target Blood Glucose Levels during Pregnancy

Recommended daily target blood glucose numbers for most pregnant women with diabetes are:

- before meals, at bedtime, and overnight: 90 or less
- one hour after eating: 130–140 or less
- two hours after eating: 120 or less

Ask your doctor what targets are right for you. If you have type 1 diabetes, your targets may be higher, so you do not develop low blood glucose, also called "hypoglycemia."

A1C Numbers

Another way to see whether you are meeting your targets is to have an A1C blood test. Results of the A1C test reflect your average blood glucose levels during the past three months. Most women with diabetes should aim for an A1C as close to normal as possible—ideally below 6.5 percent—before getting pregnant. After the first three months of pregnancy, your target may be as low as 6 percent. These targets may be different from the A1C goals you have had in the past. Your doctor can help you set A1C targets that are best for you.

Ketone Levels

When your blood glucose is too high or if you are not eating enough, your body might make ketones. Ketones in your urine or blood mean your body is using fat for energy instead of glucose. Burning large amounts of fat instead of glucose can be harmful to your health and your baby's health.

You can prevent serious health problems by checking for ketones. Your doctor might recommend you test your urine or blood daily for ketones or when your blood glucose is above a certain level, such as 200. If you use an insulin pump, your doctor might advise you to test for ketones when your blood glucose level is higher than expected. Your health-care team can teach you how and when to test your urine or blood for ketones.

Talk with your doctor about what to do if you have ketones. Your doctor might suggest making changes in the amount of insulin you take or when you take it. Your doctor may also recommend a change in meals or snacks if you need to consume more carbohydrates.

WHAT TESTS MONITOR YOUR BABY'S HEALTH DURING PREGNANCY?

You will have tests throughout your pregnancy, such as blood tests and ultrasounds, to check your baby's health. Talk with your health-care team about what prenatal tests you will have and when you might have them.[1]

---

[1] "Pregnancy If You Have Diabetes," National Institute of Diabetes and Digestive and Kidney Diseases (NIDDK), January 15, 2017. Available online. URL: www.niddk.nih.gov/health-information/diabetes/diabetes-pregnancy. Accessed May 18, 2023.

Chapter 34 | Epilepsy and Pregnancy

WHAT ARE EPILEPSIES?

Epilepsies are chronic neurological disorders in which clusters of nerve cells, or neurons, in the brain sometimes signal abnormally and cause seizures. Neurons normally generate electrical and chemical signals that act on other neurons, glands, and muscles to produce human thoughts, feelings, and actions.

During a seizure, many neurons fire (signal) at the same time—as many as 500 times per second, much faster than normal. This surge of excessive electrical activity happening at the same time causes involuntary movements, sensations, emotions, and behaviors, and the temporary disturbance of normal neuronal activity may cause a loss of awareness.

Epilepsy can be considered a spectrum disorder because of its different causes, different seizure types, its ability to vary in severity and impact from person to person, and its range of coexisting conditions. There are also many different types of epilepsies, resulting from a variety of causes. The recent adoption of the term "epilepsies" underscores the diversity of types and causes:

- Some people may have convulsions (sudden onset of repetitive general contraction of muscles) and lose consciousness.
- Others may simply stop what they are doing, have a brief lapse of awareness, and stare into space for a short period.
- Some people have seizures very infrequently, while other people may experience hundreds of seizures each day.

In general, epilepsy is diagnosed after a person has had two or more unprovoked seizures separated by at least 24 hours. In contrast, a provoked seizure is one caused by a known precipitating factor such as high fever, nervous system infections, acute traumatic brain injury (TBI), or fluctuations in blood sugar or electrolyte levels.

About 2.3 million adults and more than 450,000 children and adolescents in the United States currently live with epilepsy. Each year, an estimated 150,000 people are diagnosed with epilepsy. In the United States alone, the annual costs associated with epilepsies are estimated to be $15.5 billion in direct medical expenses and lost or reduced earnings and productivity.

WHAT CAUSES EPILEPSIES?

Anyone can develop epilepsy. Epilepsy affects both males and females of all races, ethnic backgrounds, and ages. The epilepsies have many possible causes, but about half people living with epilepsy do not know the cause. In other cases, epilepsies are clearly linked to genetic factors, developmental brain abnormalities, infection, TBI, stroke, brain tumors, or other identifiable problems. Anything that disturbs the normal pattern of neuronal activity—from illness to brain damage to abnormal brain development—can lead to seizures.

The epilepsies may develop because of an abnormality in brain wiring, an imbalance of nerve signaling in the brain (in which some cells either over-excite or over-inhibit other brain cells from sending messages), or some combination of these factors. In some pediatric conditions, abnormal brain wiring causes other problems, such as intellectual impairment.

In other people, the brain's attempt to repair itself after a head injury, stroke, or other problem may inadvertently generate abnormal nerve connections that lead to epilepsy. Brain malformations and abnormalities in brain wiring that occur during brain development may also disturb neuronal activity and lead to epilepsy.

Genetics

Genetic mutations may play a key role in the development of certain epilepsies. Many types of epilepsy affect multiple blood-related family members, pointing to a strong inherited genetic component. In other cases, gene mutations may occur spontaneously and contribute to the development of epilepsy in people with no family history of the disorder (called "de novo mutations"). Overall, researchers estimate that hundreds of genes could play a role.

Several types of epilepsy have been linked to mutations in genes that provide instructions for ion channels, the "gates" that control the flow of ions in and out of cells to help regulate neuronal signaling. For example, most infants with Dravet syndrome, a type of epilepsy associated with seizures that begin before the age of one year, carry a mutation in the *SCN1A* gene that causes seizures by affecting sodium ion channels.

Genetic mutations have been linked to disorders known as "progressive myoclonic epilepsies," which are characterized by ultra-quick muscle contractions (myoclonus) and seizures over time. For example, Lafora disease, a severe, progressive form of myoclonic epilepsy that begins in childhood, has been linked to a gene that helps break down carbohydrates in brain cells.

Mutations in genes that control neuronal migration—a critical step in brain development—can lead to areas of misplaced or abnormally formed neurons, called "cortical dysplasia," in the brain that can cause neurons to misfire and lead to epilepsy.

Other genetic mutations may not cause epilepsy but may influence the disorder in other ways. For example, one study showed that many people with certain forms of epilepsy have an abnormally active version of a gene that results in resistance to anti-seizure drugs. Genes may also control a person's susceptibility to seizures, or seizure threshold, by affecting brain development.

Other Disorders

Epilepsies may develop as a result of brain damage associated with many types of conditions that disrupt normal brain activity.

343

Seizures may stop once these conditions are treated and resolved. However, the chances of becoming seizure-free after the primary disorder is treated are uncertain and vary depending on the type of disorder, the brain region that is affected, and how much brain damage occurred prior to treatment. Examples of conditions that can lead to epilepsy include the following:

- brain tumors, including those associated with neurofibromatosis or tuberous sclerosis complex, two inherited conditions that cause benign tumors called "hamartomas" to grow in the brain
- head trauma
- alcoholism or alcohol withdrawal
- Alzheimer disease (AD)
- strokes, heart attacks, and other conditions that deprive the brain of oxygen (A significant portion of new-onset epilepsy in elderly people is due to stroke or other cerebrovascular diseases (CeVDs).)
- abnormal blood vessel formation (arteriovenous malformations) or bleeding in the brain (hemorrhage)
- inflammation of the brain
- infections such as meningitis, human immunodeficiency virus (HIV), and viral encephalitis

Cerebral palsy (CP) or other developmental neurological abnormalities may also be associated with epilepsy. About 20 percent of seizures in children can be attributed to developmental neurological conditions. Epilepsies often co-occur in people with abnormalities of brain development or other neurodevelopmental disorders. Seizures are more common, for example, among individuals with autism spectrum disorder (ASD) or intellectual impairment. In one study, a third of children with ASD had treatment-resistant epilepsy.

WHAT TRIGGERS A SEIZURE?

Seizure triggers do not cause epilepsy but can provoke "first seizures" in those who are susceptible or can cause seizures in people with epilepsy who otherwise experience good seizure control with their medication. Seizure triggers include the following:

- alcohol consumption or alcohol withdrawal
- dehydration or missing meals
- stress
- hormonal changes associated with the menstrual cycle

In surveys of people with epilepsy, stress is the most commonly reported seizure trigger. Exposure to toxins or poisons such as lead or carbon monoxide, street drugs, or even excessively large doses of antidepressants or other prescribed medications can also trigger seizures.

Sleep deprivation is a powerful trigger of seizures. Sleep disorders are common among people with epilepsies, and appropriate treatment of coexisting sleep disorders can often lead to improved control of seizures. Certain types of seizures tend to occur during sleep, while others are more common during times of wakefulness, suggesting to physicians how to best adjust a person's medication. For some people, visual stimulation can trigger seizures in a condition known as "photosensitive epilepsy." Stimulation can include such things as flashing lights or moving patterns.

IS EPILEPSY DANGEROUS IN PREGNANCY?

Females with epilepsy are often concerned about whether they can become pregnant and have a healthy child. Epilepsy itself does not interfere with the ability to become pregnant. With the right planning, supplemental vitamin use, and medication adjustments prior to pregnancy, the odds of a female with epilepsy having a healthy pregnancy and a healthy child are similar to those without a chronic medical condition.

Children of parents with epilepsy have about a 5 percent risk of developing the condition at some point during life, in comparison to about a 1 percent risk in a child in the general population. However, the risk of developing epilepsy increases if a parent has a clearly hereditary form of the disorder. Parents who are concerned that their epilepsy may be hereditary may wish to consult a genetic counselor to determine their risk of passing on the disorder.

Other potential risks to the developing child of a female with epilepsy or who takes anti-seizure medication include increased risk for major congenital malformations (also known as "birth defects") and adverse effects on the developing brain. The types of birth defects that have been most commonly reported with anti-seizure medications include the following:

- cleft lip or cleft palate
- heart problems
- stunted spinal cord development (spina bifida)
- urogenital defects
- limb-skeletal defects

Some anti-seizure medications, particularly valproate, are known to increase the risk of having a child with birth defects and/or neurodevelopmental problems, including learning disabilities, general intellectual disabilities, and ASD. It is important that parents work with a team of providers that includes a neurologist and an obstetrician to learn about any special risks associated with epilepsy and the medications the female parent may be taking.

Although planned pregnancies are essential to ensuring a healthy pregnancy, effective birth control is also essential. Some anti-seizure medications can interfere with the effectiveness of hormonal contraceptives. Females who are on these enzyme-inducing anti-seizure medications and using hormonal contraceptives may need to switch to a different kind of birth control that is more effective.

Prior to a planned pregnancy, a female with epilepsy should meet with their health-care team to reassess the current need for anti-seizure medications and to determine the following:

- the optimal medication to balance seizure control and avoid birth defects
- the lowest dose for going into a planned pregnancy

Any transitions to either a new medication or dosage should be phased in prior to the pregnancy, if possible. Discussion about the medications should occur early with the health-care professional.

Epilepsy and Pregnancy

Using supplemental folic acid prior to conception and continuing the supplement during pregnancy is an important way to lower the risk of birth defects and developmental delays. Prenatal multivitamins should also be used prior to the beginning of pregnancy. Pregnant people with epilepsy should get plenty of sleep and avoid other triggers or missed medications to avoid the worsening of seizures.

During the labor and delivery, it is important to take the same formulations and doses of anti-seizure drugs at the usual times; it is often helpful to bring medications from home. If a seizure does occur during labor and delivery, intravenous short-acting medications can be given if necessary. It is unusual for the newborns of females with epilepsy to experience symptoms of withdrawal from the anti-seizure medication (unless it is phenobarbital or a standing dose of benzodiazepines), but the symptoms resolve quickly, and there are usually no serious or long-term effects.

The use of anti-seizure medications is considered safe for breast-feeding. On very rare occasions, the baby may become excessively drowsy or feed poorly, and these problems should be closely monitored. However, experts believe the benefits of breastfeeding outweigh the risks except in rare circumstances. One large study showed that the children who were breastfed by female parents with epilepsy on anti-seizure medications performed better on learning and developmental scales than the babies who were not breastfed. It is common for the anti-seizure medication dosing to be adjusted again in the postpartum setting, especially if the dose was altered during pregnancy.

With the appropriate selection of safe anti-seizure medicines during pregnancy, the use of supplemental folic acid, and, ideally, prepregnancy planning, most people with epilepsy can have a healthy pregnancy with good outcomes for themselves and their developing child.[1]

[1] "Epilepsy and Seizures," National Institute of Neurological Disorders and Stroke (NINDS), April 6, 2023. Available online. URL: www.ninds.nih.gov/health-information/disorders/epilepsy-and-seizures. Accessed May 18, 2023.

Chapter 35 | Lupus and Pregnancy

WHAT IS LUPUS?

Lupus is a chronic (lifelong) autoimmune disease that can damage any part of the body. With autoimmune diseases, the body's immune (defense) system cannot tell the difference between viruses, bacteria, and other germs and the body's healthy cells, tissues, or organs. Because of this, the immune system attacks and destroys these healthy cells, tissues, or organs.

WHAT ARE THE DIFFERENT TYPES OF LUPUS?

There are several different types of lupus. The following are a few:

- **Systemic lupus erythematosus (SLE).** SLE is the most common and most serious type of lupus. SLE affects all parts of the body.
- **Cutaneous lupus erythematosus (CLE).** CLE affects only the skin.
- **Drug-induced lupus.** This is a short-term type of lupus caused by certain medicines.
- **Neonatal lupus.** This is a rare type of lupus that affects newborn babies.

WHO GETS LUPUS?

Anyone can get lupus. It is difficult to know how many people in the United States have lupus because the symptoms are different for every person. It is estimated that 1.5 million Americans have lupus. Other estimates range from 161,000 to 322,000 Americans with SLE. About 9 out of 10 diagnoses of lupus are in women aged 15–44.

HOW DOES LUPUS AFFECT WOMEN?

Lupus is most common in women aged 15–44 or during the years they can have children. Having lupus raises your risk of other health problems. Lupus can also make these problems happen earlier in life compared to women who do not have lupus.

These health problems include the following:

- **Heart disease.** Lupus raises the risk of the most common type of heart disease, called "coronary artery disease" (CAD). This is partly because people with lupus have more CAD risk factors, which include high blood pressure, high cholesterol, and type 2 diabetes. Lupus causes inflammation (swelling), which also increases the risk for CAD. Women with lupus may be less active because of fatigue, joint problems, and muscle pain, and this also puts them at risk for heart disease. In one study, women with lupus were 50 times more likely to have chest pain or a heart attack than other women of the same age.

- **Osteoporosis.** Medicines that treat lupus may cause bone loss. Bone loss can lead to osteoporosis, a condition that causes weak and broken bones. Also, pain and fatigue can keep women with lupus from getting physical activity. Staying active can help prevent bone loss.

- **Kidney disease.** More than half of all people with lupus have kidney problems, called "lupus nephritis." Kidney problems often begin within the first five years after lupus symptoms start to appear. This is one of the more serious complications of lupus. Also, kidney inflammation is not usually painful, so you do not know when it is happening. That is why it is important for people with lupus to get regular urine and blood tests for kidney disease. Treatment for lupus nephritis works best if caught early.[1]

---

[1] Office on Women's Health (OWH), "Lupus and Women," U.S. Department of Health and Human Services (HHS), February 18, 2021. Available online. URL: www.womenshealth.gov/lupus/lupus-and-women#8. Accessed May 18, 2023.

IS IT SAFE FOR YOU TO GET PREGNANT IF YOU HAVE LUPUS?

Yes. Women with lupus can safely become pregnant. If your disease is under control, pregnancy is unlikely to cause flares. However, you will need to start planning for pregnancy well before you get pregnant.

- **Your disease should be under control or in remission for six months before you get pregnant.** Getting pregnant when your lupus is active could result in miscarriage, stillbirth, or other serious health problems for you or your baby.
- **Pregnancy is very risky for certain groups of women with lupus.** These include women with high blood pressure, lung disease, heart failure, chronic kidney failure, kidney disease, or a history of preeclampsia. It may also include women who have had a stroke or a lupus flare within the past six months.

You will need to find an obstetrician (a doctor who is specially trained to care for women during pregnancy) who manages high-risk pregnancies and who can work closely with your regular doctor.

HOW DOES PREGNANCY AFFECT LUPUS?

Pregnant women with lupus have a higher risk for certain pregnancy complications than women who do not have lupus. You may also have other problems that happen during pregnancy:

- You may get flares during pregnancy. The flares happen most often in the first or second trimester. Most flares are mild. But some flares require medicine right away or may cause you to deliver early. Always call your doctor right away if you get the warning signs of a lupus flare.
- About 2 in 10 pregnant women with lupus get preeclampsia, a serious condition that must be treated right away. The risk of preeclampsia is higher in women with lupus who have a history of kidney disease. If you get preeclampsia, you might notice sudden weight gain, swelling of the hands and face, blurred vision,

dizziness, or stomach pain. You might have to deliver your baby early.

- Pregnancy can raise your risk for other problems, especially if you take corticosteroids. These problems include high blood pressure, diabetes, and kidney problems. Good nutrition during pregnancy can help prevent these problems during pregnancy. Regular doctor visits can help find problems such as these early, so they can be treated to keep you and your baby as healthy as possible.

HOW CAN YOU TELL IF THE CHANGES IN YOUR BODY ARE NORMAL DURING PREGNANCY OR A SIGN OF A FLARE?

You may not be able to tell the difference between changes in your body due to pregnancy and the warning signs of a lupus flare. Tell your doctor about any new symptoms. You and your doctor can figure out whether your symptoms are because of your pregnancy or your lupus. This way, you can help prevent or control any flares that do happen.

WILL YOUR BABY BE HEALTHY IF YOU HAVE LUPUS?

Most likely, yes. Most babies born to mothers with lupus are healthy. Rarely, infants are born with a condition called "neonatal lupus." Certain antibodies found in the mother can cause neonatal lupus. At birth, an infant with neonatal lupus may have a skin rash, liver problems, or low blood cell levels.

Infants with neonatal lupus can develop a serious heart defect called "congenital heart block." But, in most babies, neonatal lupus goes away after three to six months and does not come back. Your doctor will test for neonatal lupus during your pregnancy. Treatment can also begin at or before birth.

CAN YOU BREASTFEED IF YOU HAVE LUPUS?

Yes. Breastfeeding is possible for mothers with lupus. However, some medicines can pass through your breast milk to your infant.

Lupus and Pregnancy

Talk to your doctor or nurse about whether breastfeeding is safe with the medicines you use to control your lupus.

You can also enter your medicine into the LactMed® database to find out if your medicine passes through your breast milk and any possible side effects for your nursing baby.[2]

---

[2] Office on Women's Health (OWH), "Pregnancy and Lupus," U.S. Department of Health and Human Services (HHS), February 18, 2021. Available online. URL: www.womenshealth.gov/lupus/pregnancy-and-lupus. Accessed May 18, 2023.

Chapter 36 | Genetic Disorders and Pregnancy

Chapter Contents

Section 36.1 | Thalassemia and Pregnancy

WHAT IS THALASSEMIA?

Thalassemia is an inherited blood disorder, which means that it is passed from parents to children through genes. There are two main types of thalassemia: alpha thalassemia and beta thalassemia. Each of these types can be mild, moderate, or serious, depending on how much hemoglobin your body makes. Hemoglobin is a protein that helps red blood cells carry oxygen.

If you have thalassemia, your body may not make enough hemoglobin, which can lead to fewer healthy red blood cells. This can lead to a condition called "anemia."

Anemia can make you feel tired, weak, or short of breath. Or, depending on the type of thalassemia you have and how serious it is, you may have no symptoms at all. More serious types of thalassemia are usually diagnosed before a child is two years old.

Blood transfusions are used to treat thalassemia. You may need occasional or more regular blood transfusions, depending on how serious your condition is. You may also take medicine to help with complications from this treatment. It is important to talk to your health-care provider before you become pregnant. They may need to run tests or change your treatment plan.

Although thalassemia is a lifelong condition, treatments have improved over the years. People are now living with thalassemia for longer and have a better quality of life.

HOW DOES THALASSEMIA AFFECT PREGNANCY?

Thalassemia may affect your ability to become pregnant, especially if you have a moderate or serious type of thalassemia. It may also lead to a higher chance of health risks during pregnancy. There are many things you can do to minimize risks and ensure that you and your baby are safe and healthy.

Before Pregnancy

Before you and your partner conceive a child, you should meet with your health-care provider to discuss your plans. Thalassemia is an inherited condition, which means you can pass it on to your baby. You may want to meet with a genetic counselor, who can answer questions about the risk and explain the choices that are available. Depending on several factors, your health-care provider may want to do one or more of the following tests:

- **Genetics.** Because thalassemia is an inherited disorder, meaning it is passed from parents to the child through genes, your partner should be screened to see whether they carry any faulty genes related to thalassemia. If both you and your partner carry a faulty gene for thalassemia, your health-care provider may screen your baby for thalassemia before birth.

- **Iron levels.** You may have high iron levels due to regular blood transfusions. High levels of iron can be dangerous during pregnancy. Your health-care provider may use magnetic resonance imaging (MRI) to measure iron levels in your organs, including your liver and heart.

- **Heart and liver function.** Your provider may run heart tests, such as an electrocardiogram (ECG or EKG) or echocardiogram, or they may ask you to wear a Holter or event monitor. To look at your liver, your provider may use an ultrasound or MRI to check for liver disease (fibrosis).

- **Bone mineral density.** Since weak bones caused by osteoporosis are a complication of thalassemia, your health-care provider may run a test to measure your bone density. These tests are typically done using dual-energy x-ray absorptiometry (DEXA).

- **Infections.** Many viruses can lead to severe health risks during pregnancy. Your provider may test you for certain viral infections, such as hepatitis B, hepatitis C, human immunodeficiency virus (HIV), cytomegalovirus, and human Parvovirus B19. They will also recommend that you stay up-to-date on routine vaccinations.

- **Thyroid function.** Thalassemia can cause your thyroid to produce too little thyroid hormone. This can make it difficult to become pregnant. Your health-care provider can measure your levels of thyroid hormone using a blood test.

Thalassemia and iron overload associated with treatment can cause problems with fertility for both men and women. Fertility is the ability to conceive a child. Talk to your health-care provider if you are having difficulty getting pregnant with your partner. Your provider may refer you to a doctor who specializes in fertility. This specialist can work with you to make a plan that will work best for you and your family.

During Pregnancy

If you have thalassemia and become pregnant, you will need to see your health-care provider for checkups frequently—each month for the first two trimesters (28 weeks) and then every two weeks toward the end of your pregnancy.

Your provider may want to run more tests to check your heart, liver, or thyroid function. Your provider will also screen you for gestational diabetes at 16 weeks and may repeat the screening at 28 weeks, depending on the results of the first test. Finally, you may need to stop taking or switch your iron chelation medicine if you require blood transfusions throughout your pregnancy as part of your treatment.

Your provider will also monitor your baby's health and can test your baby for thalassemia. If your baby has a serious form of thalassemia, he or she may need a blood transfusion before birth to treat fetal anemia and prevent life-threatening health problems after birth. Taking precautions can help lower your risk for pregnancy complications, but they can still happen.[1]

---

[1] "Thalassemia," National Heart, Lung, and Blood Institute (NHLBI), May 31, 2022. Available online. URL: www.nhlbi.nih.gov/health/thalassemia. Accessed May 18, 2023.

Section 36.2 | Sickle Cell Disease and Pregnancy

Sickle cell disease (SCD) is a group of inherited red blood cell (RBC) disorders that affect hemoglobin, the protein that carries oxygen throughout the body. The condition affects more than 100,000 people in the United States and 20 million worldwide. Normally, RBCs (refer to Figure 36.1) are disc-shaped and flexible enough to move easily through the blood vessels.

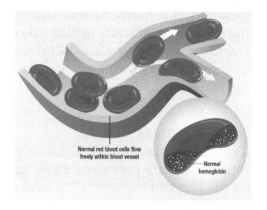

Figure 36.1. Normal Red Blood Cells

National Heart, Lung, and Blood Institute (NHLBI)

If you have SCD, your RBCs are crescent- or sickle-shaped. These cells do not bend or move easily and can block blood flow to the rest of your body (refer to Figure 36.2).

The blocked blood flow through the body can lead to serious problems, including stroke, eye problems, infections, and episodes of pain called "pain crises." SCD is a lifelong illness. A blood and bone marrow transplant is currently the only cure for SCD, but there are effective treatments that can reduce symptoms and prolong life.[2]

---

[2] "What Is Sickle Cell Disease?" National Heart, Lung, and Blood Institute (NHLBI), July 22, 2022. Available online. URL: www.nhlbi.nih.gov/health/sickle-cell-disease. Accessed June 7, 2023.

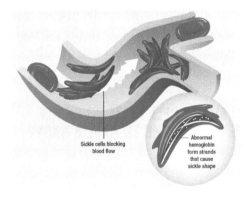

Figure 36.2. Abnormal, Sickled Red Blood Cells
(Sickle Cells)

National Heart, Lung, and Blood Institute (NHLBI)

WHAT CAUSES SICKLE CELL DISEASE AND SICKLE CELL TRAIT?

Sickle cell disease is a genetic condition that is present at birth. It is inherited when a child receives two sickle cell genes—one from each parent. A person with SCD can pass the disease on to his or her children.

Sickle cell trait (SCT) is not a disease but means that a person has inherited the sickle cell gene from one of his or her parents. People with SCT usually do not have any of the symptoms of SCD and live a normal life, but they can pass the sickle cell gene on to their children.

- When both parents have SCT, they have a 25 percent chance of having a child with SCD with every pregnancy.
- When both parents have SCT, they have a 50 percent chance of having a child with SCT with every pregnancy.

DOES SOMEONE WITH SICKLE CELL DISEASE OR SICKLE CELL TRAIT NEED TO SEE A GENETIC COUNSELOR?

The best way to find out if and how SCD runs in someone's family is for that person to see a genetic counselor. These professionals have experience with genetic blood disorders. They also specialize in prenatal genetic counseling.

The genetic counselor will look at the person's family history and discuss with him or her what is known about SCD in the person's family. It is best for a person with SCD or SCT to learn all he or she can about SCD before deciding to have children.

WHAT SHOULD SOMEONE WITH SICKLE CELL TRAIT OR SICKLE CELL DISEASE DO IF HE OR SHE IS PLANNING TO HAVE A BABY?

A woman and her partner should get tested for SCT if they are planning to have a baby.

- Testing is available at most hospitals or medical centers, from SCD community-based organizations, or at local health departments.
- If a woman or her partner has SCT, a genetic counselor can provide additional information and further discuss the risks to their children.

CAN WOMEN WITH SICKLE CELL DISEASE HAVE A HEALTHY PREGNANCY?

Yes, with early prenatal care and careful monitoring throughout the pregnancy, a woman with SCD can have a healthy pregnancy. However, women with SCD are more likely to have problems during pregnancy that can affect their health and that of their unborn baby. Therefore, they should be seen often by their obstetrician, hematologist, or primary care provider.

- During pregnancy, SCD can become more severe, and pain episodes can occur more frequently.
- A pregnant woman with SCD is at a higher risk of preterm labor and of having a low-birth-weight baby.

CAN WOMEN WITH SICKLE CELL TRAIT HAVE A HEALTHY PREGNANCY?

- Women who have SCT can also have a healthy pregnancy.
- Pregnant women with SCT should also be monitored by their obstetrician or primary care provider for the same health complications as all pregnant women.

WILL SOMEONE WITH SICKLE CELL TRAIT OR SICKLE CELL DISEASE HAVE A BABY WITH SICKLE CELL DISEASE OR SICKLE CELL TRAIT?

During pregnancy, prenatal testing can be done to find out if a baby will have SCD, SCT, or neither one.

- The prenatal tests of chorionic villus sampling (CVS) and amniocentesis are often used to find out if the baby will have the disease or carry the trait. These tests are usually conducted after the second month of pregnancy.[3]

---

[3] National Center on Birth Defects and Developmental Disabilities (NCBDDD), "What You Should Know about Sickle Cell Disease and Pregnancy," Centers for Disease Control and Prevention (CDC), September 20, 2014. Available online. URL: https://cdc.gov/ncbddd/sicklecell/documents/scd-factsheet_scd--pregnancy.pdf. Accessed June 7, 2023.

Chapter 37 | Thyroid Disease and Pregnancy

Thyroid disease is a group of disorders that affects the thyroid gland. The thyroid is a small, butterfly-shaped gland in the front of your neck that makes thyroid hormones. Thyroid hormones control how your body uses energy, so they affect the way nearly every organ in your body works—even the way your heart beats.

Sometimes, the thyroid makes too much or too little of these hormones. Too much thyroid hormone is called "hyperthyroidism" and can cause many of your body's functions to speed up. "Hyper" means the thyroid is overactive. Too little thyroid hormone is called "hypothyroidism" and can cause many of your body's functions to slow down. "Hypo" means the thyroid is underactive.

If you have thyroid problems, you can still have a healthy pregnancy and protect your baby's health by having regular thyroid function tests and taking any medicines that your doctor prescribes.

WHAT ROLE DO THYROID HORMONES PLAY IN PREGNANCY?

Thyroid hormones are crucial for normal development of your baby's brain and nervous system. During the first trimester—the first three months of pregnancy—your baby depends on your supply of thyroid hormone, which comes through the placenta. At around 12 weeks, your baby's thyroid starts to work on its own, but it does not make enough thyroid hormone until 18–20 weeks of pregnancy.

Two pregnancy-related hormones—human chorionic gonadotropin (hCG) and estrogen—cause higher measured thyroid hormone levels in your blood. The thyroid enlarges slightly in healthy women during pregnancy, but usually not enough for a health-care professional to feel during a physical exam.

Thyroid problems can be hard to diagnose in pregnancy due to higher levels of thyroid hormones and other symptoms that occur in both pregnancy and thyroid disorders. Some symptoms of hyperthyroidism or hypothyroidism are easier to spot and may prompt your doctor to test you for these thyroid diseases. Another type of thyroid disease, postpartum thyroiditis, can occur after your baby is born.

WHAT CAUSES HYPERTHYROIDISM IN PREGNANCY?

Hyperthyroidism in pregnancy is usually caused by Graves disease and occurs in 1–4 of every 1,000 pregnancies in the United States. Graves disease is an autoimmune disorder. With this disease, your immune system makes antibodies that cause the thyroid to make too much thyroid hormone. This antibody is called "thyroid stimulating immunoglobulin" (TSI).

Graves disease may first appear during pregnancy. However, if you already have Graves disease, your symptoms could improve in your second and third trimesters. Some parts of your immune system are less active later in pregnancy, so your immune system makes less TSI. This may be why symptoms improve. Graves disease often gets worse again in the first few months after your baby is born when TSI levels go up again. If you have Graves disease, your doctor will most likely test your thyroid function monthly throughout your pregnancy and may need to treat your hyperthyroidism. Thyroid hormone levels that are too high can harm your and your baby's health.

Rarely, hyperthyroidism in pregnancy is linked to hyperemesis gravidarum (HG)—severe nausea and vomiting that can lead to weight loss and dehydration. Experts believe this severe nausea and vomiting is caused by high levels of hCG early in pregnancy. High hCG levels can cause the thyroid to make too much thyroid hormone. This type of hyperthyroidism usually goes away during the second half of pregnancy. Less often, one or more nodules, or lumps in your thyroid, make too much thyroid hormone.

WHAT ARE THE SYMPTOMS OF HYPERTHYROIDISM IN PREGNANCY?

Some signs and symptoms of hyperthyroidism often occur in normal pregnancies, including faster heart rate, trouble dealing with heat, and tiredness. Other signs and symptoms can suggest hyperthyroidism:

- fast and irregular heartbeat
- shaky hands
- unexplained weight loss or failure to have normal pregnancy weight gain

HOW CAN HYPERTHYROIDISM AFFECT YOU AND YOUR BABY?

Untreated hyperthyroidism during pregnancy can lead to:

- miscarriage
- premature birth
- low birth weight
- preeclampsia—a dangerous rise in blood pressure in late pregnancy
- thyroid storm—a sudden, severe worsening of symptoms
- congestive heart failure

Rarely, Graves disease may also affect a baby's thyroid, causing it to make too much thyroid hormone. Even if your hyperthyroidism was cured by radioactive iodine treatment to destroy thyroid cells or surgery to remove your thyroid, your body still makes the TSI antibody. When levels of this antibody are high, TSI may travel to your baby's bloodstream. Just as TSI causes your own thyroid to make too much thyroid hormone, it can also cause your baby's thyroid to make too much.

Tell your doctor if you have had surgery or radioactive iodine treatment for Graves disease, so he or she can check your TSI levels. If they are very high, your doctor will monitor your baby for thyroid-related problems later in your pregnancy. An overactive thyroid in a newborn can lead to:

- a fast heart rate, which can lead to heart failure
- early closing of the soft spot in the baby's skull

- poor weight gain
- irritability

Sometimes, an enlarged thyroid can press against your baby's windpipe and make it hard for your baby to breathe. If you have Graves disease, your health-care team should closely monitor you and your newborn.

HOW DO DOCTORS DIAGNOSE HYPERTHYROIDISM IN PREGNANCY?

Your doctor will review your symptoms and do some blood tests to measure your thyroid hormone levels. Your doctor may also look for antibodies in your blood to see if Graves disease is causing your hyperthyroidism.

HOW DO DOCTORS TREAT HYPERTHYROIDISM DURING PREGNANCY?

If you have mild hyperthyroidism during pregnancy, you probably will not need treatment. If your hyperthyroidism is linked to hyperemesis gravidarum, you only need treatment for vomiting and dehydration.

If your hyperthyroidism is more severe, your doctor may prescribe antithyroid medicines, which cause your thyroid to make less thyroid hormone. This treatment prevents too much of your thyroid hormone from getting into your baby's bloodstream. You may want to see a specialist, such as an endocrinologist or expert in maternal–fetal medicine, who can carefully monitor your baby to make sure you are getting the right dose.

Doctors most often treat pregnant women with the antithyroid medicine propylthiouracil (PTU) during the first three months of pregnancy. Another type of antithyroid medicine, methimazole, is easier to take and has fewer side effects but is slightly more likely to cause serious birth defects than PTU. Birth defects with either type of medicine are rare. Sometimes, doctors switch to methimazole after the first trimester of pregnancy. Some women no longer need antithyroid medicine in the third trimester.

Small amounts of antithyroid medicine move into the baby's bloodstream and lower the amount of thyroid hormone the baby makes. If you take antithyroid medicine, your doctor will prescribe the lowest possible dose to avoid hypothyroidism in your baby but enough to treat the high thyroid hormone levels that can also affect your baby. Antithyroid medicines can cause side effects in some people, including:

- allergic reactions such as rashes and itching
- rarely, a decrease in the number of white blood cells in the body, which can make it harder for your body to fight infection
- liver failure, in rare cases

Stop your antithyroid medicine and call your doctor right away if you develop any of these symptoms while taking antithyroid medicines:

- yellowing of your skin or the whites of your eyes called "jaundice"
- dull pain in your abdomen
- constant sore throat
- fever

If you do not hear back from your doctor the same day, you should go to the nearest emergency room. You should also contact your doctor if any of these symptoms develop for the first time while you are taking antithyroid medicines:

- increased tiredness or weakness
- loss of appetite
- skin rash or itching
- easy bruising

If you are allergic to or have severe side effects from antithyroid medicines, your doctor may consider surgery to remove part or most of your thyroid gland. The best time for thyroid surgery during pregnancy is in the second trimester. Radioactive iodine treatment is not an option for pregnant women because it can damage the baby's thyroid gland.

WHAT CAUSES HYPOTHYROIDISM IN PREGNANCY?

Hypothyroidism in pregnancy is usually caused by Hashimoto disease and occurs in 2–3 out of every 100 pregnancies. Hashimoto disease is an autoimmune disorder. In Hashimoto disease, the immune system makes antibodies that attack the thyroid, causing inflammation and damage that make it less able to make thyroid hormones.

WHAT ARE THE SYMPTOMS OF HYPOTHYROIDISM IN PREGNANCY?

Symptoms of an underactive thyroid are often the same for pregnant women as for other people with hypothyroidism. Symptoms include the following:

- extreme tiredness
- trouble dealing with cold
- muscle cramps
- severe constipation
- problems with memory or concentration

Most cases of hypothyroidism in pregnancy are mild and may not have symptoms.

HOW CAN HYPOTHYROIDISM AFFECT YOU AND YOUR BABY?

Untreated hypothyroidism during pregnancy can lead to:

- preeclampsia—a dangerous rise in blood pressure in late pregnancy
- anemia
- miscarriage
- low birth weight
- stillbirth
- congestive heart failure, rarely

These problems occur most often with severe hypothyroidism.

Because thyroid hormones are so important to your baby's brain and nervous system development, untreated hypothyroidism—especially during the first trimester—can cause low IQ and problems with normal development.

HOW DO DOCTORS DIAGNOSE HYPOTHYROIDISM IN PREGNANCY?

Your doctor will review your symptoms and do some blood tests to measure your thyroid hormone levels. Your doctor may also look for certain antibodies in your blood to see if Hashimoto disease is causing your hypothyroidism.

HOW DO DOCTORS TREAT HYPOTHYROIDISM DURING PREGNANCY?

Treatment for hypothyroidism involves replacing the hormone that your own thyroid can no longer make. Your doctor will most likely prescribe levothyroxine, a thyroid hormone medicine that is the same as T4, one of the hormones the thyroid normally makes. Levothyroxine is safe for your baby and especially important until your baby can make his or her own thyroid hormone.

Your thyroid makes a second type of hormone, T3. Early in pregnancy, T3 cannot enter your baby's brain as T4 can. Instead, any T3 that your baby's brain needs is made from T4. T3 is included in a lot of thyroid medicines made with animal thyroid, such as Armour Thyroid, but it is not useful for your baby's brain development. These medicines contain too much T3 and not enough T4 and should not be used during pregnancy. Experts recommend only using levothyroxine (T4) while you are pregnant.

Some women with subclinical hypothyroidism—a mild form of the disease with no clear symptoms—may not need treatment.

If you had hypothyroidism before you became pregnant and are taking levothyroxine, you would probably need to increase your dose. Most thyroid specialists recommend taking two extra doses of thyroid medicine per week, starting right away. Contact your doctor as soon as you know you are pregnant.

Your doctor will most likely test your thyroid hormone levels every four to six weeks for the first half of your pregnancy and at least once after 30 weeks. You may need to adjust your dose a few times.

WHAT IS POSTPARTUM THYROIDITIS?

Postpartum thyroiditis is an inflammation of the thyroid that affects about 1 in 20 women during the first year after giving birth and is more common in women with type 1 diabetes. The inflammation causes stored thyroid hormone to leak out of your thyroid gland. At first, the leakage raises the hormone levels in your blood, leading to hyperthyroidism. Hyperthyroidism may last up to three months. After that, some damage to your thyroid may cause it to become underactive. Your hypothyroidism may last up to a year after your baby is born. However, in some women, hypothyroidism does not go away.

Not all women who have postpartum thyroiditis go through both phases. Some only go through the hyperthyroid phase, and some only go through the hypothyroid phase.

WHAT CAUSES POSTPARTUM THYROIDITIS?

Postpartum thyroiditis is an autoimmune condition similar to Hashimoto disease. If you have postpartum thyroiditis, you may have already had a mild form of autoimmune thyroiditis that flares up after you give birth.

WHAT ARE THE SYMPTOMS OF POSTPARTUM THYROIDITIS?

The hyperthyroid phase often has no symptoms—or only mild ones. Symptoms may include irritability, trouble dealing with heat, tiredness, trouble sleeping, and fast heartbeats.

Symptoms of the hypothyroid phase may be mistaken for the "baby blues"—the tiredness and moodiness that sometimes occur after the baby is born. Symptoms of hypothyroidism may also include trouble dealing with cold, dry skin, trouble concentrating, and tingling in your hands, arms, feet, or legs. If these symptoms occur in the first few months after your baby is born or you develop postpartum depression, talk with your doctor as soon as possible.

HOW DO DOCTORS DIAGNOSE POSTPARTUM THYROIDITIS?

If you have symptoms of postpartum thyroiditis, your doctor will order blood tests to check your thyroid hormone levels.

HOW DO DOCTORS TREAT POSTPARTUM THYROIDITIS?

The hyperthyroid stage of postpartum thyroiditis rarely needs treatment. If your symptoms are bothering you, your doctor may prescribe a beta-blocker, a medicine that slows your heart rate. Antithyroid medicines are not useful in postpartum thyroiditis, but if you have Graves disease, it may worsen after your baby is born, and you may need antithyroid medicines.

You are more likely to have symptoms during the hypothyroid stage. Your doctor may prescribe thyroid hormone medicine to help with your symptoms. If your hypothyroidism does not go away, you will need to take thyroid hormone medicine for the rest of your life.

IS IT SAFE TO BREASTFEED WHILE YOU ARE TAKING BETA-BLOCKERS, THYROID HORMONES, OR ANTITHYROID MEDICINES?

Certain beta-blockers are safe to use while you are breastfeeding because only a small amount shows up in breast milk. The lowest possible dose to relieve your symptoms is best. Only a small amount of thyroid hormone medicine reaches your baby through breast milk, so it is safe to take while you are breastfeeding. However, in the case of antithyroid drugs, your doctor will most likely limit your dose to no more than 20 mg of methimazole or, less commonly, 400 mg of PTU.

WHAT SHOULD YOU EAT DURING PREGNANCY TO HELP KEEP YOUR AND YOUR BABY'S THYROID WORKING WELL?

Because the thyroid uses iodine to make thyroid hormones, iodine is an important mineral for you while you are pregnant. During pregnancy, your baby gets iodine from your diet. You will need more iodine when you are pregnant—about 250 mcg a day. Good sources of iodine are dairy foods, seafood, eggs, meat, poultry, and iodized salt—salt with added iodine. Experts recommend taking a prenatal vitamin with 150 mcg of iodine to make sure you are getting enough, especially if you do not use iodized salt. You also need more iodine while you are breastfeeding since your baby gets iodine from breast milk. However, too much iodine from supplements such as seaweed can cause thyroid problems. Talk with your doctor about an eating plan that is right for you and what supplements you should take.[1]

[1] "Thyroid Disease & Pregnancy," National Institute of Diabetes and Digestive and Kidney Diseases (NIDDK), December 21, 2017. Available online. URL: www.niddk.nih.gov/health-information/endocrine-diseases/pregnancy-thyroid-disease. Accessed June 19, 2023.

Chapter 38 | Eating Disorders during Pregnancy

Adequate nutrition is vital during pregnancy to ensure the health and well-being of both the mother and the baby. As a result, pregnancy may present challenges for women who are struggling with or recovering from eating disorders. Pregnancy creates physical and emotional changes that can be stressful for anyone, especially for women who have preexisting mental health conditions. Even women who believe they have put their disordered eating behaviors in the past may be vulnerable to relapse due to the bodily changes associated with pregnancy. Normal weight gain during pregnancy can trigger symptoms of anorexia, for instance, while the feelings of fullness as the baby grows can create an urge to purge among people with bulimia. The food cravings that often occur during pregnancy can also be problematic for people with binge eating disorders (BED).

If left untreated during pregnancy, active eating disorders can cause serious complications that jeopardize the health of both the mother and the baby. Mothers with eating disorders are more likely to deliver by cesarean section (C-section) and experience postpartum depression. Meanwhile, babies born to mothers with eating disorders have a high risk of premature delivery, low birth weight, and small head circumference. On the other hand, some women find it easier to avoid disordered eating behavior during pregnancy as their focus shifts to protecting the health and welfare of the fetus. Given the importance of nutrition throughout pregnancy, however, women with eating disorders should seek professional advice and treatment to ensure that the condition does not interfere with the normal growth and development of the baby.

RECOGNIZING THE SIGNS OF EATING DISORDERS

Eating disorders may impact a woman's reproductive health even before she becomes pregnant. Women with anorexia or bulimia often experience irregularity or cessation of menstrual cycles, for instance, which can affect fertility and reduce the likelihood of conception. Therefore, doctors recommend that women bring eating disorders under control and maintain a healthy weight for several months before trying to get pregnant. Even in such cases, however, some women find that the bodily changes associated with pregnancy may trigger or exacerbate the symptoms of eating disorders. Some of the common signs that a woman is struggling with an eating disorder during pregnancy include:

- weight loss or very limited weight gain throughout the pregnancy
- anxiety about being overweight
- restricting food intake, skipping meals, or eliminating major food groups
- vomiting or purging to get rid of calories consumed
- extreme (to the point of exhaustion) or excessive exercising to stay thin
- chronic fatigue, dizziness, or fainting
- depression, lack of interest in socializing, or avoidance of family and friends

If these signs appear during pregnancy, it is important to seek treatment to ensure a healthy outcome for both the mother and the baby.

UNDERSTANDING THE RISKS OF EATING DISORDERS

Left untreated, eating disorders can have debilitating effects on the health of both the pregnant woman and the unborn baby. Understanding the risks posed by eating disorders may encourage expectant mothers to get the help they need to have a healthy pregnancy. Some of the potential health risks for a pregnant woman with an eating disorder include:

- severe dehydration or malnutrition
- high blood pressure (preeclampsia), gestational diabetes, or anemia
- cardiac irregularities
- miscarriage, stillbirth, or premature labor
- complications during delivery and increased risk of cesarean section
- extended time required to heal from childbirth
- postpartum depression
- difficulties breastfeeding
- low self-esteem and poor body image
- social withdrawal, isolation, and marital or family conflicts

Eating disorders also carry a number of serious risks for the developing baby, including:

- malnutrition, abnormal fetal growth, or poor development
- premature birth
- respiratory distress
- small head circumference
- low birth weight (with anorexia or bulimia)
- high birth weight (with BED)
- feeding difficulties

The seriousness of these risks, along with the natural maternal instinct to protect the developing baby, enables some women to effectively manage their eating disorders during pregnancy.

MANAGING EATING DISORDERS IN PREGNANCY

For some women, on the other hand, the physical and emotional changes that occur during pregnancy may trigger or worsen eating disorder symptoms. Those with anorexia, for instance, may struggle with their inability to fully control their eating and weight gain while pregnant.

Pregnant women who are struggling with eating disorders should see a counselor or therapist to help guide them through pregnancy-related changes, fears about weight gain, and concerns about body image. In addition, they should work with a nutritionist or dietitian to learn about nutritional requirements during pregnancy, ensure that caloric intake is sufficient to support fetal development, and create appropriate meal plans. Finally, they should inform their obstetrician about their eating disorder and make regular visits to track prenatal growth. The pregnancy may be classified as "high risk" so that the health-care provider can carefully monitor the health of both the mother and the baby. Additional tips to help alleviate concerns and manage eating disorders during pregnancy include the following:

- Remember that the source of weight gain is a growing baby.
- Avoid the scale and ask the health-care provider not to share your weight during checkups.
- Try to ignore, or at least not dwell on, comments others make about your pregnant body.
- Avoid looking at magazines that feature unrealistic postnatal weight loss stories.

MAINTAINING HEALTH AFTER CHILDBIRTH

Even when women with eating disorders manage to keep them under control during pregnancy, many tend to suffer relapses following childbirth. Women face extreme social pressure to lose pregnancy weight as quickly as possible. As a result, many women feel that they must begin a weight loss diet or exercise regimen immediately after their baby has been born. This pressure to shed pounds can trigger disordered eating behaviors. Experts recommend focusing instead on the remarkable physical accomplishment of growing and delivering a healthy baby. This focus can help women accept the changes in body shape and appearance that may have resulted from pregnancy and childbirth.

Experts also stress that it is important for women to take care of their own health following childbirth. Women with eating disorders are particularly susceptible to postnatal depression, so they should watch out for symptoms and seek professional help if they appear. Many women with eating disorders also express concerns about their ability to breastfeed. As long as the eating disorder is under control, it should not affect breastfeeding. But it is important to remember that restricting caloric intake during breastfeeding can reduce both the quantity and quality of breast milk. Adequate nutrition is also important to ensure that new mothers have the energy, health, and well-being necessary to love, care for, and enjoy their infant.

References

"Dealing with Pregnancy and Eating Disorders, What to Expect," Eating Disorder Hope, June 8, 2017. Available online. URL: www.eatingdisorderhope.com/information/ pregorexia/body-image-nutrition-change-coping. Accessed June 1, 2023.

"Eating Disorders and Pregnancy," Eating Disorders Victoria, June 24, 2015. Available online. URL: www. eatingdisorders.org.au/wp-content/uploads/2019/10/ Eating-disorders-and-pregnancy.pdf. Accessed June 1, 2023.

"Pregnancy and Eating Disorders," American Pregnancy Association, July 1, 2015. Available online. URL: https:// americanpregnancy.org/healthy-pregnancy/pregnancy-health-wellness/eating-disorders-and-pregnancy. Accessed June 1, 2023.

Chapter 39 | Do Obesity and Overweight Affect Pregnancy?

Your weight—whether too high or too low—can affect your ability to get pregnant. Being overweight or underweight can also cause problems during your pregnancy. Reaching a healthy weight can help you get pregnant and improve your chances of a healthy pregnancy and baby.

HOW DOES HAVING OVERWEIGHT OR OBESITY AFFECT YOUR ABILITY TO GET PREGNANT?

Extra weight can make it hard for you to get pregnant. For example, polycystic ovary syndrome, or PCOS, is one of the most common reasons for infertility in women and can also cause obesity. Overweight and obesity affect fertility in the following ways:

- **Preventing ovulation**. Your ovaries make the female hormone estrogen. Fat cells also make estrogen. As you gain weight, your fat cells grow and release more estrogen. Too much natural estrogen can cause your body to react as if you are taking hormonal birth control with estrogen (such as the pill, shot, or vaginal ring) or are already pregnant. This can prevent you from ovulating and having a monthly period.
- **Preventing fertility treatments from working**. Obesity may lower your chances of getting pregnant with certain fertility treatments, such as in vitro fertilization (IVF).

COULD REACHING A HEALTHY WEIGHT HELP YOU GET PREGNANT?

Yes. Every woman is different, but studies show that for women who have overweight or obesity, losing weight raises their chances of getting pregnant. Losing weight also helped menstrual cycles return to normal. Talk to your doctor or nurse about how to lose weight safely.

Women who need to gain weight before getting pregnant should gain weight gradually and talk to their doctor or nurse about how to gain weight safely.

HOW MUCH WEIGHT SHOULD YOU GAIN DURING PREGNANCY?

How much weight you should gain during pregnancy depends on your body mass index (BMI) before getting pregnant:

- **Underweight**. If you have a BMI of less than 18.5, you should gain 28–40 pounds.
- **Normal weight**. If you have a BMI of 18.5–24.9, you should gain 25–35 pounds.
- **Overweight**. If you have a BMI of 25–29.9, you should gain 15–25 pounds.
- **Obesity**. If you have a BMI of 30 or greater, you should gain no more than 11–20 pounds.

Talk to your doctor, nurse, or midwife about how much weight is safe to gain during pregnancy.

WHAT ARE THE HEALTH RISKS FOR THE MOTHER OF HAVING OVERWEIGHT OR OBESITY DURING PREGNANCY?

Having overweight or obesity during pregnancy raises your risk for problems during pregnancy. Also, even if you do not have overweight or obesity, gaining more weight than recommended can cause the same problems, including the following:

- **Gestational hypertension (high blood pressure during pregnancy)**. If not controlled during pregnancy, gestational hypertension may lead to a more serious condition called "preeclampsia."

- **Gestational diabetes (diabetes that starts during pregnancy).** Having overweight or obesity raises the risk of gestational diabetes. Women who have had gestational diabetes also have a higher lifetime risk of obesity and type 2 diabetes. Gestational diabetes can cause low blood sugar in the infant. Unborn babies may also be larger, which could injure the baby or the mother during birth.
- **Increased risk of cesarean section (C-section).** Having overweight or obesity raises the chance of having a C-section.

Talk to your doctor, nurse, or midwife about healthy weight gain during pregnancy to help lower your risk for these health problems.

HOW DOES HAVING OVERWEIGHT OR OBESITY DURING PREGNANCY AFFECT THE BABY?

Babies born to mothers with overweight or obesity are at higher risk for health problems, including:
- neural tube defects, such as spina bifida
- heart defects
- low blood sugar and larger body size, if the mother has gestational diabetes
- obesity, type 2 diabetes, and high cholesterol[1]

[1] Office on Women's Health (OWH), "Weight, Fertility, and Pregnancy," U.S. Department of Health and Human Services (HHS), February 17, 2021. Available online. URL: www.womenshealth.gov/healthy-weight/weight-fertility-and-pregnancy. Accessed June 1, 2023.

Part 5 | **Pregnancy Complications**

Chapter 40 | **Understanding Pregnancy Complications**

Chapter Contents

Section 40.1 | How Do Health Problems before Pregnancy Complicate Pregnancy?

Before pregnancy, make sure to talk to your doctor about health problems you have now or have had in the past. If you are receiving treatment for a health problem, your doctor might want to change the way your health problem is managed. Some medicines used to treat health problems could be harmful if taken during pregnancy. At the same time, stopping medicines that you need could be more harmful than the risks posed should you become pregnant. Be assured that you are likely to have a normal, healthy baby when health problems are under control and you get good prenatal care.

HEALTH PROBLEMS BEFORE PREGNANCY

Asthma

Poorly controlled asthma may increase risk of preeclampsia, poor weight gain in the fetus, preterm birth, cesarean birth, and other complications. If pregnant women stop using asthma medicine, even mild asthma can become severe.

Depression

Depression that persists during pregnancy can make it hard for a woman to care for herself and her unborn baby. Having depression before pregnancy is also a risk factor for postpartum depression.

Diabetes

High blood glucose (sugar) levels during pregnancy can harm the fetus and worsen a woman's long-term diabetes complications. Doctors advise getting diabetes under control at least three to six months before trying to conceive.

Eating Disorders

Body image changes during pregnancy can cause eating disorders to worsen. Eating disorders are linked to many pregnancy complications, including birth defects and premature birth. Women with eating disorders also have higher rates of postpartum depression.

Epilepsy and Other Seizure Disorders

Seizures during pregnancy can harm the fetus and increase the risk of miscarriage or stillbirth. But using medicine to control seizures might cause birth defects. For most pregnant women with epilepsy, using medicine poses less risk to their own health and the health of their babies than stopping medicines.

High Blood Pressure

Having chronic high blood pressure puts a pregnant woman and her baby at risk for problems. Women with high blood pressure have a higher risk of preeclampsia and placental abruption (when the placenta separates from the wall of the uterus). The likelihood of preterm birth and low birth weight is also higher.

Human Immunodeficiency Virus

Human immunodeficiency virus (HIV) can be passed from a woman to her baby during pregnancy or delivery. Yet this risk is less than 1 percent if a woman takes certain HIV medicines during pregnancy. Women who have HIV and want to become pregnant should talk to their doctors before trying to conceive. Good prenatal care will help protect a woman's baby from HIV and keep her healthy.

Migraine

Migraine symptoms tend to improve during pregnancy. Some women have no migraine attacks during pregnancy. Certain medicines commonly used to treat headaches should not be used during pregnancy. A woman who has severe headaches should speak to her doctor about ways to relieve symptoms safely.

Overweight and Obesity

Studies suggest that the heavier a woman is before she becomes pregnant, the greater her risk of a range of pregnancy complications, including preeclampsia and preterm delivery. Overweight and obese women who lose weight before pregnancy are likely to have healthier pregnancies.

Sexually Transmitted Infections

Some sexually transmitted infections (STIs) can cause early labor, a woman's water breaking too early, and infection in the uterus after birth. Some STIs can also be passed from a woman to her baby during pregnancy or delivery. Some ways STIs can harm the baby include low birth weight, dangerous infections, brain damage, blindness, deafness, liver problems, or stillbirth.

Thyroid Disease

Uncontrolled hyperthyroidism (overactive thyroid) can be dangerous to the mother and cause health problems, such as heart failure and poor weight gain in the fetus. Uncontrolled hypothyroidism (underactive thyroid) also threatens the mother's health and can cause birth defects.

Uterine Fibroids

Uterine fibroids are not uncommon, but a few cause symptoms that require treatment. Uterine fibroids rarely cause miscarriage. Sometimes, fibroids can cause preterm or breech birth. Cesarean delivery may be needed if a fibroid blocks the birth canal.[1]

---

[1] Office on Women's Health (OWH), "Pregnancy Complications," U.S. Department of Health and Human Services (HHS), January 30, 2019. Available online. URL: www.womenshealth.gov/pregnancy/youre-pregnant-now-what/pregnancy-complications. Accessed May 25, 2023.

Section 40.2 | What Are Some Common Complications during Pregnancy?

Sometimes, pregnancy problems arise—even in healthy women. Some prenatal tests done during pregnancy can help prevent these problems or spot them early. Call your doctor if you have any of the following symptoms. If a problem is found, make sure to follow your doctor's advice about treatment. Doing so will boost your chances of having a safe delivery and a strong, healthy baby.

HEALTH PROBLEMS DURING PREGNANCY
Anemia
People with anemia have a lower-than-normal number of healthy red blood cells. Symptoms may include:
- feeling tired or weak
- looking pale
- feeling faint
- shortness of breath

Treating the underlying cause of the anemia will help restore the number of healthy red blood cells. Women with pregnancy-related anemia are helped by taking iron and folic acid supplements. Your doctor will check your iron levels throughout pregnancy to be sure anemia does not happen again.

Depression
Depression is extreme sadness during pregnancy or after birth (postpartum). Symptoms may include:
- intense sadness
- helplessness and irritability
- appetite changes
- thoughts of harming self or baby

Women who are pregnant might be helped with one or a combination of treatment options, including the following:
- therapy
- support groups
- medicines

A mother's depression can affect her baby's development, so getting treatment is important for both the mother and the baby.

Ectopic Pregnancy

An ectopic pregnancy occurs when a fertilized egg implants outside of the uterus, usually in the fallopian tube. Symptoms may include:
- abdominal pain
- shoulder pain
- vaginal bleeding
- feeling dizzy or faint

With an ectopic pregnancy, the egg cannot develop. Drugs or surgery is used to remove the ectopic tissue, so your organs are not damaged.

Fetal Problems

The unborn baby has health issues, such as poor growth or heart problems. Symptoms may include:
- baby moving less than normal
- baby being smaller than normal for gestational age
- some problems that have no symptoms but are found with prenatal tests

Treatment depends on the results of tests to monitor the baby's health. If a test suggests a problem, this does not always mean the baby is in trouble. It may only mean that the mother needs special care until the baby is delivered. This can include a wide variety of things, such as bed rest, depending on the mother's condition. Sometimes, the baby has to be delivered early.

Gestational Diabetes

Some women develop too high blood sugar levels during pregnancy, which is called "gestational diabetes" (GD).

- Usually, there are no symptoms. Sometimes, there will be extreme thirst, hunger, or fatigue.
- A screening test shows high blood sugar levels.

Most women with pregnancy-related diabetes can control their blood sugar levels by following a healthy meal plan from their doctor. Some women also need insulin to keep blood sugar levels under control. Doing so is important because poorly controlled diabetes increases the risk of:

- preeclampsia
- early delivery
- cesarean birth
- having a big baby, which can complicate delivery
- baby born with low blood sugar, breathing problems, and jaundice

High Blood Pressure (Pregnancy-Related)

High blood pressure starts after 20 weeks of pregnancy and goes away after birth. There will be no other signs and symptoms of preeclampsia. The health of the mother and fetus are closely watched to make sure high blood pressure is not preeclampsia.

Hyperemesis Gravidarum

Hyperemesis gravidarum (HG) is severe, persistent nausea and vomiting during pregnancy—more extreme than "morning sickness." Symptoms may include:

- nausea that does not go away
- vomiting several times every day
- weight loss
- reduced appetite
- dehydration
- feeling faint or fainting

Dry, bland foods and fluids together are the first line of treatment. Sometimes, medicines are prescribed to help with nausea. Many women with HG have to be hospitalized, so they can be fed fluids and nutrients through a tube in their veins. Usually, women with HG begin to feel better by the 20th week of pregnancy. But some women vomit and feel nauseated throughout all three trimesters.

Miscarriage

Pregnancy loss from natural causes happens before 20 weeks. As many as 20 percent of pregnancies end in miscarriage. Often, miscarriage occurs before a woman even knows she is pregnant. Signs of a miscarriage can include:

- vaginal spotting or bleeding*
- cramping or abdominal pain
- fluid or tissue passing from the vagina

Spotting early in pregnancy does not mean miscarriage is certain. Still, contact your doctor right away if you have any bleeding.

In most cases, miscarriage cannot be prevented. Sometimes, a woman must undergo treatment to remove pregnancy tissue in the uterus. Counseling can help with emotional healing.

Placenta Previa

Placenta covers part or the entire opening of the cervix inside of the uterus. Symptoms may include:

- painless vaginal bleeding during the second or third trimester
- for some, no symptoms

If diagnosed after the 20th week of pregnancy but with no bleeding, a woman will need to cut back on her activity level and increase bed rest. If bleeding is heavy, hospitalization may be needed until the mother and baby are stable. If the bleeding stops or is light, continued bed rest is resumed until the baby is ready for delivery.

If bleeding does not stop or if preterm labor starts, the baby will be delivered by cesarean section.

Placental Abruption

Placenta separates from the uterine wall before delivery, which can mean the fetus does not get enough oxygen.

- vaginal bleeding
- cramping, abdominal pain, and uterine tenderness

When the separation is minor, bed rest for a few days usually stops the bleeding. Moderate cases may require complete bed rest. Severe cases (when more than half of the placenta separates) can require immediate medical attention and early delivery of the baby.

Preeclampsia

A condition starting after 20 weeks of pregnancy that causes high blood pressure and problems with the kidneys and other organs. It is also called "toxemia." Symptoms may include:

- high blood pressure
- swelling of hands and face
- too much protein in the urine
- stomach pain
- blurred vision
- dizziness
- headaches

The only cure is delivery, which may not be best for the baby. Labor will probably be induced if the condition is mild and the woman is near-term (37–40 weeks of pregnancy). If it is too early to deliver, the doctor will watch the health of the mother and the fetus very closely. She may need medicines and bed rest at home or in the hospital to lower her blood pressure. Medicines might also be used to prevent the mother from having seizures.

Preterm Labor

Preterm labor is going into labor before 37 weeks of pregnancy:
- increased vaginal discharge
- pelvic pressure and cramping
- back pain radiating to the abdomen
- contractions

Medicines can stop labor from progressing. Bed rest is often advised. Sometimes, a woman must deliver early. Giving birth before 37 weeks is called "preterm birth." Preterm birth is a major risk factor for future preterm births.[2]

---

[2] Office on Women's Health (OWH), "Pregnancy Complications," U.S. Department of Health and Human Services (HHS), December 29, 2022. Available online. URL: www.womenshealth.gov/pregnancy/youre-pregnant-now-what/pregnancy-complications. Accessed May 25, 2023.

Chapter 41 | Bleeding and Blood Clots in Pregnancy

Section 41.1 | Bleeding during Early Pregnancy

WHAT IS "SPOTTING" DURING PREGNANCY, AND DOES IT MEAN A PREGNANCY LOSS IS OCCURRING?

"Spotting" is the term used to describe light bleeding from the vagina. Many pregnant women have spotting and mild cramping during early pregnancy, but it does not always indicate pregnancy loss or another problem.

According to the American College of Obstetricians and Gynecologists (ACOG), up to 20 percent of pregnant women experience light bleeding in the first trimester. In many cases, spotting at this stage of pregnancy does not indicate a problem.

Research also shows that spotting may occur during the second and third trimesters. It can result from factors such as infection, or it could be a signal of labor. Heavy vaginal bleeding at any point in pregnancy can mean there is a problem. Women who experience this type of bleeding should contact their health-care provider immediately.

Likewise, pregnant women who have any of the symptoms of pregnancy loss—vaginal bleeding more than spotting, abdominal cramps, or low back pain—should also contact their health-care providers immediately.[1]

MORE THAN ONE DAY OF EARLY-PREGNANCY BLEEDING LINKED TO LOWER BIRTHWEIGHT

Women who experience vaginal bleeding for more than one day during the first trimester of pregnancy may be more likely to have a smaller baby compared to women who do not experience bleeding in the first trimester, suggest researchers at the National

---

[1] "Other FAQs about Pregnancy Loss (Before 20 Weeks of Pregnancy)," *Eunice Kennedy Shriver* National Institute of Child Health and Human Development (NICHD), September 1, 2017. Available online. URL: www.nichd.nih.gov/health/topics/pregnancyloss/more_information/faqs. Accessed May 25, 2023.

Institutes of Health (NIH). On average, full-term babies born to women with more than one day of bleeding in the first trimester were about 3 ounces lighter than those born to women with no bleeding during this time. Additionally, infants born to women with more than a day of first-trimester bleeding were roughly twice as likely to be small for gestational age, a category that includes infants who are healthy but small, as well as those whose growth has been restricted because of insufficient nutrition or oxygen or other causes.

"The good news is that only one day of bleeding was not significantly associated with reduced growth," said the study's senior author, Katherine L. Grantz, M.D., an investigator in the *Eunice Kennedy Shriver* National Institute of Child Health and Human Development (NICHD) Epidemiology Branch. "But our results suggest that even if the bleeding stops before the second trimester, a pregnancy with more than one day of bleeding is at somewhat of a greater risk for a smaller baby."

According to the study authors, first-trimester vaginal bleeding occurs in 16–25 percent of pregnancies. Earlier studies on whether bleeding is associated with adverse pregnancy outcomes have been inconclusive. The researchers analyzed data from the NICHD Fetal Growth Study, which enrolled women aged 18–40 at 12 hospitals in the United States. The study used ultrasound to track fetal growth throughout pregnancy. Of the roughly 2,300 women in the analysis, 410 (17.8%) had bleeding in the first trimester. Of these, 176 bled for one day, and 234 bled for more.

The researchers also analyzed birthweight outcomes in a secondary analysis limited to 2,116 women with birthweight data available. Compared to women with no bleeding, fetuses of women with more than one day of bleeding were 68–107 grams (approximately 2–4 ounces) lighter in weeks 35–39 of pregnancy. The average birth weight of these babies who were full-term was about 3 ounces lighter than infants born to women who did not bleed at all. Infants who were small for gestational age were delivered to 148 women in the nonbleeding group (8.5%), nine women in the one-day group (5.7%), and 33 women (15.7%) in the group that had more than a day of bleeding.

Dr. Grantz added that when ultrasound exams indicate that the fetus is small for gestational age, physicians typically increase the number of exams to monitor the pregnancy more closely.[2]

Section 41.2 | Blood Clots during Pregnancy

While everyone is at risk of developing a blood clot (also called "venous thromboembolism" (VTE)), pregnancy increases that risk fivefold.

WHY DO PREGNANT WOMEN HAVE A HIGHER RISK OF DEVELOPING A BLOOD CLOT?

Women are especially at risk of blood clots during pregnancy, childbirth, and the three-month period after delivery. Here is why:

- During pregnancy, a woman's blood clots more easily to lessen blood loss during labor and delivery.
- Pregnant women may also experience less blood flow to the legs later in pregnancy because the blood vessels around the pelvis are pressed upon by the growing baby.

Several other factors may also increase a pregnant woman's risk for a blood clot:

- a family or personal history of blood clots or a blood clotting disorder
- delivery by cesarean section (C-section)
- prolonged immobility (not moving a lot), such as during bed rest or recovery after delivery

---

[2] "More than One Day of Early-Pregnancy Bleeding Linked to Lower Birthweight," National Institutes of Health (NIH), May 9, 2018. Available online. URL: www.nih.gov/news-events/news-releases/more-one-day-early-pregnancy-bleeding-linked-lower-birthweight. Accessed May 25, 2023.

- complications of pregnancy and childbirth
- certain long-term medical conditions, such as heart or lung conditions, or diabetes

TAKE STEPS TO PROTECT YOURSELF AND YOUR BABY FROM BLOOD CLOTS DURING PREGNANCY AND AFTER DELIVERY

- Know the signs and symptoms of blood clots.
  - A blood clot occurring in the legs or arms is called "deep vein thrombosis" (DVT). Signs and symptoms of a DVT include the following:
    - swelling of the affected limb
    - pain or tenderness not caused by injury
    - skin that is warm to the touch, red, or discolored
      If you have these signs or symptoms, alert your doctor as soon as possible.
  - A blood clot in the legs or arms can break off and travel to the lungs. This is called a "pulmonary embolism" (PE) and can be life-threatening. Signs and symptoms of a PE include the following:
    - difficulty breathing
    - chest pain that worsens with a deep breath or cough
    - coughing up blood
    - faster than a normal or irregular heartbeat
      Seek immediate medical attention if you experience any of the following signs or symptoms.
- Talk with your health-care provider about factors that might increase your risk for a blood clot. Let your provider know if you or anyone else in your family has ever had a blood clot.
- Follow your health-care provider's instructions closely during pregnancy and after delivery.
  - In general, if a pregnant woman is at high risk for a blood clot or experiences a blood clot during pregnancy or after delivery, she may be prescribed a medicine called "low-molecular-weight heparin." This medicine, injected under the skin, is used to prevent or treat blood clots during and after

pregnancy. Be sure to talk with your health-care provider to understand the best course of management for you.[3]

[3] "Venous Thromboembolism (Blood Clots) and Pregnancy," Centers for Disease Control and Prevention (CDC), June 28, 2023. Available online. URL: www.nih.gov/news-events/news-releases/more-one-day-early-pregnancy-bleeding-linked-lower-birthweight. Accessed July 21, 2023.

Chapter 42 | Intrahepatic Cholestasis of Pregnancy

WHAT IS INTRAHEPATIC CHOLESTASIS OF PREGNANCY?

Intrahepatic cholestasis of pregnancy (ICP) is a liver disorder that occurs in pregnant women. Cholestasis is a condition that impairs the release of a digestive fluid called "bile" from liver cells. As a result, bile builds up in the liver, impairing liver function. Because the problems with bile release occur within the liver (intrahepatic), the condition is described as intrahepatic cholestasis. ICP usually becomes apparent in the third trimester of pregnancy. Bile flow returns to normal after delivery of the baby, and the signs and symptoms of the condition disappear. However, they can return during later pregnancies.

This condition causes severe itchiness (pruritus) in the expectant mother. The itchiness usually begins on the palms of the hands and the soles of the feet and then spreads to other parts of the body. Occasionally, affected women have yellowing of the skin and whites of the eyes (jaundice). Some studies have shown that women with ICP are more likely to develop gallstones sometime in their life than women who do not have the condition.

ICP can cause problems for the unborn baby. This condition is associated with an increased risk of premature delivery and still-birth. Additionally, some infants born to mothers with ICP have a slow heart rate and a lack of oxygen during delivery (fetal distress).

FREQUENCY OF INTRAHEPATIC CHOLESTASIS OF PREGNANCY

Intrahepatic cholestasis of pregnancy is estimated to affect 1 percent of women of Northern European ancestry. The condition is more common in certain populations, such as women of Araucanian Indian ancestry in Chile or women of Scandinavian ancestry. This condition is found less frequently in other populations.

CAUSES OF INTRAHEPATIC CHOLESTASIS OF PREGNANCY

Genetic changes in the *ABCB11* or the *ABCB4* gene can increase a woman's likelihood of developing ICP.

The *ABCB11* gene provides instructions for making a protein called the "bile salt export pump" (BSEP). This protein is found in the liver, and its main role is to move bile salts (a component of bile) out of liver cells, which is important for the normal release of bile. Changes in the *ABCB11* gene associated with ICP reduce the amount or function of the BSEP protein although enough function remains for sufficient bile secretion under most circumstances. Studies show that the hormones estrogen and progesterone (and products formed during their breakdown), which are elevated during pregnancy, further reduce the function of BSEP, resulting in impaired bile secretion and the features of ICP.

The *ABCB4* gene provides instructions for making a protein that helps move certain fats called "phospholipids across cell membranes" and release them into bile. Phospholipids attach (bind) to bile acids (another component of bile). Large amounts of bile acids can be toxic when they are not bound to phospholipids. A mutation in one copy of the *ABCB4* gene mildly reduces the production of the ABCB4 protein. Under most circumstances, though, enough protein is available to move an adequate amount of phospholipids out of liver cells to bind to bile acids. Although the mechanism is unclear, the function of the remaining ABCB4 protein appears to be impaired during pregnancy, which may further reduce the movement of phospholipids into bile. The lack of phospholipids available to bind to bile acids leads to a buildup of toxic bile acids that can impair liver function, including the regulation of bile flow.

Most women with ICP do not have a genetic change in the *ABCB11* or *ABCB4* gene. Other genetic and environmental factors likely play a role in increasing susceptibility to this condition.

INHERITANCE OF INTRAHEPATIC CHOLESTASIS OF PREGNANCY

Susceptibility to ICP is inherited in an autosomal dominant pattern, which means one copy of the altered gene in each cell is sufficient to increase the risk of developing the disorder. Some women with altered genes do not develop ICP. Many other factors likely contribute to the risk of developing this complex disorder.[1]

---

[1] MedlinePlus, "Intrahepatic Cholestasis of Pregnancy," National Institutes of Health (NIH), May1, 2015. Available online. URL: https://medlineplus.gov/genetics condition/intrahepatic-cholestasis-of-pregnancy. Accessed July 21, 2023.

Chapter 43 | Gestational Diabetes

WHAT IS GESTATIONAL DIABETES?

Gestational diabetes is a type of diabetes that can develop during pregnancy in women who do not already have diabetes. Every year, 2–10 percent of pregnancies in the United States are affected by gestational diabetes. Managing gestational diabetes will help make sure you have a healthy pregnancy and a healthy baby.

WHAT CAUSES GESTATIONAL DIABETES?

Gestational diabetes occurs when your body cannot make enough insulin during your pregnancy. Insulin is a hormone made by your pancreas that acts like a key to let blood sugar into the cells in your body for use as energy.

During pregnancy, your body makes more hormones and goes through other changes, such as weight gain. These changes cause your body's cells to use insulin less effectively, a condition called "insulin resistance." Insulin resistance increases your body's need for insulin.

All pregnant women have some insulin resistance during late pregnancy. However, some women have insulin resistance even before they get pregnant. They start pregnancy with an increased need for insulin and are more likely to have gestational diabetes.

SYMPTOMS AND RISK FACTORS OF GESTATIONAL DIABETES

Gestational diabetes typically does not have any symptoms. Your medical history and whether you have any risk factors may suggest to your doctor that you could have gestational diabetes, but you will need to be tested to know for sure.

RELATED HEALTH PROBLEMS OF GESTATIONAL DIABETES

Having gestational diabetes can increase your risk of high blood pressure during pregnancy. It can also increase your risk of having a large baby that needs to be delivered by cesarean section (C-section). If you have gestational diabetes, your baby is at higher risk of:

- being very large (nine pounds or more), which can make delivery more difficult
- being born early can cause breathing and other problems
- having low blood sugar
- developing type 2 diabetes later in life

Your blood sugar levels will usually return to normal after your baby is born. However, about 50 percent of women with gestational diabetes go on to develop type 2 diabetes. You can lower your risk by reaching a healthy body weight after delivery. Visit your doctor to have your blood sugar tested six to twelve weeks after your baby is born and then every one to three years to make sure your levels are on target.

TESTING FOR GESTATIONAL DIABETES

It is important to be tested for gestational diabetes, so you can begin treatment to protect your health and your baby's health. Gestational diabetes usually develops around the 24th week of pregnancy, so you will probably be tested between 24 and 28 weeks.

If you are at higher risk of gestational diabetes, your doctor may test you earlier. Blood sugar that is higher than normal early in your pregnancy may indicate you have type 1 or type 2 diabetes rather than gestational diabetes.

PREVENTION OF GESTATIONAL DIABETES

Before you get pregnant, you may be able to prevent gestational diabetes by losing weight if you are overweight and getting regular physical activity.

Do not try to lose weight if you are already pregnant. You will need to gain some weight—but not too quickly—for your baby to be healthy. Talk to your doctor about how much weight you should gain for a healthy pregnancy.

TREATMENT FOR GESTATIONAL DIABETES

You can do a lot to manage your gestational diabetes. Go to all your prenatal appointments and follow your treatment plan, including the following:

- **Checking your blood sugar**. This is to make sure your levels stay in a healthy range.
- **Eating healthy food**. Besides eating healthy food, it is important to have them in the right amounts at the right times. Follow a healthy eating plan created by your doctor or dietitian.
- **Being active**. Regular physical activity that is moderately intense (such as brisk walking) lowers your blood sugar and makes you more sensitive to insulin, so your body would not need as much. Make sure to check with your doctor about what kind of physical activity you can do and if there are any kinds you should avoid.
- **Monitoring your baby**. Your doctor will check your baby's growth and development.

If healthy eating and being active are not enough to manage your blood sugar, your doctor may prescribe insulin, metformin, or other medication.[1]

---

[1] "Gestational Diabetes," National Heart, Lung, and Blood Institute (NHLBI), December 30, 2022. Available online. URL: www.cdc.gov/diabetes/basics/gestational.html. Accessed May 26, 2023.

Chapter 44 | Gestational Hypertension

Some women have high blood pressure during pregnancy. This can put the mother and her baby at risk for problems during the pregnancy. High blood pressure can also cause problems during and after delivery. The good news is that high blood pressure is preventable and treatable.

High blood pressure, also called "hypertension," is very common. In the United States, high blood pressure happens in 1 in every 12–17 pregnancies among women aged 20–44. High blood pressure in pregnancy has become more common. However, with good blood pressure control, you and your baby are more likely to stay healthy.

The most important thing to do is talk with your health-care team about any blood pressure problems, so you can get the right treatment and control your blood pressure—before you get pregnant. Getting treatment for high blood pressure is important before, during, and after pregnancy.

WHAT ARE HIGH BLOOD PRESSURE COMPLICATIONS DURING PREGNANCY?

Complications from high blood pressure for the mother and infant can include the following:

- **For the mother.** Preeclampsia, eclampsia, stroke, the need for labor induction (giving medicine to start labor to give birth), and placental abruption (the placenta separating from the wall of the uterus).

- **For the baby.** Preterm delivery (birth that happens before 37 weeks of pregnancy) and low birth weight (when a baby is born weighing less than 5 pounds, 8 ounces). The mother's high blood pressure makes it more difficult for the baby to get enough oxygen and nutrients to grow, so the mother may have to deliver the baby early.

WHAT SHOULD YOU DO IF YOU HAVE HIGH BLOOD PRESSURE BEFORE, DURING, OR AFTER PREGNANCY?

Before Pregnancy

- Make a plan for pregnancy and talk with your doctor or health-care team about the following:
  - any health problems you have or had and any medicines you are taking (If you are planning to become pregnant, talk to your doctor. Your doctor or health-care team can help you find medicines that are safe to take during pregnancy.)
  - ways to keep a healthy weight through healthy eating and regular physical activity

During Pregnancy

- Get early and regular prenatal care. Go to every appointment with your doctor or health-care professional.
- Talk to your doctor about any medicines you take and which ones are safe. Do not stop or start taking any type of medicine, including over-the-counter (OTC) medicines, without first talking with your doctor.
- Keep track of your blood pressure at home with a home blood pressure monitor. Contact your doctor if your blood pressure is higher than usual or if you have symptoms of preeclampsia. Talk to your doctor or insurance company about getting a home monitor.
- Continue to choose healthy foods and keep a healthy weight.

After Pregnancy

Pay attention to how you feel after you give birth. If you have high blood pressure during pregnancy, you have higher risk of stroke and other problems after delivery. Tell your doctor or call 911 right away if you have symptoms of preeclampsia after delivery. You may need emergency medical care.

WHAT ARE TYPES OF HIGH BLOOD PRESSURE CONDITIONS BEFORE, DURING, AND AFTER PREGNANCY?

Your doctor or nurse should look for the following conditions before, during, and after pregnancy.

Chronic Hypertension

Chronic hypertension means having high blood pressure* before you get pregnant or before 20 weeks of pregnancy. Women who have chronic hypertension can also get preeclampsia in the second or third trimester of pregnancy.

Gestational Hypertension

This condition happens when you only have high blood pressure* during pregnancy and do not have protein in your urine or other heart or kidney problems. It is typically diagnosed after 20 weeks of pregnancy or close to delivery. Gestational hypertension usually goes away after you give birth. However, some women with gestational hypertension have a higher risk of developing chronic hypertension in the future.

Preeclampsia/Eclampsia

Preeclampsia happens when a woman who previously had normal blood pressure suddenly develops high blood pressure* and protein in her urine or other problems after 20 weeks of pregnancy. Women who have chronic hypertension can also get preeclampsia.

Preeclampsia happens in about 1 in 25 pregnancies in the United States. Some women with preeclampsia can develop seizures. This is called "eclampsia," which is a medical emergency. Symptoms of preeclampsia include the following:

- a headache that will not go away
- changes in vision, including blurry vision, seeing spots, or having changes in eyesight
- pain in the upper stomach area
- nausea or vomiting
- swelling of the face or hands
- sudden weight gain
- trouble breathing

Some women have no symptoms of preeclampsia, which is why it is important to visit your health-care team regularly, especially during pregnancy. You are more at risk of preeclampsia if:

- this is the first time you have given birth
- you had preeclampsia during a previous pregnancy
- you have chronic (long-term) high blood pressure, chronic kidney disease, or both
- you have a history of thrombophilia (a condition that increases risk of blood clots)
- you are pregnant with multiple babies (such as twins or triplets)
- you became pregnant using in vitro fertilization (IVF)
- you have a family history of preeclampsia
- you have type 1 or type 2 diabetes
- you have obesity
- you have lupus (an autoimmune disease)
- you are older than 40

In rare cases, preeclampsia can happen after you have given birth. This is a serious medical condition known as "postpartum preeclampsia." It can happen in women without any history of preeclampsia during pregnancy. The symptoms of postpartum preeclampsia are similar to the symptoms of preeclampsia. Postpartum preeclampsia is typically diagnosed within 48 hours after delivery but can happen up to six weeks later.

Gestational Hypertension

Tell your health-care provider or call 911 right away if you have symptoms of postpartum preeclampsia. You might need emergency medical care.

In November 2017, the American College of Cardiology (ACC) and the American Heart Association (AHA) updated the definition of chronic stage 2 hypertension to mean having blood pressure at or above 140/90 mmHg. The recommendations on hypertension in pregnancy of the American College of Obstetricians and Gynecologists (ACOG) predate the 2017 ACC/AHA's guideline and definition of hypertension and stage 2 hypertension.[1]

---

[1] "High Blood Pressure during Pregnancy," Centers for Disease Control and Prevention (CDC), June 19, 2023. Available online. URL: www.cdc.gov/bloodpressure/pregnancy.htm. Accessed June 26, 2023.

Chapter 45 | **Pregnancy and Stroke**

WHAT IS A STROKE?

A stroke, sometimes called a "brain attack," happens when blood flow to an area of the brain is blocked or when a blood vessel in the brain bursts. Blood carries oxygen to cells in the body. When brain cells are starved of blood, they die. A stroke is a medical emergency. Some treatments for stroke work only if given within the first three hours after symptoms start. A delay in treatment increases the risk of permanent brain damage or death.

WHAT PUTS WOMEN AT RISK OF STROKE?

High blood pressure, also called "hypertension," is a main risk factor for stroke. More than two in five women have blood pressure greater than or equal to 130/80 mmHg or are taking medicine to control their blood pressure. Only about one in four of those women have their blood pressure controlled to below 130/80 mmHg. Stroke risk increases with age. Because women generally live longer than men, more women have strokes over their lifetimes.

Women also have unique risk factors for stroke, including the following:

- having high blood pressure during pregnancy
- using certain types of birth control medicines, especially if they also smoke (About one in nine women smoke.)
- having higher rates of depression

HOW CAN YOU PREVENT STROKE?

Most strokes can be prevented by keeping medical conditions under control and making healthy lifestyle changes:

- Know your ABCS of heart and brain health:
  - **Aspirin.** Aspirin may help reduce your risk of stroke by preventing blood clots, but you should check with your doctor before taking aspirin to make sure it is right for you.
  - **Blood pressure.** Control your blood pressure with healthy lifestyle changes and take your blood pressure medicines as directed.
  - **Cholesterol.** Manage your cholesterol with healthy lifestyle changes and take your medicine as directed.
  - **Smoking.** Do not start smoking. If you do smoke, learn how to quit.
- Make lifestyle changes:
  - **Eat healthy.** Choose healthy foods most of the time, including foods with less salt, or sodium, to lower your blood pressure and that are rich in fiber and whole grains to manage your cholesterol.
  - **Get regular physical activity.** Regular physical activity helps you reach and maintain a healthy weight and keeps your heart and blood vessels healthier.
- Work with your health-care team:
  - **Talk to your doctor about your chances of having a stroke.** It includes your age and whether anyone in your family has had a stroke.
  - **Get other health conditions under control.** It includes diabetes or heart disease.

HOW COMMON IS STROKE DURING OR AFTER PREGNANCY?

Stroke is not common during pregnancy or during the years women can have children. But pregnancy does put women at higher risk of stroke, and the rate of pregnancy-related stroke is rising.

HOW DOES PREGNANCY INCREASE RISK OF STROKE?

Pregnancy is like a stress test; it can strain the heart and blood vessels. This is partly because the body carries more weight during pregnancy, but changing hormones also play a role.

Most women in the United States have healthy pregnancies and deliveries, but sometimes, problems that increase the risk of stroke can happen. These problems include the following:

- **High blood pressure during pregnancy**. Having high blood pressure during pregnancy is the leading cause of stroke in pregnant women or women who have recently given birth. High blood pressure happens in up to 12 percent of pregnancies in the United States. Some women who had healthy blood pressure levels before getting pregnant can develop high blood pressure during pregnancy.

- **Preeclampsia**. It is a more severe type of high blood pressure during pregnancy. Preeclampsia can cause vision problems, headaches, swelling in the hands and face, premature delivery, and a baby with low birth weight. At its most severity, preeclampsia can cause seizures (eclampsia) and lead to stroke. Women who had preeclampsia have a much higher risk of having high blood pressure, kidney disease, heart disease, and stroke later in life than women who did not have high blood pressure during pregnancy.

- **Gestational diabetes**. Some women suddenly develop problems with blood sugar (glucose) during pregnancy, a condition called "gestational diabetes." This happens in as many as 1 in 10 pregnancies in the United States. Gestational diabetes raises the risk of high blood pressure during pregnancy and for heart disease and stroke later in life.

- **Blood clots**. Pregnancy makes the blood more likely to clot, which can lead to stroke. This increased risk of clotting happens in part because swelling from pregnancy can reduce blood flow to the lower legs. When blood does not circulate well, it is more likely to

423

clot. During late pregnancy, the body also makes more of a substance that helps blood clot. This helps protect women from bleeding too much when they give birth, but it also raises the risk of stroke.

WHAT ARE THE SYMPTOMS OF STROKE DURING OR AFTER PREGNANCY?

Many women may mistake their stroke symptoms, including headaches, dizziness, or tingling arms, for issues related to pregnancy and a new baby. If your symptoms appear suddenly, that may be a clue that you are having a stroke.

Learn the key stroke symptoms:
- sudden numbness or weakness in the face, arm, or leg, especially on one side of the body
- sudden confusion, trouble speaking, or difficulty understanding speech
- sudden trouble seeing
- sudden trouble walking, dizziness, loss of balance, or lack of coordination
- sudden severe headache with no known cause

If you notice any of these symptoms in yourself or another person, call 911 right away.

WHAT SHOULD YOU DO IF YOU THINK YOU OR SOMEONE ELSE IS HAVING A STROKE?

If you think someone may be having a stroke, act fast and do the following F.A.S.T. test:
- **F—Face**. Ask the person to smile. Does one side of the face droop?
- **A—Arms**. Ask the person to raise both arms. Does one arm drift downward?
- **S—Speech**. Ask the person to repeat a simple phrase. Is the speech slurred or strange?
- **T—Time**. If you see any of these signs, call 911 right away.

Pregnancy and Stroke

Note the time when any symptoms first appear. This information helps health-care providers determine the best treatment for each person. Do not drive to the hospital or let someone else drive you. Call 911 for an ambulance so that medical personnel can begin life-saving treatment on the way to the emergency room.[1]

[1] "Women and Stroke," Centers for Disease Control and Prevention (CDC), May 4, 2023. Available online. URL: www.cdc.gov/stroke/women.htm. Accessed May 21, 2023.

Chapter 46 | Infections and Pregnancy

Chapter Contents

Section 46.1 | Fifth Disease

Fifth disease is a mild rash illness caused by Parvovirus B19. This disease is usually not a problem for pregnant women and their babies. About half of pregnant women are immune to Parvovirus B19, so they and their babies are usually protected from getting the virus and fifth disease. Pregnant women who are not immune usually have only mild illness if they are exposed to fifth disease. Also, their babies usually do not have any problems.

Rarely, a baby will develop severe anemia caused by its mother's infection with fifth disease, and the woman may have a miscarriage. But this is not common. It happens less than 5 percent of the time among all pregnant women with Parvovirus B19 infection, and it happens more commonly during the first half of pregnancy. Any pregnant woman who may have been exposed to Parvovirus B19 should contact their obstetrician or health-care provider as soon as possible.

TESTING FOR PARVOVIRUS B19 DURING PREGNANCY
A blood test for Parvovirus B19 can show if you:
- are possibly immune to this virus and have no recent serologic evidence of infection
- are not immune and have never been infected
- have had a recent infection

MONITORING PARVOVIRUS B19 INFECTION DURING PREGNANCY
Any pregnant woman who may have been exposed to Parvovirus B19 should contact their obstetrician or health-care provider as soon as possible to discuss if she:
- has been exposed to someone with fifth disease
- has an illness that might be caused by Parvovirus B19 infection
- has been recently infected with Parvovirus B19

There is no single recommended way to monitor pregnant women with Parvovirus B19 infection. Your health-care provider may recommend additional prenatal visits, blood tests, and ultrasounds.

FIFTH DISEASE OUTBREAKS IN THE WORKPLACE AND PREGNANCY

Pregnant women may choose to continue going to their workplace if there is an outbreak of fifth disease happening. However, if you are not immune to Parvovirus B19 and are not currently infected, you may want to stay away from people with the fifth disease while you are pregnant. Talk with your family, health-care provider, and employer to decide what is best for you.

Health-care providers who are pregnant should know about the potential risks to their baby and discuss this with their doctor. All health-care providers and patients should follow strict infection control practices to prevent Parvovirus B19 from spreading.[1]

Section 46.2 | Rubella

WHAT IS RUBELLA?

Rubella is a contagious disease caused by a virus. It is also called "German measles," but it is caused by a different virus than measles. Rubella was eliminated from the United States in 2004. Rubella elimination is defined as the absence of continuous disease transmission for 12 months or more in a specific geographic area. Rubella is no longer endemic (constantly present) in the United States. However, rubella remains a problem in other parts of the world. It can still be brought into the United States by people who get infected in other countries.

Rubella is very dangerous for a pregnant woman and her developing baby. Anyone who is not vaccinated against rubella is at risk

[1] "Pregnancy and Fifth Disease," Centers for Disease Control and Prevention (CDC), November 26, 2019. Available online. URL: www.cdc.gov/parvovirusb19/pregnancy.html. Accessed May 30, 2023.

of getting the disease. Although rubella was declared eliminated from the United States in 2004, cases can occur when unvaccinated people are exposed to infected people, mostly through international travel. Women should make sure they are protected from rubella before they get pregnant.

Infection with the rubella virus causes the most severe damage when the mother is infected early in pregnancy, especially in the first 12 weeks (first trimester). During 2005–2018, 15 babies with congenital rubella syndrome (CRS) have been reported in the United States.

CONGENITAL RUBELLA SYNDROME

Congenital rubella syndrome is a condition that occurs in a developing baby in the womb whose mother is infected with the rubella virus. Pregnant women who contract rubella are at risk of miscarriage or stillbirth, and their developing babies are at risk of severe birth defects with devastating, lifelong consequences. CRS can affect almost everything in the developing baby's body. The most common birth defects from CRS can include the following:

- deafness
- cataracts
- heart defects
- intellectual disabilities
- liver and spleen damage
- low birth weight
- skin rash at birth

Less common complications from CRS can include the following:

- glaucoma
- brain damage
- thyroid and other hormone problems
- inflammation of the lungs

Although specific symptoms can be treated, there is no cure for CRS. Since there is no cure, it is important for women to get vaccinated before they get pregnant.

VACCINE RECOMMENDATIONS

Women who are planning to become pregnant should check with their doctor to make sure they are vaccinated before they get pregnant.

Because the measles, mumps, and rubella (MMR) vaccine is an attenuated (weakened) live virus vaccine, pregnant women who are not vaccinated should wait to get the MMR vaccine until after they have given birth.

Adult women of childbearing age should avoid getting pregnant for at least four weeks after receiving the MMR vaccine. Pregnant women should not get the MMR vaccine. If you get rubella or are exposed to rubella while you are pregnant, contact your doctor immediately.[2]

Section 46.3 | Chickenpox

WHAT IS CHICKENPOX?

Chickenpox is a highly contagious disease caused by the varicella-zoster virus (VZV; refer to Figure 46.1). It can cause an itchy, blister-like rash, among other symptoms. The rash first appears on the chest, back, and face and then spreads over the entire body.

Chickenpox can be serious, especially during pregnancy, in babies, adolescents, adults, and people with weakened immune systems (lowered ability to fight germs and sickness). The best way to prevent chickenpox is to get the chickenpox vaccine.

SIGNS AND SYMPTOMS OF CHICKENPOX

Anyone who has not had chickenpox or gotten the chickenpox vaccine can get the disease. Chickenpox illness usually lasts about

---

[2] "Pregnancy and Rubella," Centers for Disease Control and Prevention (CDC), December 31, 2020. Available online. URL: www.cdc.gov/rubella/pregnancy.html. Accessed May 30, 2023.

four to seven days. The classic symptom of chickenpox is a rash that turns into itchy, fluid-filled blisters that eventually turn into scabs. The rash may first show up on the chest, back, and face and then spread over the entire body, including inside the mouth, eyelids, or genital area. It usually takes about one week for all of the blisters to become scabs. Other typical symptoms that may begin to appear one to two days before the rash include the following:

- fever
- tiredness
- loss of appetite
- headache

Children usually miss five to six days of school or childcare due to chickenpox.

Chickenpox in Vaccinated People (Breakthrough Chickenpox)
Some people who have been vaccinated against chickenpox can still get the disease. However, they usually have milder symptoms with fewer or no blisters (or just red spots), have a mild or no fever,

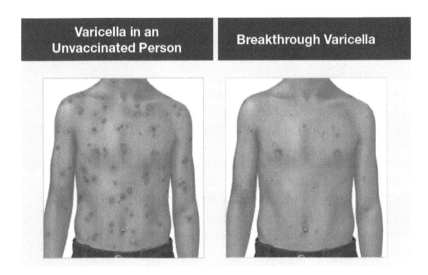

Figure 46.1. Varicella in an Unvaccinated Person and Breakthrough Varicella

Centers for Disease Control and Prevention (CDC)

and are sick for a shorter period of time than people who are not vaccinated. But some vaccinated people who get chickenpox may have a disease similar to unvaccinated people.

People at Risk of Severe Chickenpox

Some people who get chickenpox may have more severe symptoms and may be at higher risk of complications.

COMPLICATIONS OF CHICKENPOX

Complications from chickenpox can occur, but they are not common in healthy people who get the disease. People who may get a serious case of chickenpox and may be at high risk of complications include the following:

- infants
- adolescents
- adults
- people who are pregnant
- people with bodies that have a lowered ability to fight germs and sickness (weakened immune systems) because of illness or medications, for example:
  - people with human immunodeficiency virus (HIV) or acquired immunodeficiency syndrome (AIDS) or cancer
  - patients who have had transplants
  - people on chemotherapy, immunosuppressive medications, or long-term use of steroids

Serious complications from chickenpox include the following:

- bacterial infections of the skin and soft tissues in children, including group A streptococcal infections
- infection of the lungs (pneumonia)
- infection or swelling of the brain (encephalitis and cerebellar ataxia)
- bleeding problems (hemorrhagic complications)
- bloodstream infections (sepsis)
- dehydration

Some people with serious complications from chickenpox can become so sick that they need to be hospitalized. Chickenpox can also cause death.

Deaths are very rare now due to the vaccine program. However, some deaths from chickenpox continue to occur in healthy, unvaccinated children and adults. In the past, many of the healthy adults who died from chickenpox contracted the disease from their unvaccinated children.

TRANSMISSION OF CHICKENPOX

Chickenpox is a highly contagious disease caused by the VZV. The virus spreads easily from people with chickenpox to others who have never had the disease or have never been vaccinated. If one person has it, up to 90 percent of the people close to that person who are not immune will also become infected. The virus spreads mainly through close contact with someone who has chickenpox.

A person with chickenpox is considered contagious beginning one to two days before rash onset until all the chickenpox lesions have crusted (scabbed). Vaccinated people who get chickenpox may develop lesions that do not crust. These people are considered contagious until no new lesions have appeared for 24 hours.

The VZV also causes shingles. After chickenpox, the virus remains in the body (dormant). People get shingles when the VZV reactivates in their bodies after they have already had chickenpox. People with shingles can spread the VZV to people who have never had chickenpox or never received the chickenpox vaccine. This can happen through direct contact with fluid from shingles rash blisters or through breathing in virus particles that come from the blisters. If they get infected, they will develop chickenpox, not shingles.

It takes about two weeks (from 10 to 21 days) after exposure to a person with chickenpox or shingles for someone to develop chickenpox. If a vaccinated person gets the disease, they can still spread it to others. For most people, getting chickenpox once provides immunity for life. It is possible to get chickenpox more than once, but this is not common.

PREVENTION AND TREATMENT OF CHICKENPOX

Prevention of Chickenpox

The best way to prevent chickenpox is to get the chickenpox vaccine. Everyone—including children, adolescents, and adults—should get two doses of chickenpox vaccine if they have never had chickenpox or were never vaccinated.

Chickenpox vaccine is very safe and effective at preventing the disease. Most people who get the vaccine will not get chickenpox. If a vaccinated person gets chickenpox, the symptoms are usually milder, with fewer or no blisters (they may have just red spots) and low or no fever.

The chickenpox vaccine prevents almost all cases of severe illness. Since the chickenpox vaccination program began in the United States, there has been over a 97 percent decrease in chickenpox cases. Hospitalizations and deaths have become rare.

Treatments at Home for People with Chickenpox

There are several things that you can do at home to help relieve chickenpox symptoms and prevent skin infections. Calamine lotion and a cool bath with added baking soda, uncooked oatmeal, or colloidal oatmeal may help relieve some of the itching. Try to keep fingernails trimmed short and minimize scratching to prevent the virus from spreading to others and to help prevent skin infections. If you do scratch a blister by accident, wash your hands with soap and water for at least 20 seconds.

Over-the-Counter Medications

Do not use aspirin or aspirin-containing products to relieve fever from chickenpox. The use of aspirin in children with chickenpox has been associated with Reye syndrome, a severe disease that affects the liver and brain and can cause death. Instead, use nonaspirin medications, such as acetaminophen, to relieve fever from chickenpox. The American Academy of Pediatrics (AAP) recommends avoiding treatment with ibuprofen if possible because it has been associated with life-threatening bacterial skin infections.

When to Call a Health-Care Provider

For people exposed to chickenpox or shingles, call a health-care provider if the person:

- has never had chickenpox and is not vaccinated with the chickenpox vaccine
- is pregnant
- has a lowered ability to fight germs and sickness (weakened immune system) caused by disease or medication, for example:
  - a person with HIV/AIDS or cancer
  - a person who has had a transplant
  - a person on chemotherapy, immunosuppressive medications, or long-term use of steroids

If you have symptoms, call your health-care provider. Contacting a health-care provider is especially important if the person:

- is at risk of serious complications from chickenpox because they:
  - are less than one year old
  - are older than 12 years of age
  - have a weakened immune system
  - are pregnant
- develops any of the following symptoms:
  - fever that lasts longer than four days
  - fever that rises above 102 °F (38.9 °C)
  - any areas of the rash or any part of the body becoming very red, warm, or tender or beginning leaking pus (thick, discolored fluid), as these symptoms may indicate a bacterial infection
  - difficulty waking up or confused behavior
  - difficulty walking
  - stiff neck
  - frequent vomiting
  - difficulty breathing
  - severe cough
  - severe abdominal pain
  - rash with bleeding or bruising (hemorrhagic rash)

TREATMENTS PRESCRIBED BY YOUR HEALTH-CARE PROVIDER FOR PEOPLE WITH CHICKENPOX

Your health-care provider can advise you on treatment options. Antiviral medications are recommended for people with chickenpox that are more likely to develop serious illness, including the following:

- otherwise healthy people older than 12 years of age
- people with chronic skin or lung disease
- people receiving long-term salicylate therapy or steroid therapy
- people who are pregnant
- people with a weakened immune system

There are antiviral medications licensed for the treatment of chickenpox. The medication works best if it is given as early as possible, preferably within the first 24 hours after the rash starts.[3]

Section 46.4 | Cytomegalovirus

In the United States, nearly one in three children are already infected with cytomegalovirus (CMV) by age five. Over half of adults have been infected with CMV by age 40. Once CMV is in a person's body, it stays there for life and can reactivate. A person can also be reinfected with a different strain (variety) of the virus. Most people with CMV infection have no symptoms and are not aware that they have been infected.

SIGNS AND SYMPTOMS OF CYTOMEGALOVIRUS

In some cases, infection in healthy people can cause mild illnesses that may include the following:

- fever
- sore throat

---

[3] "About Chickenpox," Centers for Disease Control and Prevention (CDC), October 21, 2022. Available online. URL: www.cdc.gov/chickenpox/about/index.html. Accessed May 30, 2023.

- fatigue
- swollen glands

Occasionally, CMV can cause mononucleosis or hepatitis (liver problem). People with weakened immune systems who get CMV can have more serious symptoms affecting the eyes, lungs, liver, esophagus, stomach, and intestines.

Babies born with CMV can have brain, liver, spleen, lung, and growth problems. The most common long-term health problem in babies born with congenital CMV infection is hearing loss, which may be detected soon after birth or may develop later in childhood.

TRANSMISSION

People with CMV may pass the virus in body fluids, such as saliva, urine, blood, tears, semen, and breast milk. CMV is spread from an infected person in the following ways:

- from direct contact with saliva or urine, especially from babies and young children
- through sexual contact
- from breast milk to nursing infants
- through transplanted organs and blood transfusions

DIAGNOSIS AND TREATMENT OF CYTOMEGALOVIRUS

Blood tests can be used to diagnose CMV infection in adults who have symptoms. However, blood is not the best fluid to test newborns with suspected CMV infection. Tests of saliva or urine are preferred for newborns.

Healthy people who are infected with CMV usually do not require medical treatment. Medications are available to treat CMV infection in people who have weakened immune systems and babies with signs of congenital CMV. For babies with signs of congenital CMV infection at birth, antiviral medications, primarily valganciclovir, may improve hearing and developmental outcomes. Valganciclovir can have serious side effects and has only been studied in babies with signs of congenital CMV infection. There is limited information on the effectiveness of valganciclovir in treating infants with hearing loss alone.

BABIES BORN WITH CONGENITAL CYTOMEGALOVIRUS

When a baby is born with a CMV infection, it is called "congenital CMV." Most babies with congenital CMV never show signs or have health problems. However, some babies have health problems at birth or that develop later.

SIGNS AND SYMPTOMS OF BABIES BORN WITH CONGENITAL CYTOMEGALOVIRUS

Some babies with congenital CMV infection have signs at birth, such as:

- rash
- jaundice (yellowing of the skin or whites of the eyes)
- microcephaly (small head)
- low birth weight
- hepatosplenomegaly (enlarged liver and spleen)
- seizures
- retinitis (damaged eye retina)

Some babies with signs of congenital CMV infection at birth can have long-term health problems, such as:

- hearing loss
- developmental and motor delay
- vision loss
- microcephaly (small head)
- seizures

Some babies can have hearing loss at birth or can develop it later, even babies who passed the newborn hearing test or did not have any other signs at birth. In the most severe cases, CMV can cause pregnancy loss.

HOW DOES CYTOMEGALOVIRUS SPREAD?

Most people with CMV infection have no symptoms and are not aware that they have been infected. If you are pregnant and get infected with CMV, you can pass the virus to your baby during pregnancy. This can happen when you are infected with CMV for the first time or again during pregnancy. Young children are a common source of CMV.

By the age of five, one in three children has been infected with CMV but usually does not have symptoms. The virus can stay in a child's body fluids, such as saliva and urine, for months after the infection. People who are around young children a lot are at greater risk of CMV infection.

Parents and childcare providers can lower their risk of getting CMV in the following ways:

- reducing contact with saliva (spit) and urine from babies and young children
- not sharing food, utensils, or cups with a child
- washing hands with soap and water after changing diapers or helping a child use the toilet

DIAGNOSIS OF BABIES BORN WITH CONGENITAL CYTOMEGALOVIRUS

Congenital CMV infection can be diagnosed by testing a newborn baby's urine (preferred specimen), saliva, or blood. These specimens must be collected for testing within two to three weeks after the baby is born to confirm a diagnosis of congenital CMV infection.

TREATMENT FOR BABIES BORN WITH CONGENITAL CYTOMEGALOVIRUS

For babies with signs of congenital CMV infection at birth, antiviral medications (primarily valganciclovir) might improve hearing and developmental outcomes. Valganciclovir can have serious side effects and has only been studied in babies with signs of congenital CMV infection. There is limited information on the effectiveness of valganciclovir in treating infants with hearing loss alone.[4]

---

[4] "About Cytomegalovirus (CMV)," Centers for Disease Control and Prevention (CDC), August 18, 2020. Available online. URL: www.cdc.gov/cmv/overview.html. Accessed May 30, 2023.

Section 46.5 | **Hepatitis B**

WHAT IS HEPATITIS B?

Hepatitis B is a serious liver infection caused by the hepatitis B virus (HBV). When babies become infected with hepatitis B, they have about a 90 percent chance of developing a lifelong, chronic infection. Left untreated, about one in four children who have chronic hepatitis B will eventually die of health problems related to their infection, such as liver damage, liver disease, or liver cancer.

TEST AND VACCINATE YOUR FAMILY

Hepatitis B virus is very infectious and can also spread to other family members through contact with blood, semen, or other body fluids from an infected person. Your baby's father and everyone else who lives in your house should go to the doctor or clinic to be tested. Family members who do not have hepatitis B can get the hepatitis B vaccine to protect them from getting infected.

PROTECT YOUR BABY FROM HEPATITIS B

Your baby should get the first dose of the hepatitis B vaccine and a shot called "hepatitis B immune globulin" (HBIG) within 12 hours of being born. HBIG is a medicine that gives your baby's body a "boost" or extra help to fight the virus as soon as he or she is born. The HBIG shot is only given to babies of mothers who have hepatitis B. The HBIG and hepatitis B vaccine shots help prevent your baby from getting hepatitis B. These shots work best when they are given within 12 hours after your baby is born.

All the hepatitis B shots are necessary to help keep your baby from getting hepatitis B. Your baby will get three or four shots in all, depending on your baby's birth weight and the vaccine brand. After the first shots are given in the hospital, the next shot is usually given at one to two months of age. The last shot is given when your baby is six months old. Ask your doctor or nurse when your baby needs to come back for each shot.

Make sure your baby gets tested after completing the series of shots. After getting all the hepatitis B shots, your doctor will test your baby's blood. This blood test tells you and your doctor if your baby is protected and does not have hepatitis B. The blood test is usually done one to two months after completing the series of shots. Your baby should be at least nine months of age before getting this test.

You can breastfeed your baby if your baby gets the HBIG and hepatitis B vaccine within 12 hours of birth. You cannot give your baby hepatitis B from breast milk. Ask your doctor if you should still breastfeed if you have cracked nipples or open sores on your breast.

TAKE CARE OF YOURSELF

You may need additional tests to check the health of your liver and see if you need treatment. Medications, called "antivirals," can treat many people with hepatitis B. However, not everyone needs treatment. Ask a doctor before taking any prescription, over-the-counter medications, supplements, or vitamins because some drugs can potentially damage the liver. You may also benefit from the hepatitis A vaccine. Continue to see a doctor after giving birth to monitor your infection.[5]

PERINATAL TRANSMISSION

Hepatitis B virus infection in a pregnant woman poses a serious risk to her infant at birth. Without postexposure immunoprophylaxis, approximately 40 percent of infants born to HBV-infected mothers in the United States will develop chronic HBV infection, approximately one-fourth of whom will eventually die from chronic liver disease.

Perinatal HBV transmission can be prevented by identifying HBV-infected (i.e., hepatitis B surface antigen (HBsAg) positive)

[5] "When a Pregnant Woman Has Hepatitis B," Centers for Disease Control and Prevention (CDC), January 1, 2020. Available online. URL: www.cdc.gov/hepatitis/hbv/pdfs/hepbperinatal-protectwhenpregnant.pdf. Accessed July 17, 2023.

pregnant women and providing the HBIG and hepatitis B vaccine to their infants within 12 hours of birth. Preventing perinatal HBV transmission is an integral part of the national strategy to eliminate hepatitis B in the United States. National guidelines call for the following:

- universal screening of pregnant persons for HBsAg during each pregnancy
- HBV deoxyribonucleic acid (DNA) testing for HBsAg-positive pregnant persons at 26–28 weeks to guide the use of maternal antiviral therapy during pregnancy (The American Association for the Study of Liver Diseases (AASLD) suggests maternal antiviral therapy when HBV DNA is greater than 200,000 IU/mL.)
- case management of HBsAg-positive mothers and their infants
- provision of immunoprophylaxis for infants born to infected mothers, including the HBIG and hepatitis B vaccine within 12 hours of birth
- routine vaccination of all infants with the hepatitis B vaccine series, with the first dose administered within 24 hours of birth[6]

Section 46.6 | Zika Virus

ABOUT ZIKA AND PREGNANCY

Zika is a virus spread to people primarily through the bite of an infected mosquito. Zika infection during pregnancy can cause serious birth defects.

What We Know

- Zika virus can be passed from a pregnant woman to a fetus.

---

[6] "Perinatal Transmission," Centers for Disease Control and Prevention (CDC), February 16, 2022. Available online. URL: www.cdc.gov/hepatitis/hbv/perinatalxmtn.htm. Accessed July 17, 2023.

Infections and Pregnancy

- Infection during pregnancy can cause serious brain and eye defects. It may also cause neurodevelopmental abnormalities such as:
  - problems with hearing and vision
  - joints with a limited range of motion
  - seizures
  - too much muscle tone, restricting body movement
  - swallowing abnormalities
  - possible developmental delay
- Zika primarily spreads through bites from infected mosquitoes. You can also get Zika through sex without a condom with someone infected by Zika, even if that person does not have symptoms of Zika.
- There is no vaccine to prevent or medicine to treat Zika.
- People who are pregnant should not travel to areas with a Zika outbreak. Before traveling to other areas with risk of Zika, people considering pregnancy should talk with their doctors or other health-care providers and carefully consider risks and possible consequences of travel.

What We Have Learned about Zika and Pregnancy

When the Zika outbreak began, there were many unknowns. Since then, we have learned a lot about Zika virus infection during pregnancy because of the rich data that were collected. The Centers for Disease Control and Prevention (CDC) worked with health departments to set up systems to collect information about people exposed to Zika during pregnancy and their babies after birth. This helped us answer many questions about how the Zika virus can affect babies:

Q: How does Zika affect pregnancies?

A: Certain types of birth defects can happen from Zika virus infection during pregnancy. Several brain and eye defects were more commonly reported.

Q: How often do babies have birth defects if their mothers had Zika while pregnant?

A: About 5 percent of babies born to people with Zika while pregnant had Zika-associated birth defects. Additionally, some babies affected by Zika during pregnancy might look healthy at birth but can develop long-term health problems as they grow.

Q: When does Zika cause harm to the baby in the womb?

A: Infection during early pregnancy may be more likely to cause birth defects, but we have seen babies with birth defects born to people infected with Zika anytime during pregnancy.

Q: If a pregnant person has Zika symptoms, is her baby more likely to have birth defects?

A: We found a similar frequency of birth defects between mothers with and without Zika symptoms.

Q: Are babies getting the care they need?

A: Many babies exposed to Zika in pregnancy were not reported to receive the recommended examinations (physical and developmental exam, brain imaging, hearing test, and eye exam) during their first year of life.

What We Do Not Know

- how likely it is that a Zika infection will affect your pregnancy
- if your baby will have birth defects if you are infected while pregnant
- the full range of health effects that Zika during pregnancy might lead to

What We Are Doing to Learn More

- The CDC will collect information on some babies affected by Zika up until the children are aged five. We need to learn more about any other brain or developmental problems that children who were exposed to the Zika virus during pregnancy might experience.

ZIKA DURING PREGNANCY

The only way to completely prevent Zika infection during pregnancy is not to travel to areas with risk of Zika and to use precautions or avoid sex with someone who has recently traveled to a risk area.

We do not have accurate information on the current level of risk in specific areas. The large outbreak in the Americas is over, but Zika is and will continue to be a potential risk in many countries in the Americas and around the world. No local spread of Zika virus has been reported in the continental United States since 2017.

There is no vaccine to prevent or medicine to treat Zika. If you are considering travel to an area with risk of Zika, talk to your health-care provider first. It is important to understand the risks of Zika infection during pregnancy, ways to protect yourself, signs of Zika, and the limitations of Zika testing upon your return.

FACTORS TO CONSIDER IF YOU TRAVEL TO OR LIVE IN AN AREA WITH A ZIKA OUTBREAK OR OTHER AREAS WITH RISK OF ZIKA
During Travel or While Living in an Area with Risk of Zika

- **Protective measures**:
  - Prevent mosquito bites by using insect repellents registered with the U.S. Environmental Protection Agency (EPA) and covering skin.
  - Prevent getting Zika infection through sex by using condoms from start to finish every time you have sex (oral, vaginal, or anal) or by not having sex during your pregnancy.
- **Accommodations**. Stay in places with air conditioning, with window and door screens, or sleep under a mosquito bed net.
- **Type and length of exposure**. For extended stays, there are steps you can take to control mosquitoes inside and outside, such as removing standing water. It is important for all travelers, including those visiting friends and relatives and those with extended stays, to protect themselves against Zika infection and other mosquito-borne illnesses during the entire visit.

447

After Travel

- After any travel outside the United States during pregnancy, it is important to tell your doctor or health-care provider about your travel because of the potential risk of various infectious diseases.
- If you or your partner travel to an area with a Zika outbreak or other areas with risk of Zika, do the following:
  - Be alert for symptoms of Zika, including headache, rash, joint pain, or red eyes.
  - Take steps to prevent getting Zika through sex by using condoms from start to finish every time you have sex (oral, vaginal, or anal) or by not having sex during your entire pregnancy.

Risk of Zika Infection on Future Pregnancies

Current evidence suggests that Zika infection prior to pregnancy would not pose a risk of birth defects in a future pregnancy. From what we know about similar infections, once a person has been infected with the Zika virus, they are likely to be protected from a future Zika infection. We do not have a test to tell if someone is protected against Zika virus.

If you are thinking about having a baby in the near future and you or your partner live in or traveled to an area with a Zika outbreak or an area with risk of Zika, talk with your doctor or other health-care providers.[7]

---

[7] "What We Know about Zika and Pregnancy," Centers for Disease Control and Prevention (CDC), July 1, 2022. Available online. URL: www.cdc.gov/pregnancy/zika/pregnancy.html. Accessed May 21, 2023.

Section 46.7 | Group B *Streptococcus*

Group B *Streptococcus* (GBS) bacteria commonly live in people's bodies and usually are not harmful. Babies can be exposed to GBS bacteria during delivery. How other people are exposed to these bacteria is not completely known.

CAUSES OF GROUP B *STREPTOCOCCUS*

Group B *Streptococcus* causes GBS disease. GBS bacteria commonly live in people's gastrointestinal and genital tracts. The gastrointestinal tract is the part of the body that digests food and includes the stomach and intestines. The genital tract is the part of the body involved in reproduction and includes the vagina in women.

Most of the time, the bacteria are not harmful and do not make people feel sick or have any symptoms. Sometimes, the bacteria invade the body and cause certain infections, which are known as "GBS disease."

HOW GROUP B *STREPTOCOCCUS* SPREADS

How people spread GBS bacteria to others is generally unknown. However, experts know that pregnant women can pass the bacteria to their babies during delivery. Most babies who get GBS disease in the first week of life are exposed to the bacteria this way. It can be hard to figure out how babies who develop GBS disease later get the bacteria. The bacteria may have come from the mother during birth or from another source.

Other people who live with someone who has GBS bacteria, including other children, are not at increased risk of getting sick.

TYPES OF INFECTIONS

Group B *Streptococcus* can cause many types of infections. Some of the following infections can be life-threatening:
- bacteremia (a bloodstream infection)
- sepsis (the body's extreme response to an infection)
- bone and joint infections

449

- urinary tract infections (UTIs; an infection of the urinary tract)
- meningitis (an infection of the lining of the brain and spinal cord)
- pneumonia (a lung infection)
- skin and soft tissue infections

Most Common Infections

GBS bacteria most commonly cause bacteremia, sepsis, pneumonia, and meningitis in newborns. It is very uncommon for GBS bacteria to cause meningitis in adults.

Some of these infections are "invasive." Invasive disease means that germs invade parts of the body that are normally free from germs. When this happens, the disease is usually very severe, requiring care in a hospital and even causing death in some cases.

SIGNS AND SYMPTOMS OF GROUP B *STREPTOCOCCUS*

Group B *Streptococcus* disease can include many different types of infections. Symptoms depend on the part of the body that is infected. Symptoms of GBS disease are different in newborns compared to people of other ages who get GBS disease.

Newborns

The symptoms of GBS disease can seem like other health problems in newborns and babies. Symptoms include:

- fever
- difficulty feeding
- irritability or lethargy (limpness or hard to wake up the baby)
- difficulty breathing
- bluish color to the skin

Most newborns who get sick in the first week of life have symptoms on the day of birth. In contrast, babies who develop the disease later can appear healthy at birth and during their first week of life.

Pregnant Women Who Test Positive

Some women test positive for GBS bacteria during routine screening toward the end of their pregnancy. Those women usually do not feel sick or have any symptoms.

Others

Symptoms depend on the part of the body that is infected. The following are symptoms associated with the most common infections caused by GBS bacteria in adults:

- Symptoms of bacteremia (bloodstream infection) and sepsis (the body's extreme response to an infection) include:
  - fever
  - chills
  - low alertness
- Symptoms of pneumonia (lung infection) include:
  - fever
  - chills
  - cough
  - rapid breathing or difficulty breathing
  - chest pain
- Skin and soft tissue infections often appear as a bump or infected area on the skin that may be:
  - red
  - swollen or painful
  - warm to the touch
  - full of pus or other drainage

people with skin infections may also have a fever.
- Bone and joint infections often appear as pain in the infected area and might also include:
  - fever
  - chills
  - swelling
  - stiffness or inability to use the affected limb or joint

DIAGNOSIS, TREATMENT, AND COMPLICATIONS OF GROUP B *STREPTOCOCCUS*

Group B *Streptococcus* disease is often serious. Early diagnosis and treatment are very important.

Diagnosis of Group B *Streptococcus*

If doctors suspect someone has GBS disease, they will do the following:

- Take samples of sterile body fluids such as blood and spinal fluid. Doctors look to see if GBS bacteria grow from the samples (culture). It can take a few days to get these results since the bacteria need time to grow.
- Order a chest x-ray to help determine if someone has GBS disease. Sometimes, GBS bacteria can cause UTIs or bladder infections. Doctors use a sample of urine to diagnose UTIs.

Treatment for Group B *Streptococcus*

Doctors usually treat GBS disease with antibiotics. Sometimes, people with soft tissue and bone infections may need additional treatment, such as surgery. Treatment will depend on the kind of infection caused by GBS bacteria. It is important to start treatment as soon as possible.

Complications of Group B *Streptococcus*

BABIES

Babies may have long-term problems, such as deafness and developmental disabilities, due to having GBS disease. Babies who have meningitis are especially at risk of having long-term problems.

Even with good care, babies can still die. Care for sick babies has improved a lot in the United States. However, two to three in every 50 babies (4–6%) who develop GBS disease will die. GBS bacteria may be one of many different factors that can cause some miscarriages, stillbirths, and preterm deliveries. Most of the time, the cause of these events is not known.

ADULTS

Serious GBS infections, such as bacteremia, sepsis, and pneumonia, can also be deadly for adults. On average, about 1 in 20 nonpregnant adults with serious GBS infections die. The risk of death is lower among younger adults and adults who do not have other medical conditions.

PEOPLE AT INCREASED RISK

Anyone can get GBS disease, but some people are at greater risk than others. Being a certain age or having certain medical conditions can put you at increased risk of GBS disease.

Newborns

GBS disease is most common in newborns. There are factors that can increase a pregnant woman's risk of having a baby who will develop GBS disease, including the following:

- testing positive for GBS bacteria late in pregnancy
- developing a fever during labor
- having 18 hours or more pass between when their water breaks and when their baby is born
- about one in every four pregnant women carry GBS bacteria in their body

Adults

In adults, most cases of GBS disease are among those who have other medical conditions. Other medical conditions that put adults at increased risk include the following:

- diabetes
- heart disease
- congestive heart failure
- cancer or history of cancer
- obesity

The risk for serious GBS disease increases as people get older. Adults aged 65 or older are at increased risk compared to adults younger than 65 years of age.

PREVENTING GROUP B *STREPTOCOCCUS* DISEASE

There are currently no vaccines to prevent GBS disease, but they are under development. There are things doctors and midwives can do to prevent GBS disease during the first week of a newborn's life. Unfortunately, experts have not yet identified effective ways to prevent GBS disease in people older than one week old.

Preventing Illness in Newborns

The two best ways to prevent GBS disease during the first week of a newborn's life are:

- testing pregnant women for GBS bacteria
- giving antibiotics, during labor, to women at increased risk

TESTING PREGNANT WOMEN

The American College of Obstetricians and Gynecologists (ACOG) and the American College of Nurse-Midwives (ACNM) recommend women get tested for GBS bacteria when they are 36–37 weeks pregnant.

The test is simple and does not hurt. Doctors and midwives use a sterile swab ("Q-tip") to collect a sample from the vagina and the rectum. They send the sample to a laboratory for testing. Women who test positive for GBS bacteria are not sick. However, they are at increased risk of passing the bacteria to their babies during birth.

GBS bacteria come and go naturally in people's bodies. A woman may test positive for the bacteria at some times and not others. That is why women get tested late in their pregnancy, close to the time of delivery.

ANTIBIOTICS DURING LABOR

Doctors and midwives give antibiotics to women who are at increased risk of having a baby who will develop GBS disease. The antibiotics help protect babies from infection but only if given during labor. Antibiotics cannot be given before labor begins because the bacteria can grow back quickly.

Doctors and midwives give the antibiotic intravenously (IV; through the vein). They most commonly prescribe a type of antibiotic called "beta-lactams," which includes penicillin and ampicillin. However, they can also give other antibiotics to women who are severely allergic to these antibiotics. Antibiotics are very safe. For example, about 1 in 10 women have mild side effects from receiving penicillin. There is a rare chance (about 1 in 10,000 women) of having a severe allergic reaction that requires emergency treatment.

STRATEGIES PROVEN NOT TO WORK
The following strategies are not effective at preventing GBS disease in babies:
- taking antibiotics by mouth
- taking antibiotics before labor begins
- using birth canal washes with the disinfectant chlorhexidine

SOME FACTS ABOUT GROUP B *STREPTOCOCCUS* DISEASE
Rates of serious GBS infections are higher among newborns, but anyone can get GBS disease. The following are some other important facts about GBS disease in babies, pregnant women, and others:
- GBS disease can be very serious, especially for babies.
  - In the United States, GBS bacteria are a leading cause of meningitis and bloodstream infections in a newborn's first three months of life.
  - Newborns are at increased risk for GBS disease if their mother tests positive for the bacteria late in pregnancy.
  - Two to three in every 50 babies (4–6%) who develop GBS disease die.
- Pregnant women should get tested for GBS bacteria.
  - About one in four pregnant women carries GBS bacteria in their body.
  - Doctors and midwives should test pregnant women for GBS bacteria when they are 36–37 weeks pregnant.

- Giving pregnant women who carry GBS bacteria antibiotics through the vein (IV) during labor can prevent most cases of GBS disease in newborns during the first week of life.
- Nonpregnant adults can get serious GBS disease.
- The most common GBS infections among nonpregnant adults include bloodstream infections, pneumonia, and skin and bone infections.
- The rate of serious GBS disease increases with age.
- On average, about 1 in 20 nonpregnant adults with serious GBS infections die.[8]

Section 46.8 | Listeriosis

WHAT IS *LISTERIA MONOCYTOGENES*?

It is a harmful bacterium that can be found in refrigerated, ready-to-eat foods (meat, poultry, seafood, and dairy unpasteurized milk and milk products or foods made with unpasteurized milk) and produce harvested from soil contaminated with *Listeria monocytogenes* (*L. monocytogenes*). Many animals can carry this bacterium without appearing ill, and thus, it can be found in foods made from animals. *L. monocytogenes* is unusual because it can grow at refrigerator temperatures where most other food-borne bacteria do not. When eaten, it may cause listeriosis, an illness to which pregnant women and their unborn children are very susceptible.

HOW COULD YOU GET LISTERIOSIS?

You could get listeriosis by eating ready-to-eat meats, poultry, seafood, and dairy products that are contaminated with *L. monocytogenes*. You can also get listeriosis by eating contaminated foods

[8] "About Group B Strep," Centers for Disease Control and Prevention (CDC), October 18, 2022. Available online. URL: www.cdc.gov/groupbstrep/about/index.html. Accessed May 31, 2023.

processed or packaged in unsanitary conditions or by eating fruits and vegetables that are contaminated from the soil or from manure used as fertilizer.

HOW COULD LISTERIOSIS AFFECT YOU?

The symptoms can take a few days or even weeks to appear and may include fever, chills, muscle aches, diarrhea or upset stomach, headache, stiff neck, confusion, and loss of balance. In more serious cases, listeriosis could also lead to the mother's death.

Most of the time, pregnant women who are infected with listeriosis do not feel sick. However, they can pass the infection to their unborn babies without even knowing it. That is why prevention of listeriosis is very important. In any case, if you experience any of the above symptoms, see your doctor or health-care provider immediately.

HOW COULD LISTERIOSIS AFFECT YOUR BABY?

During the first trimester of pregnancy, listeriosis may cause miscarriage. As the pregnancy progresses to the third trimester, the mother is more at risk. Listeriosis can also lead to premature labor, the delivery of a low-birth-weight infant, or infant death. Fetuses who have a late infection may develop a wide range of health problems, including intellectual disability, paralysis, seizures, blindness, or impairments of the brain, heart, or kidney. In newborns, *L. monocytogenes* can cause blood infections and meningitis.

HOW CAN YOU PREVENT LISTERIOSIS?

The good news is that listeriosis can be prevented. Here is how.

Time to Chill

- Your refrigerator should register at 40 °F (4 °C) or below and the freezer at 0 °F (−18 °C). Place a refrigerator thermometer in the refrigerator and check the temperature periodically. During the automatic defrost cycle, the temperature may temporarily register slightly higher than 40 °F (4.4 °C). This is okay.

- Refrigerate or freeze perishables, prepared food, and leftovers within two hours of eating or preparation. Follow the 2-Hour Rule: Discard food that is left out at room temperature for longer than two hours. When temperatures are above 90 °F (32 °C), discard food after one hour.
- Use ready-to-eat, perishable foods, such as dairy, meat, poultry, seafood, and produce, as soon as possible.

Fridge Tips

- Clean your refrigerator regularly.
- Wipe up spills immediately.
- Clean the inside walls and shelves with hot water and a mild liquid dishwashing detergent; then rinse.
- Once a week, check the expiration and "use by" dates and throw out foods if the date has passed. Follow the recommended storage times for foods.

To Eat or Not to Eat?

Do not eat:

- hot dogs, deli meats, and luncheon meats—unless they were reheated until steaming hot
- soft cheeses such as Feta, Brie, and Camembert; "blue-veined cheeses"; or "queso blanco," "queso fresco," or panela—unless they were made with pasteurized milk (Make sure the label says, "made with pasteurized milk.")
- refrigerated pâtés or meat spreads
- refrigerated smoked seafood—unless it is in a cooked dish, such as a casserole (Refrigerated smoked seafood, such as salmon, trout, whitefish, cod, tuna, or mackerel, is most often labeled as "nova-style," "lox," "kippered," "smoked," or "jerky." These types of fish are found in the refrigerator section or sold at deli counters of grocery stores and delicatessens.)

- raw (unpasteurized) milk or foods that contain unpasteurized milk

It is okay to eat:
- canned or shelf-stable (able to be stored unrefrigerated on the shelf) pâtés and meat spreads
- canned or shelf-stable smoked seafood
- pasteurized milk or foods that contain pasteurized milk[9]

PEOPLE AT RISK: PREGNANT WOMEN AND NEWBORNS

The Centers for Disease Control and Prevention (CDC) estimates that *Listeria* is the third leading cause of death from food poisoning in the United States. About 1,600 people get sick from *Listeria* each year, and about 260 die.

Pregnant women and their newborns are much more likely to get a *Listeria* infection, which is called "listeriosis."
- Pregnant women are 10 times more likely than other people to get a *Listeria* infection.
- Pregnant Hispanic women are 24 times more likely than other people to get a *Listeria* infection.
- A *Listeria* infection can cause miscarriages, stillbirths, and preterm labor.
- A *Listeria* infection can cause serious illness and even death in newborns.

Food Safety Tips

- Wash your hands the right way—for 20 seconds with soap and running water.
- Use a thermometer to make sure your refrigerator is 40 °F (4.4 °C) or lower and your freezer is 0 °F (−17.78 °C) or lower.

---

[9] "Listeria from Food Safety for Moms to Be," U.S. Food and Drug Administration (FDA), September 27, 2018. Available online. URL: www.fda.gov/food/health-educators/listeria-food-safety-moms-be. Accessed May 31, 2023.

- Keep raw meat away from fresh produce and other ready-to-eat food to avoid contamination.
- Thaw or marinate foods in the refrigerator, never on the counter or in the kitchen sink.
- Wash fruits and vegetables (even if you plan to peel them) but do not wash meat, poultry, or eggs.
- Use separate cutting boards for raw produce and for raw meat, poultry, seafood, and eggs.
- Use a food thermometer to be sure food is cooked to its proper temperature.
- Refrigerate leftovers within two hours in shallow covered containers and use within three to four days.
- Know when to throw food out.[10]

Section 46.9 | Toxoplasmosis

WHAT IS TOXOPLASMOSIS?

Toxoplasmosis is an infection caused by a single-celled parasite called "*Toxoplasma gondii*." While the parasite is found throughout the world, more than 40 million people in the United States may be infected with the *Toxoplasma* parasite. The *Toxoplasma* parasite can persist for long periods of time in the bodies of humans (and other animals), possibly even for a lifetime. Of those who are infected, however, very few have symptoms because a healthy person's immune system usually keeps the parasite from causing illness. However, pregnant women and individuals who have compromised immune systems should be cautious; for them, a *Toxoplasma* infection could cause serious health problems.

---

[10] "People at Risk–Pregnant Women and Newborns," Centers for Disease Control and Prevention (CDC), October 25, 2022. Available online. URL: www.cdc.gov/listeria/risk-groups/pregnant-women.html. Accessed May 31, 2023.

HOW DO PEOPLE GET TOXOPLASMOSIS?

A *Toxoplasma* infection occurs in one of the following ways:
- eating undercooked, contaminated meat (especially pork, lamb, and venison) or shellfish (i.e., oysters, clams, or mussels)
- accidental ingestion of undercooked, contaminated meat or shellfish after handling them and not washing hands thoroughly (*Toxoplasma* cannot be absorbed through intact skin.)
- eating food that was contaminated by knives, utensils, cutting boards, and other foods that have had contact with raw, contaminated meat or shellfish
- drinking water contaminated with *T. gondii*
- accidentally swallowing the parasite through contact with cat feces that contain *Toxoplasma* that might happen by:
  - cleaning a cat's litter box when the cat has shed *Toxoplasma* in its feces
  - touching or ingesting anything that has come into contact with cat feces that contain *Toxoplasma*
  - accidentally ingesting contaminated soil (e.g., not washing hands after gardening or eating unwashed fruits or vegetables from a garden)
- mother-to-child (congenital) transmission
- receiving an infected organ transplant or infected blood via transfusion though this is rare

WHAT ARE THE SIGNS AND SYMPTOMS OF TOXOPLASMOSIS?

Symptoms of the infection vary.
- Most people who become infected with *T. gondii* are not aware of it because they have no symptoms at all.
- Some people who have toxoplasmosis may feel as if they have the "flu" with swollen lymph glands or muscle aches and pains that may last for a month or more.
- Severe toxoplasmosis, causing damage to the brain, eyes, or other organs, can develop from an acute *Toxoplasma* infection or one that had occurred earlier

461

in life and is now reactivated. Severe toxoplasmosis is more likely in individuals who have weak immune systems; though occasionally, even persons with healthy immune systems may experience eye damage from toxoplasmosis.

- Signs and symptoms of ocular toxoplasmosis can include reduced vision, blurred vision, pain (often with bright light), redness of the eye, and sometimes tearing. Ophthalmologists sometimes prescribe medicine to treat active diseases. Whether or not medication is recommended depends on the size of the eye lesion, the location, and the characteristics of the lesion (acute active versus chronic not progressing). An ophthalmologist will provide the best care for ocular toxoplasmosis.
- Most infants who are infected while still in the womb have no symptoms at birth, but they may develop symptoms later in life. A small percentage of infected newborns have serious eye or brain damage at birth.

WHO IS AT RISK OF DEVELOPING SEVERE TOXOPLASMOSIS?

People who are most likely to develop severe toxoplasmosis include the following:

- infants born to mothers who are newly infected with *T. gondii* during or just before pregnancy
- persons with severely weakened immune systems, such as individuals with acquired immunodeficiency syndrome (AIDS), those taking certain types of chemotherapy, and those who have recently received an organ transplant

WHAT SHOULD YOU DO IF YOU THINK YOU ARE AT RISK OF SEVERE TOXOPLASMOSIS?

If you are planning to become pregnant, your health-care provider may test you for *T. gondii*. If the test is positive, it means you have already been infected sometime in your life. There is usually little need to worry about passing the infection to your baby. If the test is negative, take necessary precautions to avoid infection.

If you are already pregnant, you and your health-care provider should discuss your risk for toxoplasmosis. Your health-care provider may order a blood sample for testing.

If you have a weakened immune system, ask your doctor about having your blood tested for *Toxoplasma*. If your test is positive, your doctor can tell you if and when you need to take medicine to prevent the infection from reactivating. If your test is negative, it means you need to take precautions to avoid infection.

WHAT SHOULD YOU DO IF YOU THINK YOU MAY HAVE TOXOPLASMOSIS?

If you suspect that you may have toxoplasmosis, talk to your health-care provider. Your provider may order one or more varieties of blood tests specific for toxoplasmosis. The results from the different tests can help your provider determine if you have a *T. gondii* infection and whether it is a recent (acute) infection.

WHAT IS THE TREATMENT FOR TOXOPLASMOSIS?

Once a diagnosis of toxoplasmosis is confirmed, you and your health-care provider can discuss whether treatment is necessary. In an otherwise healthy person who is not pregnant, treatment is usually not needed. If symptoms occur, they typically go away within a few weeks to months. For pregnant women or persons who have weakened immune systems, medications are available to treat toxoplasmosis.

HOW CAN YOU PREVENT TOXOPLASMOSIS?

The following are a few steps you can take to reduce your chances of becoming infected with *T. gondii*:

- Cook food to an internal temperature high enough to kill harmful pathogens such as *Toxoplasma*. The only way to tell if food is safely cooked is to use a food thermometer. You cannot tell if food is safely cooked by checking its color and texture (except for seafood).

- Use a food thermometer to ensure foods are cooked to a safe internal temperature. Learn how to place the thermometer correctly in different food to get an accurate reading.
  - whole cuts of beef, veal, lamb, and pork, including fresh ham: 145 °F (62.8 °C; then allow the meat to rest for three minutes before carving or eating)
  - fish with fins: 145 °F (62.8 °C; or cook until the flesh is opaque and separates easily with a fork)
  - ground meats, such as beef and pork: 160 °F (71.1 °C)
  - all poultry, including ground chicken and turkey: 165 °F (73.9 °C)
  - leftovers and casseroles: 165 °F (73.9 °C)
- Check the chart available at www.foodsafety.gov/food-safety-charts/safe-minimum-internal-temperatures for a detailed list of temperatures and foods.
- Freeze meat* for several days at subzero (0 °F (−17.78 °C)) temperatures before cooking to greatly reduce the chance of infection.

*Freezing does not reliably kill other parasites that may be found in meat (such as certain species of Trichinella) or harmful bacteria. Cooking meat to the U.S. Department of Agriculture (USDA) recommended internal temperatures is the safest method to destroy all parasites and other pathogens.

- Rinse fresh fruits and vegetables under running water.
- Wash your utensils, cutting boards, and countertops with hot, soapy water after preparing each food item.
- Do not eat raw or undercooked oysters, mussels, or clams (these may be contaminated with Toxoplasma that has washed into seawater).
- Do not drink unpasteurized goat's milk.
- Wear gloves when gardening and during any contact with soil or sand because it might be contaminated with cat

feces that contain *Toxoplasma*. Wash hands with soap and water after gardening or contact with soil or sand.
- Ensure that the cat litter box is changed daily. The *Toxoplasma* parasite does not become infectious until one to five days after it is shed in a cat's feces.
- Wash hands with soap and water after cleaning out a cat's litter box.
- Teach children the importance of washing hands to prevent infection.

WHEN SHOULD YOU BE CONCERNED ABOUT TOXOPLASMOSIS?

Generally, if you were infected with *Toxoplasma* before becoming pregnant, your baby is protected by your immunity. Some experts suggest waiting for six months after a recent infection to become pregnant.

HOW CAN *TOXOPLASMA* AFFECT YOUR BABY?

If you are newly infected with *Toxoplasma* while you are pregnant or just before pregnancy, then you can pass the infection on to your baby. You may not have any symptoms from the infection. Most infected infants do not have symptoms at birth but can develop serious symptoms later in life, such as blindness or mental disability. Occasionally, infected newborns have serious eye or brain damage at birth.

HOW DO YOU KNOW IF YOU HAVE BEEN INFECTED WITH *TOXOPLASMA*?

Your health-care provider may suggest one or more varieties of blood tests to check for antibodies to *Toxoplasma*.

HOW IS TOXOPLASMOSIS SPREAD?

Cats play an important role in the spread of toxoplasmosis. They become infected by eating infected rodents, birds, or other small animals. The parasite is then passed into the cat's feces. Kittens and cats can shed millions of parasites in their feces for as long as three weeks after infection. Mature cats are less likely to shed *Toxoplasma* if they have been previously infected. Cats and kittens prefer litter boxes, garden soils, and sandboxes for elimination, and you may be exposed unintentionally by touching your mouth after changing a litter box or after gardening without gloves. Fruits and vegetables may have contact with contaminated soil or water also, and you can be infected by eating fruits and vegetables if they are not cooked, washed, or peeled.

WHAT ARE THE BEST WAYS TO PROTECT YOU OR YOUR BABY AGAINST TOXOPLASMOSIS?

Cat owners and women who are exposed to cats should follow these tips to reduce exposure to *Toxoplasma*:

- Avoid changing cat litter if possible. If no one else can perform the task, wear disposable gloves and wash your hands with soap and water afterward.
- Ensure that the cat litter box is changed daily. The *Toxoplasma* parasite does not become infectious until one to five days after it is shed in a cat's feces.
- Feed your cat commercial dry or canned food, not raw or undercooked meats.
- Keep cats indoors.
- Avoid stray cats, especially kittens. Do not get a new cat while you are pregnant.
- Keep outdoor sandboxes covered.
- Wear gloves when gardening and during contact with soil or sand because it might be contaminated with cat feces that contain *Toxoplasma*. Wash hands with soap and water after gardening or contact with soil or sand.
- Wash your hands and safely diaper and feed your baby.

CAN YOU BREASTFEED YOUR BABY IF YOU CONTRACTED A *TOXOPLASMA* INFECTION DURING PREGNANCY?

Yes. Breast milk transmission of *Toxoplasma* infection is not likely. While *Toxoplasma* infection has been associated with infants who consumed unpasteurized goat's milk, there are no studies documenting breast milk transmission of *Toxoplasma* infection in humans. If a nursing woman were to experience cracked and bleeding nipples or breast inflammation within several weeks following a recent *Toxoplasma* infection (when the organism is still in her bloodstream), it is theoretically possible that she could transmit *Toxoplasma* to the infant through her breast milk. Immune-suppressed women could have *Toxoplasma* in their bloodstream for longer periods of time. However, the likelihood of human milk transmission is still very small.

IS THERE TREATMENT AVAILABLE FOR TOXOPLASMOSIS?

If you are infected during pregnancy, medication is available. You and your baby should be closely monitored during your pregnancy and after your baby is born.[11]

---

[11] "Toxoplasmosis: General FAQs," Centers for Disease Control and Prevention (CDC), December 1, 2022. Available online. URL: www.cdc.gov/parasites/toxoplasmosis/gen_info/faqs.html. Accessed June 2, 2023.

Chapter 47 | Amniotic Fluid Abnormalities

In colloquial terms, amniotic fluid is referred to as a pregnant woman's "water." This watery fluid surrounds the fetus in the uterus. Both the fluid and fetus are contained in a membrane called the "amniotic sac," which develops 12 days after conception. The fluid is clear to pale yellow in color and is made up of a combination of water, proteins, electrolytes, carbohydrates, lipids, phospholipids, and urea, with some fetal cells. The amount of fluid increases with gestational age, and the normal volume varies from 800 to 1,000 mL.

The volume is measured using a method called "amniotic fluid index" (AFI). The amniotic fluid acts as a life-support system to:

- cushion and protect the fetus
- allow room for the fetus to move and develop
- maintain a relatively constant temperature
- aid fetal lung development
- develop the fetus's digestive system (as the fetus swallows the fluid)
- act as a barrier to infections
- protect against the squeezing and compression of the umbilical cord (the cord that carries food and oxygen from the mother to the fetus)

COMMON PROBLEMS AND COMPLICATIONS
Abnormal Odor
A foul-smelling odor may be a sign of infection and may present in conjunction with a fever. A woman whose water breaks at home and who notices a foul-smelling odor should contact her doctor immediately.

469

Abnormal Color

Color that differs from clear or pale yellow is an anomaly. Green or brown fluid in near- or full-term pregnancies indicates "meconium," or the first fecal movement of the fetus, which contributes to the change in color. This is an indication that the baby is in distress or that the pregnancy has extended long enough for the fetus to pass the first stool in utero. Blood-tinged fluid during pregnancy may be an indication of cervix dilation or other placental problems. Dark-colored fluid may be an indication of the death of a fetus during pregnancy (intrauterine fetal demise (IUFD)).

"Water Breaking" Too Early

If the "water breaks" too early, this can affect both the mother and the fetus. This occurrence is called "preterm premature rupture of membranes" (PPROM/PROM). Resulting complications include impaired fetal development, early labor and delivery, and possible infection. In such cases, bed rest, intravenous (IV) antibiotics, corticosteroid administration for facilitation of fetal lung maturity, and delaying labor increase the survival chances of the fetus. If born early, the fetus will require neonatal care.

Too Little Amniotic Fluid: Oligohydramnios

Oligo means "less or scanty," and a decreased amount of the amniotic fluid in the uterus is called "oligohydramnios." The causes include:

- urinary tract malformation—a birth defect in the urinary tract causing less fetal urine output
- stunted growth of the fetus (not reaching expected growth)
- chromosomal abnormality
- placenta not functioning normally
- PROM
- post-term pregnancy (pregnancy lasting longer than 40 weeks)
- taking certain drugs, such as angiotensin-converting enzyme (ACE) inhibitors enalapril, captopril,

nonsteroidal anti-inflammatory drugs (NSAIDs), aspirin, ibuprofin, and so on during the second or third trimester

If oligohydramnios is detected in the first half of the pregnancy, then the complications are serious and include:
- potter syndrome—a combination of immature lungs and other deformities
- fetal compression that may result in a flattened nose, recessed chin, limb deformities, and other developmental abnormalities
- stillbirth or an increased chance of miscarriage

If oligohydramnios is detected in the second half of pregnancy, the complications include:
- intrauterine growth restriction (IUGR)—slower growth of the fetus than expected
- placental-cord compression and meconium-stained fluid (dark-colored amniotic fluid)
- preterm birth—the fetus becoming unable to tolerate labor (making cesarean delivery necessary)

Too Much Amniotic Fluid: Polyhydramnios

A high accumulation of the amniotic fluid is called "polyhydramnios." Most of the causes are unknown, but known causes include the following:
- maternal diabetes—elevated blood glucose levels in the mother either before getting pregnant (personal history of diabetes) or during pregnancy (diabetes that developed during gestation)
- multiple births or having more than one fetus (Twin–twin transfusion syndrome (TTTS) in identical-twin pregnancies results in one twin receiving a high amount of blood and the other receiving too little.)
- rhesus incompatibility (Rh disease)—mismatched blood types in the mother and the fetus (Rh antibodies produced by the pregnant woman enter the fetus's blood.)

- fluid buildup in the baby (hydrops fetalis)
- fetal birth defects, such as defects of the brain, spinal cord (spina bifida), heart (fetal arrhythmia), blocked esophagus, gut atresia, and others
- infection during pregnancy

Women with polyhydramnios may experience some of the following symptoms:
- heartburn
- constipation
- swelling of feet and abdominal wall
- breathlessness
- heaviness of bump with uterine contractions and discomfort
- fetal malposition such as breech presentation

The fluid accumulation stretches the uterus and puts more pressure on the pregnant woman's diaphragm, which leads to several other problems, including:
- breathing issues
- bleeding from the vagina post delivery due to a lack of uterine muscle tone
- preterm labor
- PROM
- prolapsed umbilical cord (the umbilical cord coming out of the vagina before the fetus)
- placental abruption (early detachment of the placenta from the walls of the uterus)

Intra-amniotic Infection
This infection develops when bacteria from the vagina enter the uterus and infect tissues around the fetus. Infection of these tissues (such as the amniotic fluid, placenta, the membranes around the fetus, or a combination of these) is collectively called "intra-amniotic infection." Intra-amniotic infection can cause:
- PPROM
- less oxygen in the blood around the time of delivery

- body-wide (systemic) infections, such as sepsis, pneumonia, or meningitis
- seizures
- cerebral palsy
- in certain cases, death

Amniotic Fluid Embolism

The amniotic fluid entering the woman's bloodstream causes a serious reaction and can damage the lungs and heart. A common complication is disseminated intravascular coagulation, in which small blood clots develop throughout the bloodstream. This results in widespread bleeding and a massive loss of blood and is a medical emergency.

Immediate diagnosis and treatment are essential when a pregnant woman presents with the following symptoms:

- sudden difficulty breathing
- low blood pressure
- widespread, uncontrolled bleeding

Blood transfusion and injection of a blood-clotting factor may be lifesaving. Women may require assistance with breathing or drugs to help contractions of the heart. In such cases, immediate delivery of the baby using forceps or a vacuum extractor, or even a cesarean delivery, may be done to save the fetus when it is old enough to survive outside the uterus.

Health-care providers evaluate these abnormalities with the help of ultrasound and determine the best treatment plan based on the severity of the condition.

References

Antonette T. Dulay. "Problems with Amniotic Fluid," MSD Manual, March 2018. Available online. URL www.msdmanuals.com/home/women-s-health-issues/complications-of-pregnancy/problems-with-amniotic-fluid. Accessed June 7, 2023.

Brian S. Carter. "Polyhydramnios and Oligohydramnios," Medscape, September 20, 2017. Available online. URL:

https://reference.medscape.com/article/975821-overview. Accessed June 7, 2023.

"Polyhydramnios," Mayoclinic, November 18, 2017. Available online. URL: www.mayoclinic.org/diseases-conditions/ polyhydramnios/symptoms-causes/syc-2036849. Accessed June 7, 2023.

Chapter 48 | Preeclampsia, Eclampsia, and HELLP Syndrome

Preeclampsia and eclampsia are part of the spectrum of high blood pressure, or hypertensive, disorders that can occur during pregnancy. At the mild end of the spectrum is gestational hypertension, which occurs when a woman who previously had normal blood pressure develops high blood pressure when she is more than 20 weeks pregnant and her blood pressure returns to normal within 12 weeks after delivery. This problem usually occurs without other symptoms. In many cases, gestational hypertension does not harm the mother or fetus. Severe gestational hypertension, however, may be associated with preterm birth and infants who are small for their age at birth. Some women who have gestational hypertension later develop preeclampsia.

Preeclampsia is similar to gestational hypertension because it also involves high blood pressure at or after 20 weeks of pregnancy in a woman whose blood pressure was normal before pregnancy. But preeclampsia can also include blood pressure at or greater than 140/90 mmHg, increased swelling, and protein in the urine. The condition can be serious and is a leading cause of preterm birth (before 37 weeks of pregnancy). If it is severe enough to affect brain function, causing seizures or coma, it is called "eclampsia."

A serious complication of hypertensive disorders in pregnancy is hemolysis, elevated liver enzymes, and low platelet count (HELLP) syndrome, a situation in which a pregnant woman with

475

preeclampsia or eclampsia suffers damage to the liver and blood cells. The letters in the name HELLP stand for the following problems:

- H—hemolysis, in which oxygen-carrying red blood cells break down
- EL—elevated liver enzymes, showing damage to the liver
- LP—low platelet count, meaning that the cells responsible for stopping bleeding are low

Postpartum preeclampsia describes preeclampsia that develops after the baby is delivered, usually between 48 hours and 6 weeks after delivery. Symptoms can include high blood pressure, severe headache, visual changes, upper abdominal pain, and nausea or vomiting. Postpartum preeclampsia can occur regardless of whether a woman has high blood pressure or preeclampsia during pregnancy.

Postpartum eclampsia refers to seizures that occur between 48 and 72 hours after delivery. Symptoms also include high blood pressure and difficulty breathing. About one-third of eclampsia cases occur after delivery, and nearly half of those are more than 48 hours after the birth. Postpartum preeclampsia and eclampsia can be serious and, if not treated quickly, may result in death.

WHAT CAUSES PREECLAMPSIA AND ECLAMPSIA?

The causes of preeclampsia and eclampsia are not known. These disorders previously were believed to be caused by a toxin called "toxemia" in the blood, but health-care providers now know that is not true. Nevertheless, preeclampsia is sometimes still referred to as "toxemia."

To learn more about preeclampsia and eclampsia, scientists are investigating many factors that could contribute to the development and progression of these diseases, including the following:

- placental abnormalities, such as insufficient blood flow
- genetic factors
- environmental exposures
- nutritional factors

- maternal immunology and autoimmune disorders
- cardiovascular and inflammatory changes
- hormonal imbalances

WHAT ARE THE RISKS OF PREECLAMPSIA AND ECLAMPSIA TO THE MOTHER?

Risks during Pregnancy

Preeclampsia during pregnancy is mild in the majority of cases. However, a woman can progress from mild to severe preeclampsia or to full eclampsia very quickly—even in a matter of days. Both preeclampsia and eclampsia can cause serious health problems for the mother and infant.

Women with preeclampsia are at increased risk of damage to the kidneys, liver, brain, and other organ and blood systems. Preeclampsia may also affect the placenta. The condition could lead to a separation of the placenta from the uterus (referred to as placental abruption), preterm birth, and pregnancy loss or stillbirth. In some cases, preeclampsia can lead to organ failure or stroke.

In severe cases, preeclampsia can develop into eclampsia, which includes seizures. Seizures in eclampsia may cause a woman to lose consciousness and twitch uncontrollably. If the fetus is not delivered, these conditions can cause the death of the mother and/or the fetus.

Although most pregnant women in developed countries survive preeclampsia, it is still a major cause of illness and death globally. According to the World Health Organization (WHO), preeclampsia and eclampsia cause 14 percent of maternal deaths each year, or about 50,000–75,000 women worldwide.

Risks after Pregnancy

In "uncomplicated preeclampsia," the mother's high blood pressure and other symptoms usually go back to normal within six weeks of the infant's birth. However, studies have shown that women who had preeclampsia are four times more likely to later develop hypertension (high blood pressure) and are twice as likely to later develop ischemic heart disease (reduced blood supply to the heart muscle, which can cause heart attacks), a blood clot in a vein, and stroke as are women who did not have preeclampsia.

Less commonly, mothers who have preeclampsia can experience permanent damage to their organs, such as their kidneys and liver. They can also experience fluid in the lungs. In the days following birth, women with preeclampsia remain at increased risk of developing eclampsia and seizures.

In some women, preeclampsia develops between 48 hours and 6 weeks after they deliver their baby—a condition called "postpartum preeclampsia." Postpartum preeclampsia can occur in women who had preeclampsia during pregnancy and among those who did not. One study found that slightly more than one-half of women who had postpartum preeclampsia did not have preeclampsia during pregnancy. If a woman has seizures within 72 hours of delivery, she may have postpartum eclampsia. It is important to recognize and treat postpartum preeclampsia and eclampsia because the risk of complications may be higher than if the conditions had occurred during pregnancy. Postpartum preeclampsia and eclampsia can progress very quickly if not treated and may lead to stroke or death.

WHAT ARE THE RISKS OF PREECLAMPSIA AND ECLAMPSIA TO THE FETUS?

Preeclampsia may be related to problems with the placenta early in the pregnancy. Such problems pose risks to the fetus, including the following:

- lack of oxygen and nutrients, which can impair fetal growth
- preterm birth
- stillbirth if placental abruption (separation of the placenta from the uterine wall) leads to heavy bleeding in the mother
- infant death

Stillbirths are more likely to occur when the mother has a more severe form of preeclampsia, including HELLP syndrome.

Infants whose mothers had preeclampsia are also at increased risk of later problems, even if they were born at full term (39 weeks of pregnancy). Infants born preterm due to preeclampsia face a higher risk of some long-term health issues, mostly related to being born early, including learning disorders, cerebral palsy, epilepsy, deafness, and blindness. Infants born preterm may also have to be hospitalized for a long time after birth and may be smaller than infants born full-term. Infants who have experienced poor growth in the uterus may later be at higher risk of diabetes, congestive heart failure, and high blood pressure.

WHO IS AT RISK OF PREECLAMPSIA?

Although preeclampsia occurs primarily in first pregnancies, a woman who had preeclampsia in a previous pregnancy is seven times more likely to develop preeclampsia in a later pregnancy. Other factors that can increase a woman's risk include the following:

- chronic high blood pressure or kidney disease before pregnancy
- high blood pressure or preeclampsia in an earlier pregnancy
- obesity (Women with overweight or obesity are also more likely to have preeclampsia in more than one pregnancy.)
- age (Women older than 40 are at higher risk.)
- multiple gestation (being pregnant with more than one fetus)
- African American ethnicity (Also, among women who have had preeclampsia before, non-White women are more likely than White women to develop preeclampsia again in a later pregnancy.)
- family history of preeclampsia

Preeclampsia is also more common among women who have histories of certain health conditions, such as migraines, diabetes, rheumatoid arthritis (RA), lupus, scleroderma, urinary tract infections (UTIs), gum disease, polycystic ovary syndrome (PCOS), multiple sclerosis (MS), gestational diabetes, and sickle cell disease.

Preeclampsia is also more common in pregnancies resulting from egg donation, donor insemination, or in vitro fertilization

(IVF) The U.S. Preventative Services Task Force (USPSTF) recommends that women who are at high risk of preeclampsia take low-dose aspirin starting after 12 weeks of pregnancy to prevent preeclampsia. Women who are pregnant or who are thinking about getting pregnant should talk with their health-care provider about preeclampsia risk and ways to reduce the risk.

WHAT ARE THE SYMPTOMS OF PREECLAMPSIA, ECLAMPSIA, AND HELLP SYNDROME?

Preeclampsia

Possible symptoms of preeclampsia include the following:

- high blood pressure
- too much protein in the urine
- swelling in a woman's face and hands (A woman's feet might swell too, but swollen feet are common during pregnancy and may not signal a problem.)
- systemic problems, such as headache, blurred vision, and right upper quadrant abdominal pain

Eclampsia

The following symptoms are cause for immediate concern:

- seizures
- severe headache
- vision problems, such as temporary blindness
- abdominal pain, especially in the upper right area of the belly
- nausea and vomiting
- smaller urine output or not urinating very often

HELLP Syndrome

HELLP syndrome can lead to serious complications, including liver failure and death. A pregnant woman with HELLP syndrome might bleed or bruise easily and/or experience abdominal pain, nausea or vomiting, headache, or extreme fatigue. Although most women who develop HELLP syndrome already have high blood pressure and preeclampsia, sometimes, the syndrome is the first sign. In addition, HELLP syndrome can occur without a woman having either high blood pressure or protein in her urine.

HOW DO HEALTH-CARE PROVIDERS DIAGNOSE PREECLAMPSIA, ECLAMPSIA, AND HELLP SYNDROME?

A health-care provider will check a pregnant woman's blood pressure and urine during each prenatal visit. If the blood pressure reading is considered high (140/90 mmHg or higher), especially after the 20th week of pregnancy, the health-care provider will likely perform blood tests and more extensive lab tests to look for extra protein in the urine (called "proteinuria") as well as other symptoms.

The American College of Obstetricians and Gynecologists (ACOG) provides the following criteria for a diagnosis of gestational hypertension, preeclampsia, eclampsia, and HELLP syndrome.

Gestational hypertension is diagnosed if a pregnant woman has high blood pressure but no protein in the urine. Gestational hypertension occurs when women whose blood pressure levels were normal before pregnancy develop high blood pressure after 20 weeks of pregnancy. Gestational hypertension can progress into preeclampsia. Mild preeclampsia is diagnosed when a pregnant woman has:

- Systolic blood pressure (top number) of 140 mmHg or higher or diastolic blood pressure (bottom number) of 90 mmHg or higher and either urine with 0.3 g or more of protein in a 24-hour specimen (a collection of every drop of urine within 24 hours) or a protein-to-creatinine ratio greater than 0.3 or:
  - blood tests that show kidney or liver dysfunction
  - fluid in the lungs and difficulty breathing
  - visual impairments

Severe preeclampsia occurs when a pregnant woman has any of the following:

- systolic blood pressure of 160 mmHg or higher or diastolic blood pressure of 110 mmHg or higher on two occasions at least four hours apart while the patient is on bed rest
- urine with 5 g or more of protein in a 24-hour specimen or 3 g or more of protein on two random urine samples collected at least four hours apart
- test results suggesting kidney or liver damage—for example, blood tests that reveal low numbers of platelets or high liver enzymes
- severe, unexplained stomach pain that does not respond to medication
- symptoms that include visual disturbances, difficulty breathing, or fluid buildup

Eclampsia occurs when women with preeclampsia develop seizures. The seizures can happen before or during labor or after the baby is delivered.

HELLP syndrome is diagnosed when laboratory tests show hemolysis (burst red blood cells release hemoglobin into the blood plasma), elevated liver enzymes, and low platelets. There also may or may not be extra protein in the urine.

Some women may also be diagnosed with superimposed preeclampsia—a situation in which the woman develops preeclampsia on top of high blood pressure that was present before she got pregnant. Health-care providers look for an increase in blood pressure and protein in the urine, fluid buildup, or both for a diagnosis of superimposed preeclampsia.

In addition to tests that might diagnose preeclampsia or similar problems, health-care providers may do other tests to assess the health of the mother and fetus, including:

- blood tests to see how well the mother's liver and kidneys are working

- blood tests to check blood platelet levels to see how well the mother's blood is clotting
- blood tests to count the total number of red blood cells in the mother's blood
- a maternal weight check
- an ultrasound to assess the fetus's size
- a check of the fetus's heart rate
- a physical exam to look for swelling in the mother's face, hands, or legs, as well as abdominal tenderness or an enlarged liver

WHAT ARE THE TREATMENTS FOR PREECLAMPSIA, ECLAMPSIA, AND HELLP SYNDROME?

Delivering the fetus can help resolve preeclampsia and eclampsia, but symptoms can continue even after delivery, and some of them can be serious.

Treatment decisions for preeclampsia, eclampsia, and HELLP syndrome need to take into account how severe the condition is, the potential for maternal complications, how far along the pregnancy is, and the potential risks to the fetus. Ideally, the health-care provider will minimize risks to the mother while giving the fetus as much time as possible to mature before delivery. The USPSTF recommends that women at high risk of preeclampsia take low-dose aspirin starting after 12 weeks of pregnancy to prevent the condition from occurring.

Preeclampsia Treatment

If the pregnancy is at 37 weeks or later, the health-care provider will usually want to deliver the fetus to treat preeclampsia and avoid further complications.

If the pregnancy is at less than 37 weeks, however, the woman and her health-care provider may consider treatment options that give the fetus more time to develop, depending on how severe the condition is. A health-care provider may consider the following options:

- If the preeclampsia is mild, it may be possible to wait to deliver. To help prevent further complications, the health-care provider may ask the woman to go on bed rest to try to lower blood pressure and increase blood flow to the placenta.

- Close monitoring of the woman and her fetus will be needed. Tests for the mother might include blood and urine tests to see if the preeclampsia is progressing, such as tests to assess platelet counts, liver enzymes, kidney function, and urinary protein levels. Tests for the fetus might include ultrasound, heart rate monitoring, assessment of fetal growth, and amniotic fluid assessment.
- Anticonvulsive medication, such as magnesium sulfate, might be used to prevent a seizure.
- In some cases, such as with severe preeclampsia, the woman will be admitted to the hospital, so she can be monitored closely and continuously. Treatment in the hospital might include intravenous medication to control blood pressure and prevent seizures or other complications, as well as steroid injections to help speed up the development of the fetus's lungs.

When a woman has severe preeclampsia and is at 34 weeks of pregnancy or later, the ACOG recommends delivery as soon as medically possible. If the pregnancy is at less than 34 weeks, health-care providers will probably prescribe corticosteroids to help speed up the maturation of the fetal lungs before attempting delivery.

Preterm delivery may be necessary, even if that means likely complications for the infant, because of the risk of severe maternal complications. The symptoms of preeclampsia usually go away within six weeks of delivery.

Eclampsia Treatment

Eclampsia—the onset of seizures in a woman with preeclampsia—is considered a medical emergency. Immediate treatment, usually in a hospital, is needed to stop the mother's seizures, treat blood pressure levels that are too high, and deliver the fetus.

Magnesium sulfate (a type of mineral) may be given to treat active seizures and prevent future seizures. Antihypertensive medications may be given to lower blood pressure.

Treatment for HELLP Syndrome

HELLP syndrome, a severe complication of preeclampsia and eclampsia, can lead to serious complications for the mother, including liver failure and death, as well as the fetus. The health-care provider may consider the following treatments after a diagnosis of HELLP syndrome:

* delivery of the fetus
* hospitalization to provide intravenous medication to control blood pressure and prevent seizures or other complications, as well as steroid injections to help speed up the development of the fetus's lungs

Postpartum Treatments

As mentioned earlier, some women develop preeclampsia or eclampsia after they deliver their babies. The ACOG recommends that health-care providers closely monitor women who have high blood pressure or preeclampsia during pregnancy for 72 hours after delivery, either at home or in the hospital. Because postpartum preeclampsia and eclampsia can progress quickly and can have serious effects, it is important to get treatment immediately.

Depending on a woman's specific health situation, treatment may include medications to prevent blood pressure from reaching dangerously high levels and causing stroke or other problems associated with extremely high blood pressure. It may also include medications to treat or prevent seizures.

One study looked at women who came to the emergency room with a diagnosis of postpartum preeclampsia. The most common warning symptoms in these cases were headache, vision changes, and nausea or abdominal pain. Nearly all of these women had high blood pressure when admitted, and some had already had seizures at home before coming to the hospital. Treatment for postpartum preeclampsia follows the guidelines used to treat preeclampsia during pregnancy. The women in the study received magnesium sulfate to treat or prevent seizures and, if needed, additional treatment for their high blood pressure.[1]

[1] "Preeclampsia and Eclampsia," *Eunice Kennedy Shriver* National Institute of Child Health and Human Development (NICHD), January 31, 2017. Available online. URL: www.nichd.nih.gov/health/topics/preeclampsia. Accessed June 5, 2023.

Chapter 49 | Hyperemesis Gravidarum

KNOW WHAT MORNING SICKNESS IS

Experiencing bouts of nausea and vomiting is called "morning sickness"; although unpleasant, it is considered a normal part of a healthy pregnancy. For most women, it occurs during the first trimester of pregnancy, that is, around the sixth week of pregnancy and subsequently improves or disappears around week 14. Despite the name "morning sickness," it can occur any time of the day or night. It usually needs no treatment and resolves or subsides on its own.

KNOW WHAT IS NOT NORMAL

When morning sickness becomes severe with persistent nausea and multiple episodes of vomiting per day (more than 50 times per day for some unfortunates), this medical condition needs treatment. The condition of excessive (hyper) vomiting (emesis) during pregnancy (gravidarum) is termed medically as "hyperemesis gravidarum" (HG).

ABOUT HYPEREMESIS GRAVIDARUM

This is a rare pregnancy-related condition that follows a similar timeline to morning sickness (i.e., it begins between weeks 4 and 5 and lasts throughout the entire pregnancy). Sadly, health histories say that it may continue to happen in subsequent pregnancies for women who experience it during their first pregnancy. If left untreated, it can interfere with a woman's health, as well as the fetus's ability to thrive. There are many ways to manage this condition and minimize the risk of having a low-birth-weight baby.

WHY DO SOME WOMEN GET HYPEREMESIS GRAVIDARUM, WHILE OTHERS DO NOT?

The exact etiology (cause) is still unknown, but "hormonal changes" and "hereditary reasons" are to blame. Human chorionic gonadotropin (hCG), when present at the highest level in a pregnant woman's body, can cause nausea. HG is commonly evident in a woman whose close family members, such as mothers and sisters, have had it. This is why researchers believe the condition might be hereditary. A risk factor is something that increases a person's chances of getting the disease or condition but does not mean that the person will necessarily develop that particular condition. In some cases, the following can put a woman into a high-risk category:

- carrying multiples (twins, triplets, etc.)
- history of HG in a previous pregnancy
- history of motion sickness
- history of migraine headaches with nausea and vomiting episodes

KNOW THE SYMPTOMS AND NOTICE THE SIGNS

- prolonged nausea and vomiting (increasing in severity as pregnancy progresses)
- food aversion/being unable to eat food (leading to more than 10-pound weight loss)
- feeling dizzy and lightheaded (fainting) due to hypotension (low blood pressure) when standing
- being unable to drink fluids (becoming dehydrated)
- extreme fatigue and depression (leading to confusion and headaches)

Other possible symptoms one may experience in addition to the main symptoms are:

- heightened sense of smell
- ptyalism (excessive saliva production)
- ketosis (build-up of acidic chemicals in blood and urine)

- constipation, headaches, and decrease in urination (due to dehydration)
- urinary incontinence due to bladder pressure caused by excessive vomiting in combination with relaxin hormone
- rapid heart rate
- loss of skin elasticity
- pressure sores if one is bedbound due to sickness

In addition to feeling unwell with some of the mentioned symptoms, you may also feel anxious about going out and about because of the need to vomit. This can result in feelings of isolation as some people may not fully understand what you are going through and question whether you can cope with the rest of the pregnancy.

GET IT DIAGNOSED AND TREATED

Health-care providers may take your medical history, inquire about your symptoms, perform a physical exam, and order some blood tests to diagnose HG. During the initial stage, they may recommend the following:

- **Consuming a bland diet**. Strictly avoid spicy and fatty foods.
- **Eating frequent small meals, as well as dry crackers in the morning**. High-protein snacking will help maintain nutrition.
- **Complete bed rest**. This is to provide comfort (but being bedbound for a long time should be avoided as this may cause muscle loss and bedsores).
- **Acupressure**. Applying pressure to some locations on the body gently reduces nausea. These points are located three finger lengths away from the crease of the wrist, at the middle of the inner wrist, and between the two tendons. Three-minute pressure sessions and sea bands (pressure-point wristbands available at a local drug store) can be of help.

- **Herbs.** Using ginger or peppermint, especially in tea, might help.
- **Homeopathic remedies.** These are usually effective and nontoxic medicines.
- **Hypnosis.** This is to give mental strength and reduce depression and anxiety.

Some cases of HG are severe and will not settle with the above-mentioned treatment or lifestyle modifications, requiring hospitalization. Hospital treatment includes the following:

- **Using tube feeding for a short period of time.** It means not eating by mouth to rest the gastrointestinal system. The following are the two types of tube feeding:
  - **Nasogastric tube feeding.** Nutrients will be passed through a tube that passes through the nose into the stomach.
  - **Percutaneous endoscopic gastrostomy.** Nutrients will be passed through the abdomen into the stomach via a surgical method.
- **Intravenous (IV) fluids.** This is to hydrate and restore electrolytes, nutrients, and vitamins.
- **Medications.** They include antihistamines, metoclopramide, Promethazine, Meclizine, Droperidol, and other anti-reflux medications. It is always inadvisable to self-medicate with over-the-counter (OTC) drugs and have a doctor prescribe the proper dose and remedy instead.
- **Appropriate treatment.** It can make one feel better, reduce symptoms, and sometimes completely resolve symptoms.

References

Elana Pearl Ben-Joseph. "Severe Morning Sickness (Hyperemesis Gravidarum)," KidsHealth—from Nemours, April 2014. Available online. URL: https://kidshealth.org/en/parents/hyperemesis-gravidarum.html. Accessed June 8, 2023.

"Hyperemesis Gravidarum," American Pregnancy Association—Promoting Pregnancy Wellness, July 27, 2018. Available online. URL: http://americanpregnancy. org/pregnancy-complications/hyperemesis-gravidarum. Accessed June 8, 2023.

"Hyperemesis Gravidarum (Severe Nausea and Vomiting during Pregnancy)," Cleveland Clinic, November 4, 2016. Available online. URL: https://my.clevelandclinic.org/ health/diseases/12232-hyperemesis-gravidarum-severe-nausea--vomiting-during-pregnancy. Accessed June 8, 2023.

Chapter 50 | Placental Complications

The placenta is a flat, circular organ attached to the wall of the womb (uterus) and the umbilical cord. The umbilical cord is a long muscular organ that links the fetus to the placenta. Normally, the placenta grows on the upper part of the uterus and can be seen in an ultrasound around week 18. It stays there until the fetus is delivered. Some of the significant functions of the placenta are as follows:

- It acts as a filter between the mother and fetus.
- It filters nutrients and oxygen from the mother's blood before reaching the fetus, as well as waste products, such as carbon dioxide, from the fetus to the mother's bloodstream for disposal.
- It also maintains "no blood-to-blood contact" between the mother and fetus; in other words, an intermingling of maternal and fetal blood does not occur here.
- It produces hormones that help the fetus grow and develop.
- It can protect the fetus against bacterial infections but cannot protect against viral infections.

Towards the end of the pregnancy, it also passes some of the mother's antibodies to the fetus in order to give immunity to the fetus for about three months after birth.

HOW IS THE PLACENTA DELIVERED?

If the fetus is delivered through the birth canal (vagina), it is called "vaginal/normal delivery." In such cases, the placenta will also be delivered vaginally (refer to Figure 50.1). During the last (third) stage of labor (after childbirth), the uterine contractions continue and push the placenta to the vagina. On occasions, the health-care provider might massage the lower abdomen to encourage uterine contractions in order to expel the placenta, and the mother might be asked to push again to deliver the placenta. When the placenta separates from the wall of the uterus and comes out of the vagina, it is called "afterbirth."

If the fetus is delivered by cesarean section, then the health-care provider will remove the placenta in its entirety from the uterus during the surgical procedure. They will examine the placenta to make sure it is intact, and if it is not intact, they remove any remaining fragments from the uterus completely in order to prevent bleeding and infection.

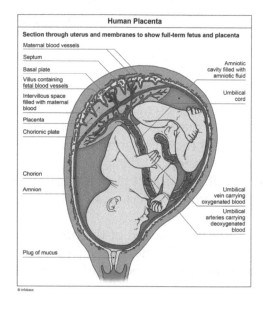

Figure 50.1. Human Placenta

Infobase

WHAT ARE THE FACTORS THAT AFFECT PLACENTAL HEALTH?

- maternal age, if older than 35 (becoming pregnant after 40 years of age)
- high blood pressure in pregnant women (developed either before pregnancy or during pregnancy)
- premature rupture of the membranes (the fluid-filled membrane that surrounds and cushions the fetus leaking or breaking before labor)
- twin or other multiple pregnancies (if carrying more than one fetus)
- substance abuse/misuse (smoking and illegal drug usage, such as cocaine, etc., during pregnancy).
- trauma to the abdomen, such as a fall
- previous surgery on the uterus, such as a cesarean section or surgery to remove fibroids
- placental problem during the previous pregnancy
- blood clotting disorders (conditions that increase the likelihood of clotting)

Some drugs, alcohol, and nicotine can cross the placenta and cause damage to the fetus when used during pregnancy. So it is best for pregnant women to be cautious and follow the health-care provider's instructions.

WHAT ARE THE MOST COMMON PLACENTAL COMPLICATIONS?

The following are the complications that can affect the placenta during pregnancy or childbirth:

- **Placenta previa**. It is also called the "low-lying placenta." This is when the placenta develops low in the uterus and obstructs the passageway of childbirth. In such cases, vaginal delivery becomes impossible, necessitating a cesarean section. Risk factors include pregnancy after the age of 35, having scarring from a previous cesarean section or abortion, smoking or tobacco use during pregnancy, and having more than one delivery. Also, women with placenta previa may have placenta accreta; therefore, seeing the placenta positioned low in an ultrasound can be a red flag for placenta previa, or placenta accreta.

- **Invasive placenta**. This is when all or part of the placenta attaches deeply to the myometrium (muscular layer of the uterine wall). Based on the depth of the attachment, it is classified into the following three grades:
  - **Placenta accreta**. The placenta attaches itself too deeply and too firmly to the uterus.
  - **Placenta increta**. The placenta attaches itself even more deeply to the muscle wall of the uterus.
  - **Placenta percreta**. The placenta attaches itself to the uterus and grows through the uterus, sometimes invading/extending itself to other organs such as the urinary bladder or rectum. This raises the complication of placenta attachment to other organs, such as the rectum, urinary bladder, and so on.

  This condition makes it difficult for the placenta to completely detach from the uterus during delivery or childbirth, leading to life-threatening excessive bleeding. During the ultrasound scan, if there is an unusually high blood flow in the uterus, it is considered a sign of placenta accreta.

- **Placental insufficiency**. This is when the placenta is not providing adequate nutrients and/or blood flow to the fetus, leading to an increased likelihood of preeclampsia/toxemia (characterized by high blood pressure that occurs after 20 weeks of pregnancy) and infant developmental issues. Blood-related conditions, such as diabetes or hypertension, in the mother increase the risk of placental insufficiency.

- **Placental abruption**. This is an early detachment of the placenta from the wall of the uterus before delivery/childbirth and causes abdominal and/or uterine pain along with bloody pregnancy discharge, contractions, and fast fetal heart rate. It commonly happens during the third trimester but can happen anytime during pregnancy. The degree of detachment can range from mild (resolves with rest and monitoring) to severe (requires emergency delivery). If vaginal bleeding is evident at any point of pregnancy, contact the health-care professional immediately.

- **Placental infarcts.** This is when areas of dead tissues called "infarcts" are present in the placenta, resulting in reduced blood flow. It is mainly caused by pregnancy-induced hypertension (gestational hypertension). In certain cases of severe hypertension, this blood flow reduction can be injurious to the fetus and, in extreme cases, leads to fetal death. Care should be taken to keep the blood pressure under control to avoid such scenarios.

HOW TO REDUCE THE RISK OF PLACENTAL COMPLICATIONS

If pregnant women experience any of the following symptoms, it may be a sign of a placental health problem:

- abdominal pain
- uterine contraction
- intolerable back pain
- vaginal bleeding

Most of the placental problems cannot be prevented directly; however, one can take steps to promote placental health as a part of achieving a healthy pregnancy. The following are a few examples:

- regular follow-ups throughout the pregnancy as instructed by the health-care provider, as they will note the position and size of the placenta in the subsequent follow-up ultrasound scans in order to rule out any abnormality and prevent further complications
- close monitoring if the mother has any ongoing health conditions, such as high blood pressure, and being compliant with the advised treatment plan
- avoidance of smoking and other illegal drug/substance usage during pregnancy
- if the mother had a placental problem during a previous pregnancy, consulting with the

health-care provider regarding ways to reduce the risk of experiencing the same problem in the current pregnancy

- keeping the health-care provider informed about any previous surgeries the mother had, especially in the abdomen or uterus

References

"Complications of the Placenta," AboutKidsHealth, September 11, 2009. Available online. URL: www.aboutkidshealth.ca/Article?contentid=354&language=English. Accessed June 8, 2023.

"Pregnancy Complications," American Pregnancy Association, April 26, 2017. Available online. URL: https://americanpregnancy.org/pregnancy-complications. Accessed June 8, 2023.

"Types of Placental Disorders," Beth Israel Deaconess Medical Center, April 22, 2011. Available online. URL: www.bidmc.org/centers-and-departments/obstetrics-and-gynecology/pregnancy/high-risk-pregnancy-maternal-fetal-medicine/new-england-center-for-placental-disorders/disorder-types. Accessed June 8, 2023.

Chapter 51 | Rhesus Incompatibility

There are four major blood types: A, B, O, and AB. The types are based on substances on the surface of the blood cells. Another blood type is called "rhesus" (Rh). Rh factor is a protein in red blood cells. Most people are Rh-positive; they have the Rh factor. Rh-negative people do not have it. The Rh factor is inherited through genes.

When you are pregnant, blood from your baby can cross into your bloodstream, especially during delivery. If you are Rh-negative and your baby is Rh-positive, your body will react to the baby's blood as a foreign substance. It will create antibodies (proteins) against the baby's blood. These antibodies usually do not cause problems during a first pregnancy.

But Rh incompatibility may cause problems in later pregnancies if the baby is Rh-positive. This is because the antibodies stay in your body once they have formed. The antibodies can cross the placenta and attack the baby's red blood cells. The baby could get Rh disease, a serious condition that can cause a serious type of anemia.

Blood tests can tell whether you have the Rh factor and whether your body has made antibodies. Injections of a medicine called "Rh immune globulin" can keep your body from making Rh antibodies. It helps prevent the problems of Rh incompatibility. If treatment is needed for the baby, it can include supplements to help the body make red blood cells and blood transfusions.[1]

[1] MedlinePlus, "Rh Incompatibility," National Institutes of Health (NIH), June 19, 2017. Available online. URL: https://medlineplus.gov/rhincompatibility.html. Accessed July 3, 2023.

Chapter 52 | Umbilical Cord Abnormalities

The umbilical cord, which is the lifeline between a mother and her baby during pregnancy, is a narrow, flexible, tube-like cord that connects the baby to the mother in her womb. This cord attaches the mother's placenta and the baby's stomach, which later on is known as the "belly button." The umbilical cord, which begins to form after five weeks of conception, continues to grow until 28 weeks of pregnancy. Reaching an average length of 22 inches, the umbilical cord contains a vein that carries oxygen- and nutrient-rich blood to the baby and two arteries that carry deoxygenated blood out from the baby's body. During the last stage of pregnancy, the placenta passes antibodies from the mother to her baby through the umbilical cord. These provide protection for the baby from infections for around three months after birth.

COMMON UMBILICAL CORD DEFECTS

The umbilical cord may be affected by a variety of conditions and is possible that the cord becomes too long or too short. It can also attach to the placenta incorrectly, or it may become knotted or compressed. Anomalies in the cord can cause issues during pregnancy, labor, or even delivery.

Though issues with the umbilical cord are normally found after the baby is born, in certain cases, abnormalities are diagnosed before birth using ultrasound. The most common umbilical cord defects and their potential effects on the baby are as follows:

- **Umbilical cord compression.** This condition is caused when pressure blocks oxygenated blood from flowing into the umbilical cord. During uterine contractions (tightening of the muscles in the uterus), minor, intermittent compressions are common. However, if the cord is compressed further than normal, the baby can suffer brain damage due to oxygen starvation, poor nutrition, or fetal acidosis (a condition caused by an accumulation of carbon dioxide in the baby's blood). Amnioinfusion is a procedure that includes injecting a room-temperature saline solution into the uterus during delivery to relieve the pressure that might cause the umbilical cord to become compressed.

- **Single umbilical artery.** An umbilical cord with just two blood vessels instead of the usual three is seen in around 1 percent of singletons and 5 percent of multiple pregnancies (twins, triplets, or more). One artery is absent in these cases. Babies affected by this condition have an increased chance of physical anomalies and birth defects, such as heart, central nervous system (CNS), and urinary tract defects, as well as chromosomal abnormalities.

- **Umbilical cord length.** The length of an umbilical cord is not something most people consider but is a significant factor in the occurrence of umbilical cord problems. A cord that is either too short or too long can cause complications. Short umbilical cords have been linked to:
  - fetal distress
  - low birth weight
  - reduced fetal activity
  - psychomotor (movement related to conscious mental activity) abnormalities
  - insufficient supply of oxygen and nutrients
  - placental abruption

Long umbilical cords are more likely to trigger emergency situations such as fetal entanglement, cord prolapse, and cord knots, all of which may lead to a lack of oxygen supply, thereby resulting in severe brain trauma.

- **Umbilical cord prolapse.** During delivery, the membranes (bag of water) rupture, and the baby descends to the birth canal. If the umbilical cord comes out through the vagina before the baby descends, such a condition is known as "umbilical cord prolapse." Around 1 in every 300 births is affected by this complication. Blood flow from the placenta to the fetus is reduced or cut off as the cord is compressed, reducing the baby's oxygen supply. If cesarean section is not performed quickly during delivery complications, umbilical cord prolapse may lead to stillbirth or lifelong disabilities, such as cerebral palsy (CP). To make it simpler to release your baby's head and reduce pressure on the umbilical cord, the practitioner may suggest you shift positions.
- **Vasa previa.** Blood vessels in the umbilical cord normally bind the fetus to the placenta's central area. Vasa previa is a condition when one or more blood vessels from the umbilical cord or placenta are trapped between the fetus and the opening of the birth canal. These vessels are at risk of rupturing during labor and childbirth due to their location. If the fetal blood vessels burst, it may result in a large amount of fetal blood loss as well as birth injury. Vasa previa occurs in 1 in 2,500 births. If a woman is diagnosed with vasa previa during pregnancy, the doctor may prescribe a cesarean section between 35 and 37 weeks of pregnancy, so they may change the kind and placement of the incision based on where the placenta and baby's blood veins are.
- **Nuchal cord.** The nuchal cord is a condition in which the umbilical cord coils around the baby's neck one or two times. The condition is quite common, affecting 15–35 percent of all pregnancies. Though nuchal cords often have little impact on pregnancy outcomes, a few situations may pose a serious risk to the baby. Normal blood level, nutrients, and oxygen exchange may be disrupted by nuchal cords. They may even cause

hypoxic ischemic encephalopathy (HIE)—a form of brain injury induced by oxygen deficiency at the time of birth.

- **Umbilical cord knots.** In a few pregnancy complications, the umbilical cord twists and tangles, forming into a knot. Knots are most common in identical twin births and also when the umbilical cord is too long. The majority of the cord knots turn out to be relatively weak and quickly undone. Some umbilical knots, on the other hand, can become very tight and dangerous, blocking the supply of oxygen and nutrients from reaching the baby. Umbilical cord knots are seen in less than 2 percent of pregnancies. The practitioner will be able to detect a reduction in the baby's heart rate if a loose knot tightens during delivery and will make the necessary decisions to ensure the baby's safe delivery into the world.

- **Umbilical cord cyst.** The umbilical cord cyst refers to cystic lesions that are present on the umbilical cord. This can cause birth defects as well as issues in the kidney. The umbilical cord cyst may develop as a result of incomplete embryonic growth or swelling of Wharton jelly (a tissue that protects blood vessels). Although umbilical cord cysts are relatively common, they could cause concern, prompting the doctor to recommend an amniocentesis (amniotic fluid is removed from the uterus for testing) to ensure there are no symptoms of a birth defect. According to certain studies, small cysts can be detected in up to 3 percent of first-trimester pregnancies.

PREVENTING UMBILICAL CORD PROBLEMS

When the umbilical cord is affected, there will be signs of fetal distresses, such as vaginal bleeding, maternal cramps, a decrease in fetal movements, and abnormal heart rate. These signs should be taken seriously, and the distresses can be detected by fetal heart rate control and other prenatal examinations. Early maternal care should ensure that the mother is as safe as possible during the pregnancy to prevent any complications. Smoking, alcohol, and other recreational substances can interfere with a fetus's development and should be prevented to avoid placental insufficiency and other pregnancy complications. Most complications faced by the mother or infant during delivery are immediately solved by a cesarean section.

References

"Pregnancy Complications: Umbilical Cord Abnormalities," Apollo Cradle, September 28, 2018. Available online. URL: www.apollocradle.com/pregnancy-complications-umbilical-cord-abnormalities. Accessed June 8, 2023.

"Types of Umbilical Cord Problems," American Baby and Child Law Centers, March 18, 2019. Available online. URL: www.abclawcenters.com/umbilical-cord-problems. Accessed June 8, 2023.

"Umbilical Cord Abnormalities," March of Dimes, June 24, 2016. Available online. URL: www.marchofdimes.org/pregnancy/umbilical-cord-abnormalities.aspx. Accessed June 8, 2023.

"Umbilical Cord Problems," Birth Injury Help Center, January 18, 2019. Available online. URL: www.birthinjuryhelpcenter.org/umbilical-cord-problems.html. Accessed June 8, 2023.

Chapter 53 | Sexually Transmitted Diseases during Pregnancy

Section 53.1 | Sexually Transmitted Diseases and Pregnancy

If you are pregnant, you can become infected with the same sexually transmitted diseases (Stds) as women who are not pregnant. Pregnant women should ask their doctors about getting tested for STDs since some doctors do not routinely perform these tests. The content below answers basic questions about STDs during pregnancy.

I AM PREGNANT. CAN I GET AN STD?

Yes, you can. Women who are pregnant can become infected with the same STDs as women who are not pregnant. Pregnancy does not provide women or their babies any additional protection against STDs. Many STDs are "silent," or have no symptoms, so you may not know if you are infected. If you are pregnant, you should be tested for STDs, including human immunodeficiency virus (HIV; the virus that causes acquired immunodeficiency syndrome (AIDS)), as a part of your medical care during pregnancy. The results of an STD can be more serious, even life-threatening, for you and your baby if you become infected while pregnant. It is important that you are aware of the harmful effects of STDs and how to protect yourself and your unborn baby against infection. If you are diagnosed with an STD while pregnant, your sex partner(s) should also be tested and treated.

HOW CAN STDS AFFECT YOU AND YOUR UNBORN BABY?

Sexually transmitted diseases can complicate your pregnancy and may have serious effects on both you and your developing baby. Some of these problems may be seen at birth; others may not be discovered until months or years later. In addition, it is well-known that infection with an STD can make it easier for a person to get infected with HIV. Most of these problems can be prevented if you receive regular medical care during pregnancy. This includes tests for STDs starting early in pregnancy and repeated close to delivery, as needed.

SHOULD YOU BE TESTED FOR STDS DURING YOUR PREGNANCY?

Yes. Testing and treating pregnant women for STDs is a vital way to prevent serious health complications to both the mother and the baby that may otherwise happen with infection. The sooner you begin receiving medical care during pregnancy, the better the health outcomes will be for you and your unborn baby. The 2015 STD Treatment Guidelines of the Centers for Disease Control and Prevention (CDC) recommend screening pregnant women for STDs.

Be sure to ask your doctor about getting tested for STDs. It is also important that you have an open, honest conversation with your provider and discuss any symptoms you are experiencing and any high-risk sexual behavior that you engage in since some doctors do not routinely perform these tests. Even if you have been tested in the past, you should be tested again when you become pregnant.

CAN YOU GET TREATED FOR AN STD WHILE PREGNANT?

It depends. STDs such as chlamydia, gonorrhea, syphilis, trichomoniasis, and bacterial vaginosis (BV) can all be treated and cured with antibiotics that are safe to take during pregnancy. STDs that are caused by viruses, such as genital herpes, hepatitis B, or HIV, cannot be cured. However, in some cases, these infections can be treated with antiviral medications or other preventive measures to reduce the risk of passing the infection to your baby. If you are pregnant or considering pregnancy, you should be tested, so you can take steps to protect yourself and your baby.

HOW CAN YOU REDUCE YOUR RISK OF GETTING AN STD WHILE PREGNANT?

The only way to avoid STDs is not to have vaginal, anal, or oral sex. If you are sexually active, you can do the following things to lower your chances of getting chlamydia:

- being in a long-term mutually monogamous relationship with a partner who has been tested and has negative STD test results

- using latex condoms the right way every time you have sex[1]

Section 53.2 | Sexually Transmitted Diseases Complicating Pregnancy

Sexually transmitted diseases (STDs) can complicate pregnancy and may have serious consequences for both a woman and her developing baby. As a health-care provider caring for pregnant women, you play a key role in safeguarding the health of both a mother and her unborn child.

A critical component of appropriate prenatal care is ensuring that pregnant patients are tested for STDs. Test your pregnant patients for STDs starting early in their pregnancy and repeat close to delivery, as needed. To ensure that the correct tests are being performed, we encourage you to have open, honest conversations with your pregnant patients and, when possible, their sex partners about symptoms they have experienced or are currently experiencing and any high-risk sexual behaviors in which they engage. Table 53.1 includes the Centers for Disease Control and Prevention's (CDC) screening recommendations for pregnant women.

BACTERIAL VAGINOSIS

Bacterial vaginosis (BV), a common cause of vaginal discharge in women of childbearing age, is a polymicrobial clinical syndrome resulting from a change in the vaginal community of bacteria. Although BV is often not considered an STD, it has been linked to sexual activity. Women may have no symptoms or may complain of a foul-smelling, fishy vaginal discharge. BV during pregnancy has been associated with serious pregnancy complications, including premature rupture of the membranes surrounding the baby in the

---

[1] "STDs during Pregnancy—CDC Detailed Fact Sheet," Centers for Disease Control and Prevention (CDC), April 12, 2022. Available online. URL: https://cdc.gov/std/pregnancy/stdfact-pregnancy.htm. Accessed May 31, 2023.

uterus, preterm labor, premature birth, chorioamnionitis, as well as endometritis. While there is no evidence to support screening for BV in pregnant women at high risk for preterm delivery, symptomatic women should be evaluated and treated. There are no known direct effects of BV on the newborn.

Table 53.1. Screening Recommendations for Pregnant Women

Disease	The CDC Recommendation
Chlamydia	**First prenatal visit.** Screen all pregnant women under 25 years of age and older pregnant women at increased risk for infection. **Third trimester.** Rescreen if under 25 years of age or at continued high risk. **Risk factors:** • new or multiple sex partners • sex partner with concurrent partners • sex partner who has a sexually transmitted disease (STD) *Note: Pregnant women found to have chlamydial infection should have a test-of-cure three to four weeks after treatment and then be retested within three months.*
Gonorrhea	**First prenatal visit.** Screen all pregnant women under 25 years of age and older pregnant women at increased risk for gonorrhea at the first prenatal visit. **Third trimester.** Rescreen for women at continued high risk. **Risk factors:** • living in a high-morbidity area • previous or coexisting sexually transmitted infection (STI) • new or multiple sex partners • inconsistent condom use among persons not in mutually monogamous relationships • exchanging sex for money or drugs
Syphilis	**First prenatal visit.** Screen all pregnant women. **Third trimester (28 weeks and at delivery).** Rescreen women who: • are at risk of syphilis during pregnancy (e.g., misuses drugs, has had another STI during pregnancy, or has had multiple sex partners, a new partner, or a partner with an STI) • live in areas with high numbers of syphilis cases • were not previously tested or had a positive test in the first trimester
Bacterial vaginosis (BV)	Evidence does not support routine screening for BV in asymptomatic pregnant women at high or low risk for preterm delivery.

Table 53.1. Continued

Disease	The CDC Recommendation
Trichomoniasis	Evidence does not support routine screening for trichomoniasis in asymptomatic pregnant women.
Herpes virus (HSV)	Evidence does not support routine HSV-2 serologic testing among asymptomatic pregnant women.
Human immunodeficiency virus (HIV)	**First prenatal visit.** Screen all pregnant women. **Third trimester.** Rescreen women at high risk for acquiring HIV infection.
Hepatitis B virus (HBV)	**First prenatal visit.** Screen all pregnant women. **Third trimester.** Test those who were not screened prenatally, those who engage in behaviors that put them at high risk for infection, and those with signs or symptoms of hepatitis at the time of admission to the hospital for delivery. **Risk factors:** • having had more than one sex partner in the previous six months • evaluation or treatment for an STD • recent or current injection drug use • an HBsAg-positive sex partner
Human papillomavirus (HPV)	There are no screening recommendations for HPV.
Hepatitis C virus (HCV)	**First prenatal visit.** Screen all pregnant women during each pregnancy, except in a setting where the prevalence of HCV infection is (HCV RNA-positivity) less than 0.1 percent.

CHLAMYDIA

Chlamydia is the most common sexually transmitted bacterium in the United States. Although the majority of chlamydial infections (including those in pregnant women) do not have symptoms, infected women may have abnormal vaginal discharge, bleeding after sex, or itching/burning with urination. Untreated chlamydial infection has been linked to problems during pregnancy, including preterm labor, premature rupture of membranes, and low birth weight. The newborn may also become infected during delivery as the baby passes through the birth canal. Exposed newborns can develop eye and lung infections.

GONORRHEA

Gonorrhea is a common STD in the United States. Untreated gonococcal infection in pregnancy has been linked to miscarriages, premature birth, low birth weight, premature rupture of membranes, and chorioamnionitis. Gonorrhea can also infect an infant during delivery as the infant passes through the birth canal. If untreated, infants can develop eye infections. Because gonorrhea can cause problems in both the mother and her baby, it is important for providers to accurately identify the infection, treat it with effective antibiotics, and closely follow up to make sure that the infection has been cured.

HEPATITIS B

Hepatitis B is a liver infection caused by the hepatitis B virus (HBV). A mother can transmit the infection to her baby during pregnancy. While the risk of an infected mother passing HBV to her baby varies, depending on when she becomes infected, the greatest risk happens when mothers become infected close to the time of delivery. Infected newborns also have a high risk (up to 90%) of becoming chronic HBV carriers themselves. Infants who have a lifelong infection with HBV are at an increased risk of developing chronic liver disease or liver cancer later in life. Approximately 25 percent of infants who develop chronic HBV infection will eventually die from chronic liver disease. By screening your pregnant patients for the infection and providing treatment to at-risk infants shortly after birth, you can help prevent mother-to-child transmission of HBV.

HEPATITIS C

Hepatitis C is a liver infection caused by the hepatitis C virus (HCV) and can be passed from an infected mother to her child during pregnancy. In general, an infected mother will transmit the infection to her baby 10 percent of the time, but the chances are higher in certain subgroups, such as women who are also infected with HIV. In some studies, infants born to HCV-infected women have been shown to have an increased risk of being small for gestational age, premature, and having a low birth weight. Newborn infants with HCV infection usually do not have symptoms, and a majority will clear the infection without any medical help.

HERPES SIMPLEX VIRUS

Herpes simplex virus (HSV) has two distinct virus types that can infect the human genital tract: HSV-1 and HSV-2. Infections of the newborn can be of either type, but most are caused by HSV-2. Generally, the symptoms of genital herpes are similar in pregnant and nonpregnant women; however, the major concern regarding HSV infection relates to complications linked to infection of the newborn. Although transmission may occur during pregnancy and after delivery, the risk of transmission to the neonate from an infected mother is high among women who acquire genital herpes near the time of delivery and low among women with recurrent herpes or who acquire the infection during the first half of pregnancy. HSV infection can have very serious effects on newborns, especially if the mother's first outbreak occurred during the third trimester. Cesarean section is recommended for all women in labor with active genital herpes lesions or early symptoms, such as vulvar pain and itching.

HUMAN IMMUNODEFICIENCY VIRUS

Human immunodeficiency virus (HIV) is the virus that causes acquired immunodeficiency syndrome (AIDS). HIV destroys specific blood cells that are crucial to helping the body fight diseases. According to the CDC's HIV surveillance data, women make up 19 percent of all new HIV diagnoses in the United States and dependent areas. The most common ways that HIV passes from mother to child are during pregnancy, childbirth, or breast-feeding. However, when HIV is diagnosed before or early during pregnancy and appropriate steps are taken, the risk of mother-to-child transmission can be less than 1 percent. A mother who knows early in her pregnancy that she has HIV has more time to consult with her health-care provider and decide on effective ways to protect her health and that of her unborn baby.

HUMAN PAPILLOMAVIRUS

Human papillomaviruses (HPV) are viruses that most commonly involve the lower genital tract, including the cervix, vagina, and external genitalia. Genital warts frequently increase in number and size during pregnancy. Genital warts often appear as small cauliflower-like clusters, which may burn or itch. If a woman has genital warts during pregnancy, you may elect to delay treatment until after delivery. When large or spread out, genital warts can complicate a vaginal delivery. In cases where there are large genital warts that are blocking the birth canal, a cesarean section may be recommended. Infection of the mother may be linked to the development of laryngeal papillomatosis in the newborn—a rare, noncancerous growth in the larynx.

SYPHILIS

Syphilis is primarily an STD, but it may be transmitted to a baby by an infected mother during pregnancy. Transmission of syphilis to a developing baby can lead to a serious multisystem infection known as "congenital syphilis." Recently, there has been a sharp increase in the number of congenital syphilis cases in the United States. Syphilis has been linked to premature births, stillbirths, and, in some cases, death shortly after birth. Untreated infants that survive tend to develop problems in multiple organs, including the brain, eyes, ears, heart, skin, teeth, and bones.

TRICHOMONIASIS

Vaginal infection due to the sexually transmitted parasite *Trichomonas vaginalis* is very common. Although most people report no symptoms, others complain of itching, irritation, unusual odor, discharge, and pain during urination or sex. If you have a pregnant patient with symptoms of trichomoniasis, she should be evaluated for *T. vaginalis* and treated appropriately. Infection in pregnancy has been linked to premature rupture of membranes, preterm birth, and low birth weight infants. Rarely, the female newborn can acquire the infection when passing through the birth canal during delivery and have vaginal discharge after birth.

Screening and prompt treatment are recommended at least annually for all HIV-infected women, based on the high prevalence of *T. vaginalis* infection, the increased risk of pelvic inflammatory disease (PID) associated with this infection, and the ability of treatment to reduce genital tract viral load and vaginal HIV shedding. This includes HIV-infected women who are pregnant, as *T. vaginalis* infection is a risk factor for vertical transmission of HIV. For other pregnant women, screening may be considered at the discretion of the treating clinician, as the benefit of routine screening for pregnant women has not been established. Screening might be considered for persons receiving care in high-prevalence settings (e.g., STD clinics or correctional facilities) and for asymptomatic persons at high risk for infection. Decisions about screening might be informed by local epidemiology of *T. vaginalis* infection. However, data are lacking on whether screening and treatment for asymptomatic trichomoniasis in high-prevalence settings or persons at high risk can reduce any adverse health events and health disparities or reduce the community burden of infection.

SEXUALLY TRANSMITTED DISEASE TREATMENT DURING PREGNANCY

Sexually transmitted diseases such as chlamydia, gonorrhea, syphilis, and trichomoniasis can all be treated and cured with antibiotics that are safe to take during pregnancy. Viral STDs, such as genital herpes, hepatitis B, and HIV, cannot be cured. However, in some cases, these infections can be treated with antiviral medications or other preventive measures to reduce the risk of passing the infection to the baby.

SEXUALLY TRANSMITTED DISEASE PREVENTION DURING PREGNANCY

The most reliable way to avoid transmission of STDs is to abstain from oral, vaginal, and anal sex or to be in a long-term, mutually monogamous relationship with a partner known to be uninfected. For patients who are being treated for an STD other than HIV (or whose partners are undergoing treatment), counseling that encourages abstinence from sexual intercourse until completion of the entire course of medication is crucial.[2]

[2] "STDs during Pregnancy—CDC Detailed Fact Sheet," Centers for Disease Control and Prevention (CDC), April 11, 2023. Available online. URL: https://cdc.gov/std/pregnancy/stdfact-pregnancy-detailed.htm. Accessed May 31, 2023.

Chapter 54 | Human Immunodeficiency Virus during Pregnancy, Labor and Delivery, and Birth

CAN A PREGNANT PERSON TRANSMIT HIV TO THEIR BABY?

Yes, however, treatment with a combination of human immunodeficiency virus (HIV) medicines (called "antiretroviral therapy" (ART)) can prevent transmission of HIV to your baby and protect your health.

HOW CAN YOU PREVENT TRANSMITTING HIV TO YOUR BABY?

If you have HIV, there are several steps you can take to reduce your risk of transmitting HIV to your baby.

Get Tested for HIV as Soon as Possible to Know Your Status

- If you are pregnant or planning to get pregnant, get tested for HIV as early as possible during each pregnancy. Knowing your HIV status gives you powerful information.
- If you learn you have HIV, the sooner you start treatment, the better—for your health and your baby's health and to prevent transmitting HIV to your partner.

- If you learn you do not have HIV but are at increased risk of acquiring it, get tested again in your third trimester.
- Know your HIV status. Encourage your partner to get tested for HIV.

HIV-Negative but at Risk? Take Medicine to Prevent HIV

- If you have a partner with HIV and you are considering getting pregnant, talk to your health-care provider about pre-exposure prophylaxis (PrEP).
- PrEP is medicine people at risk of HIV take to prevent getting HIV from sex or injection drug use. PrEP can stop HIV from taking hold and spreading throughout your body.
- PrEP may be an option to help protect you and your baby from getting HIV while you try to get pregnant, during pregnancy, or while breastfeeding. Find out if PrEP is right for you.
- If your partner has HIV, also encourage them to get and stay on HIV medicine. This will keep them healthy and help prevent them from transmitting HIV to you.

HIV-Positive? Take Medicine to Treat HIV

- Taking HIV medicine reduces the amount of HIV in your body (your viral load) to a very low level, called "viral suppression." If your viral load is so low that a standard lab test cannot detect it, this is called having an undetectable viral load. Taking HIV medicine and getting and keeping an undetectable viral load is the best thing you can do to stay healthy and prevent transmission to your baby.
- If you have HIV and take HIV medicine as prescribed throughout your pregnancy and childbirth and give HIV medicine to your baby for two to six weeks after giving birth, your risk of transmitting HIV to your baby can be less than 1 percent.
- As long as your viral load remains undetectable, you can have a normal delivery.

- Taking HIV medicine reduces the risk of transmitting HIV to your baby through breastfeeding* to less than 1 percent. However, the risk is not zero.
- Taking HIV medicine also protects your HIV-negative partner. People with HIV who take HIV medicine as prescribed and get and keep an undetectable viral load can live long and healthy lives and will not transmit HIV to their HIV-negative partners through sex.

*Following the current recommendation, the term "breastfeeding" is used to describe feeding a child one's own milk (either direct feeding or with expressed milk). Some transgender men and gender-diverse individuals may prefer using the term "chestfeeding" rather than "breastfeeding." The recommendations advise health-care providers to assess and use an individual's preferred terminology and to support all pregnant individuals with HIV, regardless of gender identity, in their infant feeding options.

ARE HIV MEDICINES SAFE FOR YOU TO USE DURING PREGNANCY?

Most HIV medicines are safe to use during pregnancy. Talk with your health-care provider about the benefits and risks of specific HIV medicines when deciding which HIV medicines to use during pregnancy or while you are trying to get pregnant.

CAN YOU BREASTFEED IF YOU HAVE HIV?

The current recommendation in the United States supports shared decision-making between you and your health-care provider regarding infant feeding. Taking HIV medicine and keeping an undetectable viral load substantially decreases your risk of transmitting HIV to your baby through breastfeeding to less than 1 percent. However, the risk is not zero. Properly prepared infant formula or banked donor human breast milk are alternative options that eliminate the risk of transmission through breastfeeding. If you are pregnant or thinking of becoming pregnant, talk to your health-care provider as early as possible about what infant feeding choice is right for you.

WHAT SHOULD YOU ASK YOUR HEALTH-CARE PROVIDER ABOUT HAVING A BABY?

You might ask your health-care provider some of the following questions:

- What is the safest way to conceive?
- Will HIV cause problems for me during pregnancy or delivery?
- Will my HIV treatment cause problems for my baby?
- What are the pros and cons of taking HIV medicine while I am pregnant?
- What infant feeding option is the best choice for me and my baby?
- Is my viral load undetectable?
- How do I avoid transmitting HIV to my partner(s), surrogate, or baby during conception, pregnancy, and delivery?
- What medical and community programs and support groups can help me and my baby?
- What birth control methods are best for me?

Adopting a baby is also an option for people who want to begin or expand their families.[1]

SHOULD WOMEN WITH HIV TAKE HIV MEDICINES DURING PREGNANCY?

Yes. All pregnant women with HIV should take HIV medicines throughout pregnancy for their own health and to prevent perinatal transmission of HIV. (HIV medicines are called "antiretrovirals"). Perinatal transmission of HIV is also called "mother-to-child transmission of HIV."

HIV medicines, when taken as prescribed, prevent HIV from multiplying and reduce the amount of HIV in the body (called the

---

[1] HIV.gov, "Preventing Perinatal Transmission of HIV," U.S. Department of Health and Human Services (HHS), April 10, 2023. Available online. URL: https://hiv.gov/hiv-basics/hiv-prevention/reducing-mother-to-child-risk/preventing-mother-to-child-transmission-of-hiv. Accessed June 12, 2023.

"viral load"). An undetectable viral load is when the level of HIV in the blood is too low to be detected by a viral load test. The risk of perinatal transmission of HIV during pregnancy and childbirth is lowest when a woman with HIV has an undetectable viral load. Maintaining an undetectable viral load also helps keep the mother-to-be healthy.

ARE HIV MEDICINES SAFE TO USE DURING PREGNANCY?

Most HIV medicines are safe to use during pregnancy. In general, HIV medicines do not increase the risk of birth defects. When recommending HIV medicines to use during pregnancy, health-care providers consider the benefits and risks of specific HIV medicines for women and their unborn babies.

WHEN SHOULD PREGNANT WOMEN WITH HIV START TAKING HIV MEDICINES?

All pregnant women with HIV should start taking HIV medicines as soon as possible during pregnancy. In most cases, women who are already on an effective HIV treatment regimen when they become pregnant should continue using the same regimen throughout their pregnancies.

WHAT HIV MEDICINES SHOULD A PREGNANT WOMAN WITH HIV TAKE?

The choice of an HIV treatment regimen to use during pregnancy depends on several factors, including a woman's current or past use of HIV medicines, other medical conditions she may have, and the results of drug-resistance testing. In general, pregnant women with HIV can use the same HIV treatment regimens recommended for nonpregnant adults—unless the risk of any known side effects to a pregnant woman or her baby outweighs the benefits of a treatment regimen.

Sometimes, a woman's HIV treatment regimen may change during pregnancy. Women and their health-care providers should discuss whether any changes need to be made to an HIV treatment regimen during pregnancy.

DO WOMEN WITH HIV CONTINUE TO TAKE HIV MEDICINES DURING CHILDBIRTH?

Yes. A baby is exposed to any HIV in the mother's blood and other fluids while passing through the birth canal. During childbirth, HIV medicines that pass from mother to baby across the placenta prevent perinatal transmission of HIV, especially near delivery. Women who are already taking HIV medicines when they go into labor should continue taking their HIV medicines on schedule as much as possible during childbirth.

DO WOMEN WITH HIV CONTINUE TO TAKE HIV MEDICINES AFTER CHILDBIRTH?

Prenatal care for women with HIV includes counseling on the benefits of continuing HIV medicines after childbirth. HIV medicines help people with HIV live longer, healthier lives and reduce the risk of HIV transmission. Together with their health-care providers, women with HIV make decisions about continuing or changing their HIV medicines after childbirth. After birth, babies born to women with HIV receive HIV medicine to reduce the risk of perinatal transmission of HIV. Several factors determine what HIV medicine they receive and how long they receive the medicine.[2]

---

[2] HIV.gov, "HIV Medicines during Pregnancy and Childbirth," U.S. Department of Health and Human Services (HHS), August 18, 2021. Available online. URL: https://hivinfo.nih.gov/understanding-hiv/fact-sheets/hiv-medicines-during-pregnancy-and-childbirth. Accessed June 12, 2023.

Chapter 55 | Pregnancy Loss: Ectopic Pregnancy, Miscarriage, and Stillbirth

Section 55.1 | Ectopic Pregnancy

WHAT IS AN ECTOPIC PREGNANCY?

Normally, a fertilized egg gets implanted and develops in the main uterine cavity. However, sometimes, a fertilized egg implants itself in another place, often the fallopian tubes (the structures leading from the ovaries to the uterus). This is called an "ectopic" or "tubular pregnancy." Ectopic pregnancies can also occur in the ovaries, cervix, or abdominal cavity. Since these other anatomical structures lack the space and nourishing environment of the uterus, an ectopic pregnancy will not be viable. Also, ectopic pregnancies must be removed immediately because, if not treated, the growing embryonic tissue will damage the mother's reproductive organs, resulting in serious and potentially life-threatening blood loss.

WHAT ARE THE RISK FACTORS FOR AN ECTOPIC PREGNANCY?

All women have a slight risk of ectopic pregnancy. However, the risk increases with the following factors:
- becoming pregnant over the age of 35
- history of:
  - ectopic pregnancy
  - endometriosis
  - pelvic surgery, abdominal surgery, or multiple abortions
  - sexually transmitted diseases (STDs)
- structural abnormalities in the fallopian tubes that restrict the movement of eggs
- conception that occurs in spite of tubal ligation or intrauterine device
- conception assisted by fertility drugs or procedures
- hormonal imbalances
- smoking
- abnormal development of a fertilized egg

WHAT ARE THE SYMPTOMS OF AN ECTOPIC PREGNANCY?

The symptoms of an ectopic pregnancy are similar to those in the early stages of a normal pregnancy. As with a normal pregnancy, a woman will experience a missed period, nausea, and tenderness in the breasts. A pregnancy test will be positive. However, an ectopic pregnancy does not proceed normally. The first indication is slight vaginal bleeding or brown watery discharge accompanied by dull pelvic pain. However, the pain in the pelvis may spread to the abdomen and become sharp and stabbing. A woman may also experience shoulder pain or an urge to move her bowels if blood has leaked from the fallopian tube and pooled in the abdominal cavity, where it irritates related nerves. If the fallopian tube is completely ruptured, heavy bleeding in the abdominal cavity, light-headedness, fainting, and shock will occur.

WHEN SHOULD YOU CALL FOR EMERGENCY HELP?

Given the potentially life-threatening complications of an ectopic pregnancy, emergency help should be sought out immediately should you experience:

- severe pain in the abdomen and pelvic areas accompanied by vaginal bleeding
- fainting and light-headedness
- pain in the shoulders

HOW IS AN ECTOPIC PREGNANCY DIAGNOSED?

The doctor will perform an initial pregnancy test and pelvic examination. Since an ectopic pregnancy cannot be detected by a physical examination alone, the doctor will also order an ultrasound test. When the pregnancy is too early to see via imaging, the doctor will monitor the patient using blood tests until the condition can be confirmed using ultrasound. One of the ultrasound tests frequently used is a transvaginal ultrasound, which uses a wand-like device placed in the vagina to produce images of the uterus and fallopian tubes to detect an ectopic pregnancy.

HOW IS AN ECTOPIC PREGNANCY TREATED?

An ectopic pregnancy is treated by removing the implanted embryo via the following methods:

- **Medication.** If the ectopic pregnancy has been detected early, doctors will inject methotrexate into the embryo to stop cell growth and dissolve the tissue. They will then monitor levels of the pregnancy hormone human chorionic gonadotropin (hCG) in the patient's blood. If the levels are high, indicating that the fetal tissue has not been completely removed, the doctor will administer a second injection of the same drug.
- **Surgery.** Doctors can also use laparoscopic surgery to remove an ectopic embryo. An incision is made in or near the naval, and a tube is inserted with surgical tools and a camera with a light source. The embryo is then removed, and any damage to the fallopian tube is repaired. If heavy bleeding and heavy damage to the fallopian tube have occurred, the surgeon may remove the fallopian tube as well. After surgery, the patient is monitored for levels of the hCG hormone to confirm that all ectopic tissue was removed. Otherwise, a methotrexate injection is administered.

HOW CAN AN ECTOPIC PREGNANCY BE PREVENTED?

An ectopic pregnancy cannot be prevented, but the risk factors can be controlled.

- Limit the number of sexual partners.
- Do not engage in unprotected sex.
- Quit smoking.

WHAT IS THE OUTLOOK AFTER AN ECTOPIC PREGNANCY?

The outlook after an ectopic pregnancy depends on what effect it has had on the fallopian tubes or other reproductive organs. If the fallopian tubes are intact and damage has been minimal, the chances of having a normal pregnancy in the future are good. You will be advised to wait for two to three months before trying to get pregnant again. About 65 percent of women who have undergone treatment for ectopic pregnancy successfully become pregnant within 18 months of treatment. In some cases, in vitro fertilization (IVF) treatment may be necessary. The risk for a repeat ectopic pregnancy exists but is significantly less at 10 percent.

HOW CAN YOU COPE AFTER AN ECTOPIC PREGNANCY?

The loss of a pregnancy is devastating. It is important to recognize the loss and give yourself time to grieve. Seek the support of your partner, friend, or loved one. Contact a support group, grief counselor, or mental health provider for support if needed.

Women who have been treated for ectopic pregnancies often go on to have healthy pregnancies later. If one fallopian tube was removed during treatment, the other fallopian tube could still function as part of a normal pregnancy. IVF treatment could be an option for women who have lost both fallopian tubes due to ectopic pregnancies. Plan your pregnancy ahead of time and discuss it with your doctor. You can be reassured of a normal pregnancy with the help of blood tests and ultrasound imaging early in your pregnancy.

References

"Ectopic Pregnancy," Mayo Foundation for Medical Education and Research (MFMER), March 12, 2022. Available online. URL: http://mayoclinic.org/diseases-conditions/ectopic-pregnancy/basics/definition/con-20024262. Accessed June 8, 2023.

"Ectopic Pregnancy," NHS Choices, August 23, 2022. Available online. URL: http://nhs.uk/conditions/ectopic-pregnancy/pages/introduction.aspx. Accessed June 8, 2023.

Marissa Selner. "Ectopic Pregnancy," Healthline, January 8, 2018. Available online. URL: http://healthline.com/health/pregnancy/ectopic-pregnancy. Accessed June 8, 2023.

Shishira Sreenivas. "Ectopic Pregnancy: What to Know,"
WebMD, LLC, January 20, 2023. Available online. URL:
http://webmd.com/baby/pregnancy-ectopic-pregnancy.
Accessed June 8, 2023.

Section 55.2 | What Is a Miscarriage?

Pregnancy loss is the unexpected loss of a fetus before the 20th week of pregnancy. It is sometimes called "miscarriage," early pregnancy loss, midtrimester pregnancy loss, fetal demise, or spontaneous abortion.

Health-care providers use a different term—stillbirth—to describe the loss of a fetus after 20 weeks of pregnancy. Pregnancy loss may occur so early that a woman may not know she is pregnant.

Researchers can only estimate the number of women who experience pregnancy loss because some losses occur before a woman's pregnancy is confirmed by a health-care provider or pregnancy test. But the American College of Obstetricians and Gynecologists (ACOG) estimates that early pregnancy loss is common, occurring in about 10 percent of confirmed pregnancies.

WHAT ARE THE SYMPTOMS OF PREGNANCY LOSS (BEFORE 20 WEEKS OF PREGNANCY)?

Symptoms of pregnancy loss may include:
- bleeding from the vagina
- pain or cramps in the lower stomach area (abdomen)
- low back pain
- fluid, tissue, or clot-like material coming out of the vagina

However, bleeding from the vagina during pregnancy does not always mean a miscarriage. Many pregnant women have spotting and cramping in early pregnancy but do not miscarry. Your health-care provider might call this pregnancy "threatened." In any case, pregnant women who have any of the symptoms of miscarriage should contact their health-care provider immediately.

Some women do not experience any symptoms of pregnancy loss. Although this is rare in the United States, some women who have a miscarriage may get an infection in the uterus, which can be life-threatening. Women who have the following symptoms for more than 24 hours should call 911:

- a fever higher than 100.4 °F (38 °C) on more than two occasions
- severe pain in the lower abdomen
- bloody discharge from the vagina (which can include pus and be foul smelling)

WHAT ARE THE CAUSES OF PREGNANCY LOSS (BEFORE 20 WEEKS OF PREGNANCY)?

Pregnancy loss may occur for many reasons, and sometimes, the cause remains unknown even after additional tests are completed.

Possible Causes

Pregnancy loss often happens when a pregnancy does not develop normally. In many cases, miscarriages result from a problem with the chromosomes in the fetus. The number of chromosomes the fetus has—too many or too few—can affect survival. Other possible causes of pregnancy loss include the following:

- being exposed to toxins in the environment
- problems of the placenta, cervix, or uterus
- problems with the father's sperm

In many cases, though, health-care providers cannot identify a cause or causes for pregnancy loss.

RISK FACTORS FOR PREGNANCY LOSS

Problems with chromosomes happen more often in the fetuses of older parents, particularly among women who are older than 35.

For this reason, risk of pregnancy loss increases as the parents age; it is much higher at age 45 than at age 35.

Women who have had previous miscarriages are also at higher risk of pregnancy loss. Health issues, such as chronic diseases, in the mother that can also increase risk of pregnancy loss include the following:

- chronic diseases, such as high blood pressure, diabetes, thyroid disease, or polycystic ovary syndrome (PCOS)
- problems with the immune system, such as an autoimmune disorder
- infections (such as untreated gonorrhea or Zika)
- hormone problems
- extremes in weight, such as obesity or being too thin
- lifestyle factors, such as using drugs or alcohol, smoking, or consuming more than 200 mg of caffeine per day (equal to about one 12-ounce cup of coffee)

HOW DO HEALTH-CARE PROVIDERS DIAGNOSE AND TREAT PREGNANCY LOSS (BEFORE 20 WEEKS OF PREGNANCY)?

If a pregnant woman has any of the symptoms of pregnancy loss, such as abdominal cramps, back pain, light spotting, or bleeding, she should contact her health-care provider immediately. Remember that vaginal bleeding during pregnancy does not definitely mean a pregnancy loss is occurring.

Diagnosing Pregnancy Loss

Depending on how far along the pregnancy is, health-care providers may use different methods to determine whether a pregnancy loss has occurred:

- a blood test to check the level of human chorionic gonadotropin (hCG), the pregnancy hormone
- a pelvic exam to see whether the woman's cervix is dilated or thinned, which can be a sign of pregnancy loss
- an ultrasound test, which allows the provider to look at the pregnancy, uterus, and placenta

If a woman has had more than one miscarriage, she may want to have a health-care provider check her blood for chromosome problems, hormone problems, or immune system disorders that may be contributing to pregnancy loss.

Treating Pregnancy Loss

Treatments for pregnancy loss focus on ensuring that the nonviable pregnancy leaves the woman's body safely and completely. Women going through pregnancy loss are at risk of bleeding, pain, and infection, especially if some of the pregnancy tissue remains behind in the uterus.

The specific treatment used depends on how far along the pregnancy is, the woman's overall health, her age, and other factors.

In many cases, pregnancy loss before 20 weeks may not require any special treatment. The bleeding that occurs with pregnancy loss empties the uterus without any further problems. Women who have heavy bleeding during pregnancy loss should contact a health-care provider immediately. For reference, heavy bleeding refers to soaking at least two maxi pads an hour for at least two hours in a row.

Some women may need a surgical procedure called a "dilation and curettage" (D&C) to remove any pregnancy tissue that is still in the uterus. A D&C is recommended if a woman is bleeding heavily or if an ultrasound shows pregnancy tissue is still in the uterus. D&C may also be used if a woman has any signs of infection, such as a fever, or if she has other health problems, such as cardiovascular disease or a bleeding disorder.

Some women are treated with a medication called "misoprostol," which helps the tissue pass out of the uterus and controls the resulting bleeding. Research shows that misoprostol is safe and effective in most cases. Women who lose a pregnancy may also need other treatments to control mild-to-moderate bleeding, prevent infection, relieve pain, and help with emotional support.

Although this is rare in the United States, some women who have a miscarriage may get an infection in the uterus, which can be life-threatening. Women who have the following symptoms more than 24 hours after treatment should call 911:

- a fever higher than 100.4 °F (38 °C) on more than two occasions
- severe pain in the lower abdomen
- bloody discharge from the vagina that includes pus or foul smelling

IS THERE A WAY TO PREVENT PREGNANCY LOSS (BEFORE 20 WEEKS OF PREGNANCY)?

There is currently no known way to prevent pregnancy loss before 20 weeks from occurring, nor is there a way to stop pregnancy loss once it has started.

There are ways to lower the risk of general pregnancy complications, but none of them definitely prevent pregnancy loss. Some ways to lower overall risk include the following:

- staying in good health before becoming pregnant and getting regular care during pregnancy
- diagnosing any health conditions, such as diabetes or thyroid disorders, and taking steps to manage or treat the condition before getting pregnant
- avoiding environmental hazards, such as exposure to radiation, pollution, or toxic chemicals
- avoiding alcohol and drugs, including high levels of caffeine in both partners
- protecting yourself from certain infections by not traveling to certain areas and by preventing mosquito bites[1]

---

[1] "About Pregnancy Loss (before 20 Weeks of Pregnancy)," *Eunice Kennedy Shriver* National Institute of Child Health and Human Development (NICHD), September 1, 2017. Available online. URL: https://nichd.nih.gov/health/topics/pregnancyloss/conditioninfo. Accessed May 31, 2023.

Section 55.3 | What Is a Stillbirth?

The loss of a baby due to stillbirth remains a sad reality for many families and takes a serious toll on families' health and well-being.

A stillbirth is the death or loss of a baby before or during delivery. Both miscarriage and stillbirth describe pregnancy loss, but they differ according to when the loss occurs. In the United States, a miscarriage is usually defined as loss of a baby before the 20th week of pregnancy, and a stillbirth is loss of a baby at or after 20 weeks of pregnancy. Stillbirth is further classified as early, late, or term stillbirth:

- An early stillbirth is a fetal death occurring between 20 and 27 completed weeks of pregnancy.
- A late stillbirth occurs between 28 and 36 completed pregnancy weeks.
- A term stillbirth occurs between 37 or more completed pregnancy weeks.

HOW MANY BABIES ARE STILLBORN?

Stillbirth affects about 1 in 175 births, and each year about 21,000 babies are stillborn in the United States. That is about the same as the number of babies that die during the first year of life. Because of advances in medical technology over the past 30 years, prenatal care (medical care during pregnancy) has improved, which has dramatically reduced the number of late and term stillbirths. However, the rate of early stillbirth has remained about the same over time.

WHAT INCREASES THE RISK OF STILLBIRTH?

Stillbirth with an unknown cause is called "unexplained stillbirth." The further along a woman is in her pregnancy, the more likely it is that the stillbirth will be unexplained. Having an autopsy on the baby and other laboratory tests is important in trying to understand why the baby died before birth. Your health-care provider can share more information about this.

Stillbirth occurs in families of all races, ethnicities, and income levels and to women of all ages. However, stillbirth occurs more commonly among certain groups of people including women who:

- are of Black race
- are 35 years of age or older
- are of low socioeconomic status
- smoke cigarettes during pregnancy
- have certain medical conditions, such as high blood pressure, diabetes, and obesity
- have multiple pregnancies, such as triplets or quadruplets
- have had a previous pregnancy loss

This does not mean that every individual of Black race or older age is at higher risk of having a stillbirth. It simply means that overall as a group, more stillbirths occur among all mothers of Black race or older age when compared to White mothers and mothers under 35 years of age. Some factors that might contribute to these stillbirth disparities include differences in maternal preconception health, socioeconomic status, access to quality health care, and stress.[2]

Section 55.4 | Stillbirths due to Placental Complications

Half of all stillbirths result from pregnancy disorders and conditions that affect the placenta, according to a new report. Risk factors already known at the start of pregnancy—such as previous pregnancy loss or obesity—accounted for only a small proportion of the overall risk of stillbirth.

Stillbirth is the death of a baby during the second half of pregnancy—at or after the 20th week of gestation. It occurs in 1 out

---

[2] National Center on Birth Defects and Developmental Disabilities (NCBDDD), "What Is Stillbirth?" Centers for Disease Control and Prevention (CDC), September 29, 2022. Available online. URL: https://cdc.gov/ncbddd/stillbirth/facts.html. Accessed May 31, 2023.

of 160 pregnancies nationwide. Some risk factors had previously been linked to stillbirth, including maternal diabetes or high blood pressure. But the underlying causes of stillbirth remained unknown in as many as half of stillbirths.

To learn more about the origins and prevention of stillbirth, the National Institutes of Health (NIH) created the Stillbirth Collaborative Research Network. With support from the NIH *Eunice Kennedy Shriver* National Institute of Child Health and Human Development (NICHD), the network enrolled more than 600 women who delivered a stillbirth in certain regions of the country. The findings were reported in a pair of papers published in the *Journal of the American Medical Association* on December 14, 2011.

In one of the studies, the researchers compared 614 stillbirths with 1,816 live births. They searched for factors at the start of pregnancy that might raise the risk of stillbirth. The analysis strongly linked stillbirth with several reproductive features, including being a first-time mother or having a stillbirth or miscarriage in earlier pregnancies. Other maternal factors linked with stillbirth include being overweight or obese, age 40 or older, AB blood type, a history of drug addiction, and smoking three months prior to pregnancy. Still, these early risk factors represented little of the overall risk, and so they have limited usefulness as predictors of stillbirth.

The analysis confirmed earlier findings that African American women are at greater risk of stillbirth compared with White or Hispanic women. The stillbirth risk for African Americans was greatest for deliveries before the 24th week of pregnancy. Further analyses of early pregnancy may yield insights for reducing the racial disparity in stillbirth rates.

In the other study, researchers completed comprehensive medical evaluations of 512 stillborn babies to identify the causes of death. The evaluation included an autopsy of the fetus, an examination of the placenta, a karyotype test to check for abnormalities in the baby's chromosomes, and a review of the medical records.

The detailed medical evaluations allowed scientists to identify a probable cause of death in 61 percent of cases and a probable or possible cause of death in 76 percent of cases. Earlier studies, which typically were limited to analyzing medical records, could identify a cause of death in only about half of cases.

The researchers found that pregnancy or birth-related complications contributed to the largest proportion of stillbirths (29%). These complications include preterm labor or premature rupture of membranes that hold the amniotic fluid. Another such complication is abruption of the placenta, in which the placenta separates from the wall of the uterus. Other identified causes included abnormalities of the placenta (24% of cases), genetic conditions or birth defects (14%), infection (13%), problems with the umbilical cord (10%), and maternal high blood pressure (9%).

"Our study showed that a probable cause of death—more than 60 percent—could be found by a thorough medical evaluation," says study co-author Dr. Uma M. Reddy M.D., M.P.H. of the NICHD, the vice chair of research and a professor of obstetrics and gynecology in the Department of Obstetrics and Gynecology at Columbia University Irving Medical Center. "Greater availability of medical evaluation of stillborn infants, particularly autopsy, placental exam, and karyotype, would provide information to better understand the causes of stillbirth."[3]

Section 55.5 | Coping with Pregnancy Loss

WHY DOES PREGNANCY LOSS HAPPEN?

As many as 10–15 percent of confirmed pregnancies are lost. The true percentage of pregnancy losses might even be higher as many take place before a woman even knows that she is pregnant. Most losses occur very early on—before eight weeks. A pregnancy that ends before 20 weeks is called a "miscarriage." Miscarriage usually happens because of genetic problems in the fetus. Sometimes, problems with the uterus or cervix may play a role in miscarriage. Health problems, such as polycystic ovary syndrome, may also be a factor.

---

[3] "Most Stillbirths Caused by Placental, Pregnancy Conditions," National Institutes of Health (NIH), December 19, 2011. Available online. URL: https://nih.gov/news-events/nih-research-matters/most-still-births-caused-placental-pregnancy-conditions. Accessed May 31, 2023.

After 20 weeks, losing a pregnancy is called "stillbirth." Stillbirth is much less common. Some reasons stillbirth occurs include problems with the placenta, genetic problems in the fetus, poor fetal growth, and infections. Almost half of the time, the reason for stillbirth is not known.

COPING WITH LOSS

After the loss, you might be stunned or shocked. You might be asking, "Why me?" You might feel guilty that you did or did not do something to cause your pregnancy to end. You might feel cheated and angry. Or you might feel extremely sad as you come to terms with the baby that will never be. These emotions are all normal reactions to loss. With time, you will be able to accept the loss and move on. You will never forget your baby. But you will be able to put this chapter behind you and look forward to life ahead. To help get you through this difficult time, try some of the following ideas:

- turn to loved ones and friends for support and share your feelings and ask for help when you need it
- talk to your partner about your loss and keep in mind that men and women cope with loss in different ways
- take care of yourself: eat healthy foods, keep active, and get enough sleep to restore energy and well-being
- join a support group, which might help you feel less alone
- do something in remembrance of your baby
- seek help from a grief counselor, especially if your grief does not ease with time

TRYING AGAIN

Give yourself plenty of time to heal emotionally. It could take a few months or even a year. Once you and your partner are emotionally ready to try again, confirm with your doctor that you are in good physical health and that your body is ready for pregnancy. Following a miscarriage, most healthy women do not need to wait before trying to conceive again. You might worry that pregnancy loss could happen again. But take heart in knowing that most women who have gone through pregnancy loss go on to have healthy babies.[4]

[4] Office on Women's Health (OWH), "Pregnancy Loss," U.S. Department of Health and Human Services (HHS), February 22, 2021. Available online. URL: https://womenshealth.gov/pregnancy/youre-pregnant-now-what/pregnancy-loss. Accessed May 31, 2023.

Chapter 56 | Molar Pregnancy

Molar pregnancy, also known as "hydatidiform moles," is a rare complication that involves an unusual growth of tissues during fertilization of the egg and sperm. This mass of abnormal tissues resembles a cluster of grapes and grows rapidly compared to a fetus's growth.

TYPES OF MOLAR PREGNANCY
The following are the two types of molar pregnancies:
- **Complete molar pregnancy.** A complete molar pregnancy is when there is no fetus at all. Instead, there is only a growth of abnormal tissues. This kind of pregnancy occurs when an empty egg gets fertilized.
- **Partial molar pregnancy.** A partial molar pregnancy is when a fetus is formed along with an abnormal mass of tissues. The mass proliferates and deprives the fetus of its requirements, causing the death of the fetus.

CAUSES OF MOLAR PREGNANCY
An imbalance of chromosomes causes molar pregnancies. Generally, of the 23 pairs of chromosomes present, each pair contains one from the father and one from the mother in normal fertilization. However, in complete molar pregnancy, the chromosomes from the mother's egg are missing, and only the father's chromosomes are copied. In a partial molar pregnancy, the mother's chromosomes are present, but there are two sets of chromosomes from the father

since two sperm fertilize the egg. This results in the embryo having 69 chromosomes instead of 46.

SIGNS AND SYMPTOMS OF MOLAR PREGNANCY

Most molar pregnancies seem normal at first. Later, the following symptoms begin to develop:

- severe nausea and vomiting
- pelvic pressure or pain
- vaginal spotting and bleeding
- high blood pressure
- swelling of feet and ankles
- rapidly growing uterus
- no movement of the fetus

On visiting the health-care provider, the following signs may also be detected:

- no fetal heart rate
- increased human chorionic gonadotropin (hCG) levels
- ovarian cysts
- hyperthyroidism and anemia

RISK FACTORS OF MOLAR PREGNANCY

It is essential to know who is at risk. Women of the following categories are more prone to facing challenges:

- women over the age of 40 or below the age of 15
- women who have had two or more miscarriages in the past
- women who have had a prior molar pregnancy
- White women who are more at risk than Black in the United States

DIAGNOSIS OF MOLAR PREGNANCY

Molar pregnancy can be detected during routine prenatal tests, usually in the first trimester. An ultrasound reveals a "cluster of grapes" like appearance instead of a normal fetus. The level of hCG

hormones produced during pregnancy is abnormally high in molar pregnancies. A blood test can detect the high levels present. The following additional tests may also be taken:
- ultrasound of the pelvis
- complete blood count
- blood clotting tests
- computed tomography (CT) or magnetic resonance imaging (MRI) of the abdomen
- kidney and liver functions
- chest x-ray

TREATMENT FOR MOLAR PREGNANCY

Medication is given to contract the uterus and expel the mass of abnormal tissues, ending the pregnancy. The hCG levels are frequently checked to ensure that the entire mass has left the body. Serious complications may be involved if any remains of the abnormal tissues are present in the uterus. The doctor may check the hCG levels even after six months after treatment to ensure no tissues are left behind.

In severe cases, the molar pregnancy must be removed surgically. For this, anesthesia is given, and dilation and curettage (D& C) is done. In rare cases, a hysterectomy is performed, meaning the uterus is removed surgically.

COMPLICATIONS IN MOLAR PREGNANCY

The abnormal tissues may remain in the uterus after surgery. This condition may cause the cells to grow around the uterus, known as the "invasive mole." However, it is quite rare and happens in less than 15 percent of molar pregnancy cases.

In rare cases, molar pregnancy can lead to choriocarcinoma, a cancer that forms in the uterus and spreads to other body parts. This treatment would require chemotherapy or radiation.

Other complications may involve sepsis (blood infection), uterine infection, preeclampsia (very high blood pressure), or shock (very low blood pressure).

PREVENTION OF MOLAR PREGNANCY

There is no way to prevent this condition, but if a person has had a previous molar pregnancy, it is advisable not to conceive for at least a year since the diagnosis. It is best to take advice on this from a doctor.

References

"Hydatidiform Mole," John D. Jacobson, David C. Dugdale, October 11, 2022. Available online. URL: https://medlineplus.gov/ency/article/000909.htm. Accessed July 12, 2023.

"Molar Pregnancy," Cleveland Clinic, December 26, 2022. Available online. URL: https://my.clevelandclinic.org/health/diseases/17889-molar-pregnancy. Accessed July 12, 2023.

"Molar Pregnancy," Mayo Foundation for Medical Education and Research, November 12, 2022. Available online. URL: www.mayoclinic.org/diseases-conditions/molar-pregnancy/symptoms-causes/syc-20375175. Accessed July 12, 2023.

"Molar Pregnancy: Symptoms, Risks & Treatment," American Pregnancy Association, May 30, 2007. Available online. URL: https://americanpregnancy.org/healthy-pregnancy/birth-defects/molar-pregnancy. Accessed July 12, 2023.

Chapter 57 | Preterm and Postterm Labor and Birth

Chapter Contents

Section 57.1 | What Is Preterm Labor?

ABOUT PRETERM LABOR AND BIRTH

In general, a normal human pregnancy is about 40 weeks long (9.2 months). Health-care providers now define "full-term" birth as birth that occurs between 39 and 40 weeks and 6 days of pregnancy. Infants born during this time are considered full-term infants.

Infants born in the 37th and 38th weeks of pregnancy—previously called "term" but now referred to as "early term"—face more health risks than do those born at 39 or 40 weeks. Deliveries before 37 weeks of pregnancy are considered "preterm" or premature:

- Labor that begins before 37 weeks of pregnancy is preterm or premature labor.
- A birth that occurs before 37 weeks of pregnancy is preterm or premature birth.
- An infant born before 37 weeks in the womb is a preterm or premature infant. (These infants are commonly called "preemies" as a reference to being born prematurely.)

"Late preterm" refers to 34–36 weeks of pregnancy. Infants born during this time are considered late-preterm infants, but they face many of the same health challenges as preterm infants. More than 70 percent of preterm infants are born during the late-preterm time frame.

Preterm birth is the most common cause of infant death and is the leading cause of long-term disability in children. Many organs, including the brain, lungs, and liver, are still developing in the final weeks of pregnancy. The earlier the delivery, the higher the risk of serious disability or death.

Infants born prematurely are at risk of cerebral palsy (a group of nervous system disorders that affect control of movement and posture and limit activity), developmental delays, and vision and hearing problems. Late-preterm infants typically have better health outcomes than those born earlier, but they are still three times more likely to die in the first year of life than full-term infants. Preterm births can also take a heavy emotional and economic toll on families.

549

WHAT ARE THE SYMPTOMS OF PRETERM LABOR?

Preterm labor is any labor that occurs from 20 weeks through 36 weeks of pregnancy. Here are the symptoms:

- contractions (tightening of stomach muscles or birth pains) every 10 minutes or more often
- change in vaginal discharge (leaking fluid or bleeding from the vagina)
- feeling of pressure in the pelvis (hip) area
- low, dull backache
- cramps that feel like menstrual cramps
- abdominal cramps with or without diarrhea

It is normal for pregnant women to have uterine contractions throughout the day. It is not normal to have frequent uterine contractions, such as six or more in one hour. Frequent uterine contractions, or tightening, may cause the cervix to begin to open. If a woman thinks that she might be having preterm labor, she should call her doctor or go to the hospital to be evaluated.

WHAT CAUSES PRETERM LABOR AND BIRTH?

The causes of preterm labor and premature birth are numerous, complex, and only partly understood. Medical, psychosocial, and biological factors may all play a role in preterm labor and birth. The following are the three main situations in which preterm labor and premature birth may occur:

- **Spontaneous preterm labor and birth**. This term refers to unintentional, unplanned delivery before the 37th week of pregnancy. This type of preterm birth can result from a number of causes, such as infection or inflammation, although the cause of spontaneous preterm labor and delivery is usually not known. A history of delivering preterm is one of the strongest predictors for subsequent preterm births.
- **Medically indicated preterm birth**. If a serious medical condition—such as preeclampsia—exists, the health-care provider might recommend a preterm delivery. In these cases, health-care providers often take

steps to keep the baby in the womb as long as possible to allow for additional growth and development while also monitoring the mother and fetus for health issues. Providers also use additional interventions, such as steroids, to help improve outcomes for the baby.

- **Nonmedically indicated (elective) preterm delivery.** Some late-preterm births result from inducing labor or having a cesarean delivery, even though there is not a medical reason to do so, even though this practice is not recommended. Research indicates that even babies born at 37 or 38 weeks of pregnancy are at higher risk of poor health outcomes than babies born at 39 weeks of pregnancy or later. Therefore, unless there are medical problems, health-care providers should wait until at least 39 weeks of pregnancy to induce labor or perform a cesarean delivery to prevent possible health problems.

The National Child and Maternal Health Education Program (NCMHEP), led by *Eunice Kennedy Shriver* National Institute of Child Health and Human Development (NICHD) in collaboration with 33 other agencies, organizations, and groups focused on maternal and child health, offers videos and other information about why it is best to wait until at least 39 weeks of pregnancy to deliver unless there is a medical reason.

WHAT ARE THE RISK FACTORS FOR PRETERM LABOR AND BIRTH?

There are several risk factors for preterm labor and premature birth, including ones that researchers have not yet identified. Some of these risk factors are "modifiable," meaning they can be changed to help reduce the risk. Other factors cannot be changed. Health-care providers consider the following factors to put women at high risk of preterm labor or birth:

- Women who have delivered preterm before or who have experienced preterm labor before are considered to be at high risk of preterm labor and birth.
- Being pregnant with twins, triplets, or more (called "multiple gestations") or the use of assisted

reproductive technology is associated with a higher risk of preterm labor and birth. One study showed that more than 50 percent of twin births occurred preterm, compared with only 10 percent of births of single infants.

- Women with certain anomalies of the reproductive organs are at greater risk of preterm labor and birth than women who do not have these anomalies. For instance, women who have a short cervix (the lower part of the uterus) or whose cervix shortens in the second trimester (fourth through sixth months) of pregnancy instead of the third trimester are at high risk of preterm delivery.

Certain medical conditions, including some that occur only during pregnancy, also place a woman at higher risk of preterm labor and delivery. Some of these conditions include the following:

- urinary tract infections (UTIs)
- sexually transmitted infections (STIs)
- certain vaginal infections, such as bacterial vaginosis (BV) and trichomoniasis
- high blood pressure
- bleeding from the vagina
- certain developmental anomalies in the fetus
- pregnancy resulting from in vitro fertilization (IVF)
- being underweight or obese before pregnancy
- the short time period between pregnancies (less than six months between a birth and the beginning of the next pregnancy)
- placenta previa, a condition in which the placenta grows in the lowest part of the uterus and covers all or part of the opening to the cervix
- being at risk of rupture of the uterus (when the wall of the uterus rips open; rupture of the uterus is more likely if you have had a prior cesarean delivery or have had a uterine fibroid removed)

- diabetes (high blood sugar) and gestational diabetes (which occurs only during pregnancy)
- blood clotting problems

Other factors that may increase risk of preterm labor and premature birth include the following:

- **Ethnicity.** Preterm labor and birth occur more often among certain racial and ethnic groups. For example, infants of African American mothers are more likely to be born preterm than infants of White mothers. American Indian/Alaska Native mothers are also more likely to give birth preterm than White mothers.
- **Age of the mother:**
  - Women younger than age 18 are more likely to have a preterm delivery.
  - Women older than age 35 are also at risk of having preterm infants because they are more likely to have other conditions (such as high blood pressure and diabetes) that can cause complications requiring preterm delivery.
- **Certain lifestyle and environmental factors:** They include:
  - late or no health care during pregnancy
  - smoking
  - drinking alcohol
  - using illegal drugs
  - domestic violence, including physical, sexual, or emotional abuse
  - lack of social support
  - stress
  - long working hours with long periods of standing
  - exposure to certain environmental pollutants[1]

[1] "Preterm Labor and Birth," *Eunice Kennedy Shriver* National Institute of Child Health and Human Development (NICHD), May 9, 2023. Available online. URL: www.nichd.nih.gov/health/topics/preterm. Accessed June 13, 2023.

Section 57.2 | Preterm Labor Prediction and Prevention

CAN WE PREDICT WHO IS MORE LIKELY TO EXPERIENCE PRETERM LABOR AND BIRTH?

Currently, there is no definitive way to predict preterm labor or premature birth. Many research studies are focusing on this important issue. By identifying which women are at increased risk, health-care providers may be able to provide early interventions, treatments, and close monitoring of these pregnancies to prevent preterm delivery or to improve health outcomes.

However, in some situations, health-care providers know that a preterm delivery is very likely. Some of these situations are described in the following sections.

Shortened Cervix

As preparation for birth, the cervix (the lower part of the uterus) naturally shortens late in pregnancy. However, in some women, the cervix shortens prematurely, around the fourth or fifth month of pregnancy, increasing the risk for preterm delivery.

In some cases, a health-care provider may recommend measuring a pregnant woman's cervical length, especially if she previously had preterm labor or a preterm birth. Ultrasound scans may be used to measure cervical length and identify women with a shortened cervix.

Incompetent Cervix

The cervix normally remains closed during pregnancy. In some cases, the cervix starts to open early, before a fetus is ready to be born. Health-care providers may refer to a cervix that begins to open as an "incompetent" cervix. The process of cervical opening is painless and unnoticeable, without labor contractions or cramping.

To try to prevent preterm birth, a doctor may place a stitch around the cervix to keep it closed. This procedure is called "cervical cerclage." The research supported by the National Institute of Child Health and Human Development (NICHD) has found that in women with a prior preterm birth who have a short cervix, cerclage may improve the likelihood of full-term delivery.

HOW DO HEALTH-CARE PROVIDERS DIAGNOSE PRETERM LABOR?
If a woman is concerned that she could be showing signs of preterm labor, she should call her health-care provider or go to the hospital to be evaluated. In particular, a woman should call if she has more than six contractions in an hour or if fluid or blood is leaking from the vagina.

Physical Exam
If a woman is experiencing signs of labor, the health-care provider may perform a pelvic exam to see if:
• the membranes have ruptured
• the cervix is beginning to get thinner (efface)
• the cervix is beginning to open (dilate)

Any of these situations could mean the woman is in preterm labor. Providers may also do an ultrasound exam and use a monitor to electronically record contractions and the fetal heart rate.

Fetal Fibronectin Test
The fetal fibronectin (fFN) test is used to detect whether the protein fetal fibronectin is being produced. fFN is like a biological "glue" between the uterine lining and the membrane that surrounds the fetus.

Normally, fFN is detectable in the pregnant woman's secretions from the vagina and cervix early in the pregnancy (up to 22 weeks, or about five months) and again toward the end of the pregnancy (one to three weeks before labor begins). It is usually not present between 24 and 34 weeks of pregnancy (5½–8½ months). If fFN is detected during this time, it may be a sign that the woman may be at risk of preterm labor and birth.

In most cases, the fFN test is performed on women who are showing signs of preterm labor. Testing for fFN can help predict which pregnant women showing signs of preterm labor will have a preterm delivery. It is typically used for its negative predictive value, meaning that if it is negative, it is unlikely that a woman will deliver within the next seven days.

WHAT TREATMENTS ARE USED TO PREVENT PRETERM LABOR AND BIRTH?

Currently, treatment options for preventing preterm labor or birth are somewhat limited, in part because the cause of preterm labor or birth is often unknown. But the following are a few options:

- **Hormone treatment.** Progesterone, a hormone produced by the body during pregnancy, was thought to prevent preterm birth in certain groups at high risk of preterm birth, such as those with prior preterm birth. The NICHD's Maternal-Fetal Medicine Units Network found that progesterone given to women at risk of preterm birth due to a prior preterm birth reduces chances of a subsequent preterm birth by one-third when started at 16 weeks of gestation and continued to 37 weeks of gestation. Because subsequent research did not show the same effect, the use of progesterone to prevent preterm birth is now under review by the U.S. Food and Drug Administration (FDA).

- **Cerclage.** A surgical procedure called "cervical cerclage" is sometimes used to try to prevent early labor in women who have an incompetent (weak) cervix and have experienced early pregnancy loss accompanied by a painless opening (dilation) of the cervix (the bottom part of the uterus). In the cerclage procedure, a doctor stitches the cervix closed. The stitch is then removed closer to the woman's due date.

- **Bed rest.** Contrary to expectations, confining the mother to bed rest does not help prevent preterm birth. In fact, bed rest can make preterm birth even more likely among some women.

Women should discuss all of their treatment options—including the risks and benefits—with their health-care providers. If possible, these discussions should occur during regular prenatal care visits, before there is any urgency, to allow for a complete discussion of all the issues.[2]

Section 57.3 | Preterm Labor Risk Reduction Methods That Work and Do Not Work

If a pregnant woman is showing signs of preterm labor, her doctor will often try treatments to stop labor and prolong the pregnancy until the fetus is more fully developed. Treatments include therapies to try to stop labor (tocolytics) and medications administered before birth to improve outcomes for the infant if born preterm (antenatal steroids to improve the respiratory outcomes and neuroprotective medications such as magnesium sulfate).

MEDICATIONS TO DELAY LABOR
Drugs called "tocolytics" can be given to many women with symptoms of preterm labor. These drugs can slow or stop contractions of the uterus and may prevent labor for two to seven days. One common treatment for delaying labor is magnesium sulfate, given to the pregnant woman intravenously through a needle inserted in an arm vein.

MEDICATIONS TO SPEED DEVELOPMENT OF THE FETUS
Tocolytics may provide extra time for treatment with corticosteroids to speed up the development of the fetus's lungs and

---

[2] "Preterm Labor and Birth," *Eunice Kennedy Shriver* National Institute of Child Health and Human Development (NICHD), September 27, 2018. Available online. URL: www.nichd.nih.gov/health/topics/preterm. Accessed June 5, 2023.

some other organs or for the pregnant woman to get to a hospital that offers specialized care for preterm infants. Corticosteroids can be particularly effective if the pregnancy is between 24 and 34 weeks (between 5½ and 7¾ months) and the woman's health-care provider suspects that the birth may occur within the next week. Intravenously delivered magnesium sulfate may also reduce the risk of cerebral palsy (CP) if the child is born early.

WHAT METHODS DO NOT WORK TO PREVENT PRETERM LABOR?
Researchers have found that some methods for trying to stop preterm labor are not as effective as once thought. These include:
- home uterine monitors
- routine screening of all asymptomatic women for bacterial vaginosis (BV; *Trichomonas vaginalis*) infection (Routine screening and treatment with antibiotics did not reduce preterm birth; in fact, the latter increased the risk of preterm birth.)[3]

Section 57.4 | Overdue/Postdue Pregnancy

The actual due date for childbirth is between the 39th week and the end of the 40th week. This is known as a "full-term pregnancy." Birth before 37 weeks is known as "preterm," and pregnancy beyond 42 weeks is called "overdue" or "postdue pregnancy." Birth in the 41st week of pregnancy is known as "late-term." Post the 40th week, the midwife or doctor checks on the mother daily to ensure the baby is normal and safe.

Only 5 percent of women give birth on the exact date of their due date. Sixty percent of women give birth before their due date, and 35 percent give birth beyond their due date.

---

[3] "What Treatments Can Reduce the Chances of Preterm Labor & Birth?" *Eunice Kennedy Shriver* National Institute of Child Health and Human Development (NICHD), January 31, 2017. Available online. URL: https://nichd.nih.gov/health/topics/preterm/conditioninfo/reduce. Accessed May 30, 2023.

CAUSES OF OVERDUE PREGNANCY

A few of the reasons for overdue pregnancy are as follows:

- **First-time pregnancy.** If this is the mother's first birth, there is a higher chance of an overdue pregnancy.
- **Overweight mother.** Excess weight with a body mass index over 30 can cause hormonal changes resulting in late delivery.
- **Prior history.** An overdue pregnancy is likely to occur if the mother's previous birth occurred beyond the due date.
- **Size and position of the baby.** If the baby has a large head or has not turned to the head-down position, it will not be easy for childbirth as the foot-down position can cause complications.
- **Diseases.** Conditions related to the liver, endocrine system, or sexually transmitted diseases can cause late deliveries.
- **Hereditary.** It is possible that overdue pregnancies run in the family.

GETTING LABOR STARTED

When the onset of labor is delayed, the midwife and/or doctor closely monitor the mother and baby to ensure everything is normal. Depending on the current stage and condition, they recommend the following:

- **Breaking the water.** If the amniotic sac remains intact, the fluid is released by rupturing the sac.
- **Medicine.** Oxytocin is given to speed up contractions and expand the cervix.
- **Cervical ripening.** A small inflatable balloon attached at the end of the catheter is used to soften and ripen the cervix.
- **Moving around and staying active.** Walking and doing exercises such as the butterfly stretch, pelvic tilts, and lunges may help initiate labor.
- **Relaxation techniques.** Gentle circular stroking of the abdomen and massage of feet, back, and shoulders may help.

• **Inducing labor.** Prostaglandin gel is inserted intravaginally to ripen the cervix, and oral oxytocin tablets are taken to help in contractions and induce labor.

TESTS TO BE DONE

An ultrasound and a cardiotocograph are recommended twice weekly from the 41st week onward. If the results show a risk, an induction is done immediately, and if the baby is healthy and all other signs are normal, the doctor waits for natural labor to begin.

RISKS INVOLVED IN OVERDUE PREGNANCY

When the baby remains in the womb beyond 41 weeks, it creates increased risks for the mother and the baby. Common risks that affect the baby are as follows:

• Toward the end of pregnancy, the placenta is aged and is unable to carry out its normal functions, such as providing oxygen and nutrients to the baby. The lack of oxygen causes an overdue pregnancy to end in a stillbirth (the baby dies before birth).
• Vernix caseosa is a layer of skin that protects the baby's skin while it is in the womb. Toward the end of pregnancy, the vernix caseosa starts wearing off, and the baby is exposed to the amniotic fluid. This causes wrinkles and peeling skin in overdue babies.
• The baby's first stool (meconium) could enter the lungs and cause serious respiratory issues.
• The umbilical cord gets compressed during contractions, affecting the baby's heart rate and oxygen flow to the lungs.

Risks that affect the mother are:
• infections in the uterus
• a long labor and difficult birth
• severe vaginal tears
• postpartum bleeding resulting in heavy blood loss

It is best to keep the doctor informed if one finds no signs of labor while nearing the due date. Follow the physical exercises recommended by the midwife or doctor and ensure to get checked frequently to avoid complications.

References

"The Evidence On: Due Dates," Evidence Based Birth, November 24, 2019. Available online. URL: https://evidencebasedbirth.com/evidence-on-due-dates. Accessed July 17, 2023.

"Pregnancy and Birth: When Your Baby's Due Date Has Passed," National Library of Medicine, March 22, 2018. Available online. URL: www.ncbi.nlm.nih.gov/books/NBK279571. Accessed July 12, 2023.

"Slow Progress in Labor," Health Direct Australia, July 2022. Available online. URL: www.pregnancybirthbaby.org. au/slow-progress-in-labour. Accessed July 12, 2023.

Chapter 58 | Birth Defects and Developmental Disabilities

Chapter Contents

Section 58.1 | Birth Defects That May Be Diagnosed during Pregnancy

Birth defects are common, costly, and critical conditions that affect 1 in every 33 babies born in the United States each year. This section provides information about birth defects and how women can improve their chances of having a baby born without a birth defect.

BIRTH DEFECTS ARE COMMON
Every 4½ minutes, a baby is born with a birth defect in the United States. That means nearly 120,000 babies are affected by birth defects each year.

Birth defects are structural changes present at birth that can affect almost any part or parts of the body (e.g., heart, brain, foot). They may affect how the body looks, works, or both. Birth defects can vary from mild to severe. The well-being of each child affected with a birth defect depends mostly on which organ or body part is involved and how much it is affected. Depending on the severity of the defect and what body part is affected, the expected lifespan of a person with a birth defect may or may not be affected.

IDENTIFYING BIRTH DEFECTS
A birth defect can be found before birth, at birth, or any time after birth. Most birth defects are found within the first year of life. Some birth defects (such as cleft lip) are easy to see, but others (such as heart defects or hearing loss) are found using special tests, such as an echocardiogram (an ultrasound picture of the heart), x-rays, or hearing tests.

CAUSES OF BIRTH DEFECTS
Birth defects can occur during any stage of pregnancy. Most birth defects occur in the first three months of pregnancy when the

organs of the baby are forming. This is a very important stage of development. However, some birth defects occur later in pregnancy. During the last six months of pregnancy, the tissues and organs continue to grow and develop.

For some birth defects, such as fetal alcohol syndrome, we know the cause. But, for most birth defects, we do not know what causes them. For most birth defects, we think they are caused by a complex mix of factors. These factors include our genes (information inherited from our parents), our behaviors, and things in the environment. But we do not fully understand how these factors might work together to cause birth defects.

While we still have more work to do, we have learned a lot about birth defects through past research. For example, some things might increase the chances of having a baby with a birth defect, such as:

- smoking, drinking alcohol, or taking certain drugs during pregnancy
- having certain medical conditions, such as being obese or having uncontrolled diabetes before and during pregnancy
- taking certain medications, such as isotretinoin (a drug used to treat severe acne)
- having someone in your family with a birth defect (To learn more about your risk of having a baby with a birth defect, you can talk with a clinical geneticist or a genetic counselor.)
- having certain infections during pregnancy, such as Zika virus and cytomegalovirus
- experiencing a fever greater than 101 °F (38.3 °C) or having an elevated body temperature due to heat exposure
- being an older mother as the risk of chromosomal abnormalities increases with age

Having one or more of these risks does not mean you will have a pregnancy affected by a birth defect. Also, women can have a baby born with a birth defect even when they do not have any of these risks. It is important to talk to your doctor about what you can do to lower your risk.[1]

DIAGNOSIS OF BIRTH DEFECTS DURING PREGNANCY: PRENATAL TESTING

Birth defects can be diagnosed during pregnancy or after the baby is born, depending on the specific type of birth defect.

Screening Tests

A screening test is a procedure or test that is done to see if a woman or her baby might have certain problems. A screening test does not provide a specific diagnosis—that requires a diagnostic test. A screening test can sometimes give an abnormal result even when there is nothing wrong with the mother or her baby. Less often, a screening test result can be normal and miss a problem that does exist. During pregnancy, women are usually offered these screening tests to check for birth defects or other problems for the woman or her baby. Talk to your doctor about any concerns you have about prenatal testing.

First Trimester Screening

First trimester screening is a combination of tests completed between weeks 11 and 13 of pregnancy. It is used to look for certain birth defects related to the baby's heart or chromosomal disorders, such as Down syndrome. This screen includes a maternal blood test and an ultrasound.

- **Maternal blood screen.** The maternal blood screen is a simple blood test. It measures the levels of two proteins, human chorionic gonadotropin (hCG) and pregnancy-associated plasma protein A (PAPP-A). If the protein

---

[1] National Center on Birth Defects and Developmental Disabilities (NCBDDD), "What Are Birth Defects?" Centers for Disease Control and Prevention (CDC), June 28, 2023. Available online. URL: https://cdc.gov/ncbddd/birthdefects/facts.html. Accessed July 24, 2023.

levels are abnormally high or low, there could be a chromosomal disorder in the baby.

- **Ultrasound**. An ultrasound creates pictures of the baby. The ultrasound for the first trimester screen looks for extra fluid behind the baby's neck. If there is increased fluid found on the ultrasound, there could be a chromosomal disorder or heart defect in the baby.

Second Trimester Screening

Second trimester screening tests are completed between weeks 15 and 20 of pregnancy. They are used to look for certain birth defects in the baby. Second trimester screening tests include a maternal serum screen and a comprehensive ultrasound evaluation of the baby, looking for the presence of structural anomalies (also known as an "anomaly ultrasound").

- **Maternal serum screen**. The maternal serum screen is a simple blood test used to identify if a woman is at increased risk of having a baby with certain birth defects, such as neural tube defects, or chromosomal disorders, such as Down syndrome. It is also known as a "triple screen" or "quad screen," depending on the number of proteins measured in the mother's blood. For example, a quad screen tests the levels of four proteins: alpha-fetoprotein (AFP), hCG, estriol, and inhibin A. Generally, the maternal serum screen is completed during the second trimester.

- **Fetal echocardiogram**. A fetal echocardiogram is a test that uses sound waves to evaluate the baby's heart for heart defects before birth. This test can provide a more detailed image of the baby's heart than a regular pregnancy ultrasound. Some heart defects cannot be seen before birth, even with a fetal echocardiogram. If your health-care provider finds a problem in the structure of the baby's heart, a detailed ultrasound may be done to look for other problems with the developing baby.

- **Anomaly ultrasound**. An ultrasound creates pictures of the baby. This test is usually completed around 18–20 weeks of pregnancy. The ultrasound is used to check the size of the baby and looks for birth defects or other problems with the baby.

DIAGNOSTIC TESTS

If the result of a screening test is abnormal, doctors usually offer further diagnostic tests to determine if birth defects or other possible problems with the baby are present. These diagnostic tests are also offered to women with higher-risk pregnancies, which may include women who are 35 years of age or older; women who have had a previous pregnancy affected by a birth defect; women who have chronic diseases such as lupus, high blood pressure, diabetes, or epilepsy; or women who use certain medications.

High-Resolution Ultrasound

An ultrasound creates pictures of the baby. This ultrasound, also known as a "level II ultrasound," is used to look in more detail for possible birth defects or other problems with the baby that were suggested in the previous screening tests. It is usually completed between weeks 18 and 22 of pregnancy.

Chorionic Villus Sampling

Chorionic villus sampling (CVS) is a test where the doctor collects a tiny piece of the placenta, called "chorionic villus," which is then tested to check for chromosomal or genetic disorders in the baby. Generally, a CVS test is offered to women who received an abnormal result on a first trimester screening test or to women who could be at higher risk. It is completed between 10 and 12 weeks of pregnancy, earlier than an amniocentesis.

Amniocentesis

An amniocentesis is a test where the doctor collects a small amount of amniotic fluid from the area surrounding the baby. The fluid is then tested to measure the baby's protein levels, which might indicate certain birth defects. Cells in the amniotic fluid can be tested for chromosomal disorders, such as Down syndrome, and genetic problems, such as cystic fibrosis (CF) or Tay-Sachs disease. Generally, an amniocentesis is offered to women who received an abnormal result on a screening test or to women who might be at higher risk. It is completed between 15 and 18 weeks of pregnancy. The following are some of the proteins for which an amniocentesis tests:

- **Alpha-fetoprotein.** AFP is a protein that the baby produces. A high level of AFP in the amniotic fluid might mean that the baby has a defect indicating an opening in the tissue, such as a neural tube defect (anencephaly or spina bifida), or a body wall defect, such as omphalocele or gastroschisis.
- **Acetylcholinesterase (AChE).** AChE is an enzyme that the baby produces. This enzyme can pass from the baby to the fluid surrounding the baby if there is an opening in the neural tube.

AFTER THE BABY IS BORN

Certain birth defects might not be diagnosed until after the baby is born. Sometimes, the birth defect is immediately seen at birth. For other birth defects, including some heart defects, the birth defect might not be diagnosed until later in life.

When there is a health problem with a child, the primary care provider might look for birth defects by taking a medical and family history, doing a physical exam, and sometimes recommending further tests. If a diagnosis cannot be made after the exam, the primary care provider might refer the child to a specialist in birth defects and genetics. A clinical geneticist is a doctor with special training to evaluate patients who may have genetic conditions or birth defects. Even if a child sees a specialist, an exact diagnosis might not be reached.[2]

---

[2] National Center on Birth Defects and Developmental Disabilities (NCBDDD), "Diagnosis of Birth Defects," Centersfor Disease Control and Prevention (CDC), June 28, 2023. Available online. URL: https://cdc.gov/ncbddd/birthdefects/diagnosis.html. Accessed July 24, 2023.

PREVENTION OF BIRTH DEFECTS

Not all birth defects can be prevented. But there are things that a woman can do before and during pregnancy to increase her chance of having a healthy baby:

- Be sure to see your health-care provider regularly and start prenatal care as soon as you think you might be pregnant.
- Get 400 mcg of folic acid every day, starting at least one month before getting pregnant.
- Do not drink alcohol or smoke.
- Talk to a health-care provider about any medications you are taking or thinking about taking. This includes prescription and over-the-counter (OTC) medications and dietary or herbal supplements. Do not stop or start taking any type of medication without first talking with a doctor.
- Know how to prevent infections during pregnancy.
- Be proactive in identifying and treating fever when ill or after getting a vaccine. Treat fevers higher than 101 °F (38.3 °C) with Tylenol® (or store-brand acetaminophen) and avoid hot tubs, saunas, or other environments that might cause overheating.
- If possible, be sure any medical conditions are under control before becoming pregnant. Some conditions, such as diabetes, can increase the risk of birth defects.[3]

---

[3] See footnote [1].

Section 58.2 | Developmental Disabilities

Developmental disabilities are a group of conditions due to an impairment in physical, learning, language, or behavior areas. These conditions begin during the developmental period, may impact day-to-day functioning, and usually last throughout a person's lifetime.

DEVELOPMENTAL MILESTONES

Developmental monitoring is an active, ongoing process of watching a child grow and encouraging conversations between parents and providers about a child's skills and abilities. Developmental monitoring involves observing how your child grows and whether your child meets the typical developmental milestones or gains skills that most children reach by a certain age in playing, learning, speaking, behaving, and moving.

Parents, grandparents, early childhood education providers, and other caregivers can participate in developmental monitoring. If you notice that your child is not meeting milestones, talk with your doctor or nurse about your concerns and ask about developmental screening.

When you take your child to a well-child visit, your doctor or nurse will also do developmental monitoring. The doctor or nurse might ask you questions about your child's development or will talk and play with your child to see if they are developing and meeting milestones.

DEVELOPMENTAL MONITORING AND SCREENING

Developmental screening takes a closer look at how your child is developing. Developmental screening is more formal than developmental monitoring. It is a regular part of some well-child visits, even if there is not a known concern.

The American Academy of Pediatrics (AAP) recommends developmental and behavioral screening for all children during regular well-child visits at the following ages:
- 9 months
- 18 months
- 30 months

In addition, the AAP recommends that all children be screened specifically for autism spectrum disorder (ASD) during regular well-child visits at the following ages:
- 18 months
- 24 months

Screening questionnaires and checklists are based on research that compares your child to other children of the same age. Questions may ask about language, movement, and thinking skills, as well as behaviors and emotions. Developmental screening can be done by a doctor or nurse or other professionals in health care, community, or school settings. Your doctor may ask you to complete a questionnaire as part of the screening process. Screening at times other than the recommended ages should be done if you or your doctor have a concern. Additional screening should also be done if a child is at high risk for ASD (e.g., having a sibling or other family member with ASD) or if behaviors sometimes associated with ASD are present. If your child's health-care provider does not periodically check your child with a developmental screening test, you can ask that it be done.

CAUSES AND RISK FACTORS OF DEVELOPMENTAL DISABILITIES

Developmental disabilities begin anytime during the developmental period and usually last throughout a person's lifetime. Most developmental disabilities begin before a baby is born, but some can happen after birth because of injury, infection, or other factors.

Most developmental disabilities are thought to be caused by a complex mix of factors. These factors include genetics, parental health and behaviors (such as smoking and drinking) during pregnancy, complications during birth, infections the mother might have during pregnancy or the baby might have very early in life, and exposure of the mother or child to high levels of environmental toxins, such as lead. For some developmental disabilities, such as fetal alcohol syndrome (FAS), which is caused by drinking alcohol during pregnancy, we know the cause. But, for most, we do not.

The following are some examples of what we know about specific developmental disabilities:

- At least 25 percent of hearing loss among babies is due to maternal infections during pregnancy, such as cytomegalovirus (CMV) infection, complications after birth, and head trauma.
- Some of the most commonly known causes of intellectual disability include fetal alcohol syndrome disorder (FASD); genetic and chromosomal conditions, such as Down syndrome and fragile X syndrome; and certain infections during pregnancy.
- Children who have a sibling with ASD are at higher risk of also having ASD.
- Low birth weight, premature birth, multiple birth, and infections during pregnancy are associated with an increased risk of many developmental disabilities.
- Untreated newborn jaundice (high levels of bilirubin in the blood during the first few days after birth) can cause a type of brain damage known as "kernicterus." Children with kernicterus are more likely to have cerebral palsy, hearing and vision problems, and problems with their teeth. Early detection and treatment of newborn jaundice can prevent kernicterus.

The Study to Explore Early Development (SEED) is a multiyear study funded by the Centers for Disease Control and Prevention (CDC). It is currently the largest study in the United States to help identify factors that may put children at risk for ASDs and other developmental disabilities.

WHO IS MORE LIKELY TO GET AFFECTED?
Developmental disabilities occur among all racial, ethnic, and socioeconomic groups. Recent estimates in the United States show that about one in six, or about 17 percent, of children aged 3 through 17 have one or more of the following developmental disabilities:

- attention deficit hyperactivity disorder (ADHD)
- ASD
- cerebral palsy (CP)
- hearing loss
- intellectual disability
- learning disability
- vision impairment and
- other developmental delays

LIVING WITH A DEVELOPMENTAL DISABILITY

Children and adults with disabilities need health care and health programs for the same reasons anyone else does—to stay well and active and be a part of the community.

Having a disability does not mean a person is not healthy or that he or she cannot be healthy. Being healthy means the same thing for all of us—getting and staying well, so we can lead full, active lives. That includes having the tools and information to make healthy choices and knowing how to prevent illness. Some health conditions, such as asthma, gastrointestinal symptoms, eczema and skin allergies, and migraine headaches, have been found to be more common among children with developmental disabilities. Thus, it is especially important for children with developmental disabilities to see a health-care provider regularly.[4]

[4] National Center on Birth Defects and Developmental Disabilities (NCBDDD), "Facts about Developmental Disabilities," Centers for Disease Control and Prevention (CDC), April 27, 2022. Available online. URL: https://cdc.gov/ncbddd/developmentaldisabilities/facts.html. Accessed May 30, 2023.

Part 6 | **Labor and Delivery**

Chapter 59 | **All about Labor and Delivery**

Chapter Contents

Section 59.1 | Signs of Labor

For most women, labor begins sometime between week 37 and week 42 of pregnancy. Labor that occurs before 37 weeks of pregnancy is considered premature, or preterm. Just as pregnancy is different for every woman, the start of labor, the signs of labor, and the length of time it takes to go through labor vary from woman to woman and even from pregnancy to pregnancy.

The primary sign of labor is a series of contractions (tightening and relaxing of the uterus) that arrive regularly. Over time, they become stronger, last longer, and are more frequent. Some women may experience false labor when contractions are weak or irregular or stop when the woman changes positions. Women who have regular contractions every 5–10 minutes for an hour should let their health-care provider know.

It is important to discuss labor and signs of labor with a health-care provider early in pregnancy before labor begins. Some providers may want a woman to wait until she has multiple signs of labor or is in "active" labor before coming to the hospital or birthing center. Other signs of labor include the following:

- **Lightening**. This term refers to when the fetus "drops," or moves lower in the uterus. This may happen several weeks or only a few hours before labor begins. Not all fetuses drop before birth. Lightening gets its name from the feeling of lightness or relief that some women experience when the fetus moves from the rib cage to the pelvic area. It allows some women to breathe more easily and more deeply and may provide relief from heartburn.
- **Increase in vaginal discharge**. Also called "show" or the "bloody show," the discharge can be clear, pink, or slightly bloody. This discharge occurs as the cervix begins to open (dilate) and can happen several days before labor or just as labor begins.

Labor contractions before 37 weeks of pregnancy are a sign of preterm labor. Women who notice regular, frequent contractions at any point in pregnancy should notify a provider or go to the hospital. Providers can check for changes in the cervix to see whether labor has begun. As needed, providers can also give women in preterm labor specialized care. Among women who experience preterm labor, only about 10 percent go on to give birth within a week.

Other signs of labor include the following:
- change in vaginal discharge
- pain or pressure around the front of the pelvis or the rectum
- low, dull backache
- cramps that feel like menstrual cramps, with or without diarrhea
- a gush or trickle of fluid, which is a sign of water breaking

Sometimes, if the health of the mother or the fetus is at risk, a woman's health-care provider will recommend inducing or causing labor using medically supervised methods, such as medication.

Unless earlier delivery is medically necessary or occurs on its own, waiting until at least 39 weeks before delivering gives the mother and baby the best chance for healthy outcomes. During the last few weeks of pregnancy, the fetus's lungs, brain, and liver are still developing.[1]

[1] "When Does Labor Usually Start?" *Eunice Kennedy Shriver* National Institute of Child Health and Human Development (NICHD), September 1, 2017. Available online. URL: www.nichd.nih.gov/health/topics/labor-delivery/topicinfo/start-of-labor. Accessed May 19, 2023.

Section 59.2 | What Are False Labor and Braxton Hicks Contractions?

WHAT IS FALSE LABOR, AND WHAT ARE BRAXTON HICKS CONTRACTIONS?

"False labor" refers to irregular contractions that sometimes happen before true labor begins. These contractions are also called "Braxton Hicks contractions." It can be hard to tell the difference between Braxton Hicks contractions and true labor contractions.

Table 59.1, from the American Congress of Obstetricians and Gynecologists (ACOG), shows some ways that Braxton Hicks contractions differ from true labor contractions.

Table 59.1. Difference between True and False Labor

Type of Change	False Labor	True Labor
Timing of contractions	Contractions do not come regularly and do not get closer together.	Contractions come at regular times and get closer together over time. Each lasts about 30–70 seconds.
Effect of movement	Contractions may stop when the woman walks or rests, or they may stop when the woman changes position.	Contractions continue despite movement.
Strength of contractions	Contractions are usually weak and do not get much stronger, or they may start strong and get weaker.	Contractions get steadily stronger.
Pain of contractions	The woman usually feels pain only in the front.	Pain usually starts in the back and moves to the front.

HOW ARE LABOR AND DELIVERY DIFFERENT FOR A WOMAN HAVING MULTIPLES?

When women carry multiple fetuses—twins, triplets, or quadruplets, for example—labor and delivery proceed through the same stages as with a single infant. But labor and delivery with multiples have some important differences. For example, women having multiples are more likely to have certain complications. The most common are preterm labor and preterm birth.

Preterm labor is labor that starts before 37 weeks of pregnancy. It can result in preterm birth. More than half of all twins are born preterm. Preterm infants can have problems with breathing and eating and may have to stay in the hospital longer than other infants.

In a pregnancy with multiples, providers look to see whether the woman has one or more than one placenta, which direction(s) the fetuses are facing, and where the umbilical cords lie. In addition, they closely monitor the woman's health because carrying multiples can increase a woman's risk of gestational diabetes and preeclampsia. These factors can all affect when and how a provider recommends delivering the babies. Some of these complications may require a cesarean delivery to resolve. Multiples are about 2.5 times more likely to be delivered by cesarean section (C-section) than singletons are.

WHAT IS THE APGAR TEST?

The Apgar test, performed one minute and five minutes after birth, gauges an infant's overall health. A health-care provider assesses the following aspects of an infant's health:

- skin color
- heart rate
- reflexes (response to stimulation, such as a mild pinch)
- muscle tone
- breathing

Based on this examination, the health-care provider gives the infant an Apgar score of 1–10. The higher the score, the better the infant is doing.

ARE THERE ADDED LABOR AND DELIVERY RISKS FOR OLDER WOMEN?

Women older than 35 are at higher risk for preterm labor and preterm birth. Preterm infants can have serious short- and long-term health problems.

Older women are also more likely to have a stillbirth, which is when a fetus dies in the uterus after 20 weeks of pregnancy. Women in their 30s are also more likely than younger women to need a cesarean delivery.

WHAT SHOULD WOMEN CONSIDER WHEN CHOOSING WHERE TO DELIVER?

Although most women give birth in hospitals, some families choose a home birth or birth in an out-of-hospital birthing center. The American Academy of Pediatrics (AAP) and the ACOG recommend births in hospitals or birthing centers as the safest options.

Talk to your health-care provider about where you want to deliver your baby. If possible, schedule a time to visit the hospital, birthing center, or other setting before you make your decision. Consider the risks and benefits of each as you make your decision. Women who are good candidates for home birth:

- are generally in good health
- have not had a previous cesarean delivery
- do not have pregnancy-related health problems or illnesses
- do not have multiples
- have a fetus with good size and health
- have a fetus in the head-down position
- go into labor at 37 weeks or later

Planned home births benefit from having the following resources in place:

- a certified nurse-midwife, certified midwife, or practicing physician
- at least one appropriately trained individual whose primary responsibility is the care of the newborn infant
- quick access to health-care providers who can provide consultation if complications happen
- a reliable plan for safe and fast transportation to a nearby hospital in case of an emergency

IS GIVING BIRTH IN WATER BENEFICIAL?

Some women report that being immersed in water during early labor shortened their labor and reduced their pain. However, these and other benefits of giving birth in water are unconfirmed by research evidence. Also, water births carry risks, including infections and drowning. The ACOG notes that allowing women to labor in a birthing pool may have benefits, but it recommends against giving birth in water.[2]

[2] "Other Labor and Delivery FAQs," *Eunice Kennedy Shriver* National Institute of Child Health and Human Development (NICHD), September 1, 2017. Available online. URL: www.nichd.nih.gov/health/topics/labor-delivery/topicinfo/more_information/questions. Accessed June 8, 2023.

Chapter 60 | Maternity Care Practices

In the United States, nearly all infants are born in a hospital. Their stay is typically very short, but events during this time have lasting effects. Experiences with breastfeeding in the first hours and days of life significantly influence an infant's later feeding. Several key supportive hospital practices can improve breastfeeding outcomes. Birth facility policies and practices that create a supportive environment for breastfeeding begin prenatally and continue through discharge and include the following:

- **Hospital policies.** Written hospital policies support breastfeeding and are communicated to staff and patients.
- **Staff training.** The hospital requires breastfeeding education, clinical training, and competency verification for all maternity staff who work with breastfeeding families.
- **Immediate skin-to-skin contact.** Newborns are placed skin-to-skin with their mothers immediately after birth, with no bedding or clothing between them, allowing enough uninterrupted time (at least one hour) for the mother and the baby to start breastfeeding well.
- **Early and frequent breastfeeding.** Hospital staff help mothers and babies start breastfeeding as soon as possible after birth, with many opportunities to practice throughout the hospital stay.
- **Teaching about breastfeeding.** Hospital staff teach mothers and babies how to breastfeed and to recognize and respond to feeding cues.

- **Exclusive breastfeeding.** Hospital staff follow current evidence-based protocols for breastfeeding infants and provide supplementary feedings only when medically necessary.
- **Rooming-in.** Hospital staff encourage mothers and babies to room together and teach families the benefits of this kind of close contact, including more opportunities to practice breastfeeding and learn their infant's feeding cues.
- **Follow-up after discharge.** Hospital staff schedule follow-up visits for mothers and babies after they go home and connect families to community breastfeeding resources.[1]

---

[1] "Overview: Maternity Care Practices," Centers for Disease Control and Prevention (CDC), May 25, 2023. Available online. URL: www.cdc.gov/breastfeeding/data/mpinc/maternity-care-practices.htm. Accessed June 8, 2023.

Chapter 61 | Birth Partners

Chapter Contents

Section 61.1 | Tip Card for Expectant Dads

When dads are involved as supportive partners during pregnancy, it is good for their babies, good for moms, and good for dads.

- When their partner supports them, pregnant women are more likely to get regular prenatal care and eat and live healthily, which increases the likelihood of positive health outcomes for their babies.
- Dads who are there for mom and baby during the pregnancy are better prepared for their role as new dads. They feel more involved, and their baby has more opportunities to get to know their dad.
- Moms who have calm and supportive birth partners have better labor experiences.

WHAT YOU CAN DO

Be involved, be encouraging, and be there.

- Talk with your partner about expectations and feelings: What is she expecting from you as a dad? What are you feeling and expecting?
- Take a childbirth class; go to prenatal and doctor visits with your partner: Get to know the people who are going to be delivering your baby.
- Recognize that pregnancy can be stressful for you and your partner. Besides supporting and helping her, you also need to find time to focus on yourself.
- Talk with other dads and ask how they prepared for the birth of their children.
- Start taking on extra responsibilities around the house: Pick things up, clean the house, make some meals, and go shopping.
- Prepare for the birth.
  - Get things ready for your new baby: You will need a crib, diapers, a car seat, and a stroller.
  - Map out a route to the hospital.

- Help your partner prepare a bag that will be ready with a change of clothes and other essentials to take with you.
- If you are employed, talk with your employer about taking family leave or working flexible time after birth, so you can help care for your new baby.[1]

Section 61.2 | Doula Services

Doulas provide services to other women during pregnancy, childbirth, and the postpartum period. The content of their services are composed of continuous nonmedical social, physical, and emotional support, and Doulas' roles are recognized as "sister-like," "woman-to-woman," "mother-to-daughter," or "friend-to-friend" relationship. Doulas often encourage young mothers to explore their goals.

In traditional societies, relatives and elderly women (e.g., mothers and grandmothers) are acknowledged as young mothers' role models to teach childbearing skills from one generation to another. Contrary to traditional societies, in individualistic cultures, the help of family members is barely available to young mothers.

Due to the lack of partners of family members, doulas take the role of these extended family members in individualistic cultures. For example, doulas help mothers by providing 24-hour call availability during pre-birth, labor, delivery, and the postpartum period; individual counseling; and transportation provision to mothers. While providing services and accompanying mothers, all doulas respect each woman's uniqueness and diverse religious and cultural beliefs.

[1] "Tip Card for Expectant Dads," National Responsible Fatherhood Clearinghouse (NRFC), September 25, 2020. Available online. URL: www.fatherhood.gov/sites/default/files/resource_files/nrfc_tip_card_for_expectant_dads_release_508.pdf. Accessed May 19, 2023.

THE ROLE OF DOULAS

The main role of doulas is a caring process for mothers in early pregnancy through the transition of motherhood. Doulas professionally assist the mother through all of her child's development and meet their needs. The role of doulas is to help women have a safe and empowering birthing experience. Doulas accompany women throughout labor and delivery at home and in a hospital setting. Furthermore, doulas educate mothers, their partners, and family members about childbirth preparation and breastfeeding.

The following are the three types of doulas:

- **Prenatal doula.** The first one is called a "prenatal doula." Prenatal doulas promote health, build healthy relationships, encourage receiving good medical care, educate mothers about the baby, and teach about labor and delivery.
- **Birth doula.** The other one is called a "birth doula" (intrapartum) who provides comfort, assists in the birth progress, and nurtures family interaction. After the birth, doulas make home visits to teach breastfeeding techniques, nurture the family connection, educate the new parents on childbearing, and help new mothers with transportation.
- **Postpartum doula.** The third one is classified as a postpartum doula. These doulas accompany mothers to take care of their newborn babies, teaching baby care basics.

Although there are three types of doulas, sometimes, doulas can carry out all roles.[2]

---

[2] "Doulas' Perceptions on Single Mothers' Risk and Protective Factors, and Aspirations Relative to Child-Birth," U.S. Department of Education (ED), April 30, 2017. Available online. URL: https://files.eric.ed.gov/fulltext/EJ1005000.pdf. Accessed May 19, 2023.

Chapter 62 | Vaginal and Cesarean Childbirths

Chapter Contents

Section 62.1 | Vaginal/Natural Childbirth

SPOT THE SIGNS OF LABOR

As you approach your due date, you will be looking for any little sign that labor is about to start. You might notice that your baby has "dropped" or moved lower into your pelvis. This is called "lightening." If you have a pelvic exam during your prenatal visit, your doctor might report changes in your cervix that you cannot feel, but that suggest your body is getting ready. For some women, a flurry of energy and the impulse to cook or clean, called "nesting," are signs that labor is approaching.

Some signs suggest that labor will begin very soon. Call your doctor or midwife if you have any of the following signs of labor. Call your doctor even if it is weeks before your due date—you might be going into preterm labor. Your doctor or midwife can decide if it is time to go to the hospital or if you should be seen at the office first.

- You have contractions that become stronger at regular and increasingly shorter intervals.
- You have lower back pain and cramping that do not go away.
- Your water breaks (can be a large gush or a continuous trickle).
- You have a bloody (brownish or red-tinged) mucus discharge. This is probably the mucus plug that blocks the cervix. Losing your mucus plug usually means your cervix is dilating (opening up) and becoming thinner and softer (effacing). Labor could start right away or may still be days away.

Did Your Water Break?

It is not always easy to know. If your water breaks, it could be a gush or a slow trickle of amniotic fluid. Rupture of membranes is the medical term for your water breaking. Let your doctor know the time your water breaks and any color or odor. Also, call your doctor if you think your water broke but are not sure. An easy test can tell your doctor if the leaking fluid is urine (many pregnant women leak urine) or amniotic fluid. Often, a woman will go into labor soon after her water breaks. When this does not happen, her doctor may want to induce (bring about) labor. This is because once your water breaks, your risk of getting an infection goes up as labor is delayed.

FALSE LABOR

Many women, especially first-time mothers-to-be, think they are in labor when they are not. This is called "false labor." "Practice" contractions called "Braxton Hicks contractions" are common in the last weeks of pregnancy or earlier. The tightening of your uterus might startle you. Some might even be painful or take your breath away. It is no wonder that many women mistake Braxton Hicks contractions for the real thing. So do not feel embarrassed if you go to the hospital thinking you are in labor, only to be sent home.

So how can you tell if your contractions are true labor? Time them. Use a watch or clock to keep track of the time one contraction starts to the time the next contraction starts, as well as how long each contraction lasts. With true labor, contractions become regular, stronger, and more frequent. Braxton Hicks contractions are not in a regular pattern, and they taper off and go away. Some women find that a change in activity, such as walking or lying down, makes Braxton Hicks contractions go away. This will not happen with true labor. Even with these guidelines, it can be hard to tell if labor is real. If you ever are unsure if contractions are true labor, call your doctor.

STAGES OF LABOR

Labor occurs in three stages. When regular contractions begin, the baby moves down into the pelvis as the cervix both effaces (thins) and dilates (opens). How labor progresses and how long it lasts are different for every woman. But each stage features some milestones that are true for every woman.

First Stage

Most babies' heads enter the pelvis facing to one side and then rotate to face down.

The first stage begins with the onset of labor and ends when the cervix is fully opened. It is the longest stage of labor, usually lasting about 12–19 hours. Many women spend the early part of this first stage at home. You might want to rest, watch TV, hang out with family, or even go for a walk. Most women can drink and eat during labor, which can provide needed energy later. Yet some doctors advise laboring women to avoid solid food as a precaution should a cesarean delivery be needed. Ask your doctor about eating during labor. While at home, time your contractions and keep your doctor up to date on your progress. Your doctor will tell you when to go to the hospital or birthing center.

At the hospital, your doctor will monitor the progress of your labor by periodically checking your cervix, as well as the baby's position and station (location in the birth canal). Most babies' heads enter the pelvis facing to one side and then rotate to face down. Sometimes, a baby will be facing up toward the mother's abdomen. Intense back labor often goes along with this position. Your doctor might try to rotate the baby, or the baby might turn on its own.

As you near the end of the first stage of labor, contractions become longer, stronger, and closer together. Many of the positioning and relaxation tips you learned in childbirth class can help now. Try to find the most comfortable position during contractions and let your muscles go limp between contractions. Let your support person know how he or she can be helpful, such as by rubbing your lower back, giving you ice chips to suck, or putting a cold washcloth on your forehead.

Sometimes, medicines and other methods are used to help speed up labor that is progressing slowly. Many doctors will rupture the membranes. Although this practice is widely used, studies show that doing so during labor does not help shorten the length of labor.

Your doctor might want to use an electronic fetal monitor to see if the blood supply to your baby is okay. For most women, this involves putting two straps around the mother's abdomen.

One strap measures the strength and frequency of your contractions. The other strap records how the baby's heartbeat reacts to the contraction.

The most difficult phase of this first stage is the transition. Contractions are very powerful, with very little time to relax in between, as the cervix stretches the last few centimeters (cm). Many women feel shaky or nauseated. The cervix is fully dilated when it reaches 10 cm.

Second Stage

The baby twists and turns through the birth canal.

The second stage involves the pushing and delivery of your baby. It usually lasts 20 minutes to 2 hours. You will push hard during contractions and rest between contractions. Pushing is hard work, and a support person can really help keep you focused. A woman can give birth in many positions, such as squatting, sitting, kneeling, or lying back. Giving birth in an upright position, such as squatting, appears to have some benefits, including shortening this stage of labor and helping to keep the tissue near the birth canal intact. You might find pushing to be easier or more comfortable one way, and you should be allowed to choose the birth position that feels best to you.

When the top of your baby's head fully appears (crowning), your doctor will tell you when to push and deliver your baby. Your doctor may make a small cut, called an "episiotomy," to enlarge the vaginal opening. Most women in childbirth do not need episiotomy. Sometimes, forceps (tool shaped like salad tongs) or suction is used to help guide the baby through the birth canal. This is called "assisted vaginal delivery." After your baby is born, the umbilical cord is cut. Make sure to tell your doctor if you or your partner would like to cut the umbilical cord.

Third Stage

The third stage involves delivery of the placenta (afterbirth). It is the shortest stage, lasting 5–30 minutes. Contractions will begin 5–30 minutes after birth, signaling that it is time to deliver the placenta.

You might have chills or shakiness. Labor is over once the placenta is delivered. Your doctor will repair the episiotomy and any tears you might have. Now you can rest and enjoy your newborn!

MANAGING LABOR PAIN

Virtually all women worry about how they will cope with the pain of labor and delivery. Childbirth is different for everyone. So no one can predict how you will feel. The amount of pain a woman feels during labor depends partly on the size and position of her baby, the size of her pelvis, her emotions, the strength of the contractions, and her outlook.

Some women do fine with natural methods of pain relief alone. Many women blend natural methods with medications that relieve pain. Building a positive outlook on childbirth and managing fear may also help some women cope with the pain. It is important to realize that labor pain is not like pain due to illness or injury. Instead, it is caused by contractions of the uterus that are pushing your baby down and out of the birth canal. In other words, labor pain has a purpose.

Try the following to help you feel positive about childbirth:
- Take a childbirth class. Call the doctor, midwife, hospital, or birthing center for class information.
- Get information from your doctor or midwife. Write down your questions and talk about them at your regular visits.
- Share your fears and emotions with friends, family, and your partner.[1]

[1] Office on Women's Health (OWH), "Labor and Birth," U.S. Department of Health and Human Services (HHS), February 22, 2021. Available online. URL: www.womenshealth.gov/pregnancy/childbirth-and-beyond/labor-and-birth. Accessed May 22, 2023.

Section 62.2 | Cesarean Section

Cesarean delivery, also called "C-section," is surgery to deliver a baby. The baby is taken out through the mother's abdomen. Most cesarean births result in healthy babies and mothers. But a C-section is major surgery and carries risks. Healing also takes longer than with vaginal birth.

Most healthy pregnant women with no risk factors for problems during labor or delivery have their babies vaginally. Still, the cesarean birth rate in the United States has risen greatly in recent decades. Today, nearly one in three women has babies by C-section in this country. The rate was one in five in 1995.

Public health experts think that many C-sections are unnecessary. So it is important for pregnant women to get the facts about C-sections before they deliver. Women should find out what C-sections are, why they are performed, and the pros and cons of this surgery.

REASONS FOR CESAREAN SECTIONS

Your doctor might recommend a C-section if he or she thinks it is safer for you or your baby than vaginal birth. Some C-sections are planned. But most C-sections are done when unexpected problems happen during delivery. Even so, there are risks of delivering by C-section. Limited studies show that the benefits of having a C-section may outweigh the risks when:

- the mother is carrying more than one baby (twins, triplets, etc.)
- the mother has health problems, including human immunodeficiency virus (HIV) infection, herpes infection, and heart disease
- the mother has dangerously high blood pressure
- the mother has problems with the shape of her pelvis
- there are problems with the placenta
- there are problems with the umbilical cord
- there are problems with the position of the baby, such as breech

- the baby shows signs of distress, such as a slowed heart rate
- the mother has had a previous C-section

PATIENT-REQUESTED CESAREAN SECTION: CAN A WOMAN CHOOSE?

A growing number of women are asking their doctors for C-sections when there is no medical reason. Some women want a C-section because they fear the pain of childbirth. Others like the convenience of being able to decide when and how to deliver their baby. Still, others fear the risks of vaginal delivery, including tearing and sexual problems.

But is it safe and ethical for doctors to allow women to choose C-sections? The answer is unclear. Only more research on both types of deliveries will provide the answer. In the meantime, many obstetricians feel it is their ethical obligation to talk women out of elective C-sections. Others believe that women should be able to choose a C-section if they understand the risks and benefits.

Experts who believe C-sections should only be performed for medical reasons point to the risks. These include infection, dangerous bleeding, blood transfusions, and blood clots. Babies born by C-sections have more breathing problems right after birth. Women who have C-sections stay at the hospital for longer than women who have vaginal births. Plus, recovery from this surgery takes longer and is often more painful than that after a vaginal birth. C-sections also increase the risk of problems in future pregnancies. Women who have had C-sections have a higher risk of uterine rupture. If the uterus ruptures, the life of the baby and mother is in danger.

Supporters of elective C-sections say that this surgery may protect a woman's pelvic organs, reduces the risk of bowel and bladder problems, and is as safe for the baby as vaginal delivery.

The National Institutes of Health (NIH) and the American College of Obstetricians (ACOG) agree that a doctor's decision to perform a C-section at the request of a patient should be made on a case-by-case basis and be consistent with ethical principles. The ACOG states that "if the physician believes that (cesarean) delivery promotes the overall health and welfare of the woman and her fetus more than vaginal birth, she or he is ethically justified in performing" a C-section. Both organizations also say that a C-section should never be scheduled before a pregnancy is 39 weeks or the lungs are mature unless there is a medical need.

THE CESAREAN SECTION EXPERIENCE

Most C-sections are unplanned. So learning about C-sections is important for all women who are pregnant. Whether a C-section is planned or comes up during labor, it can be a positive birth experience for many women. The overview that follows will help you know what to expect during a nonemergency C-section and what questions to ask.

Before Surgery

Cesarean delivery takes about 45–60 minutes. It takes place in an operating room. So, if you were in a labor and delivery room, you would be moved to an operating room. Often, the mood of the operating room is unhurried and relaxed. A doctor will give you medicine through an epidural or spinal block, which will block the feeling of pain in part of your body but allow you to stay awake and alert. The spinal block works right away and completely numbs your body from the chest down. The epidural takes away the pain, but you might be aware of some tugging or pushing. Medicine that makes you fall asleep and lose all awareness is usually only used in emergency situations. Your abdomen will be cleaned and prepped. You will have an intravenous line for fluids and medicines. A nurse will insert a catheter to drain urine from your bladder. This is to protect the bladder from harm during surgery. Your heart rate, blood pressure, and breathing will also be monitored. The following are a few questions to ask:

- Can I have a support person with me during the operation?
- What are my options for blocking pain?
- Can I have music played during the surgery?
- Will I be able to watch the surgery if I want?

During Surgery

The doctor will make two incisions. The first is about six inches long and goes through the skin, fat, and muscle. Most incisions are made side to side and low on the abdomen, called a "bikini incision." Next, the doctor will make an incision to open the uterus. The opening is made just wide enough for the baby to fit through. One doctor will use a hand to support the baby while another doctor pushes the uterus to help push that baby out. Fluid will be suctioned out of your baby's mouth and nose. The doctor will hold up your baby for you to see. Once your baby is delivered, the umbilical cord is cut, and the placenta is removed. Then the doctor cleans and stitches up the uterus and abdomen. The repair takes up most of the surgery time. The following are a few questions to ask:

- Can my partner cut the umbilical cord?
- What happens to my baby right after delivery?
- Can I hold and touch my baby during the surgery repair?
- When is it okay for me to try to breastfeed?
- When can my partner take pictures or videos?

After Surgery

You will be moved to a recovery room and monitored for a few hours. You might feel shaky, nauseated, and very sleepy. Later, you will be brought to a hospital room. When you and your baby are ready, you can hold, snuggle, and nurse your baby. Many people will be excited to see you. But do not accept too many visitors. Use your time in the hospital, usually about four days, to rest and bond with your baby. C-section is major surgery, and recovery takes about six weeks (not counting the fatigue of new motherhood). In the weeks ahead, you will need to focus on healing, getting as much rest as possible, and bonding with your baby—nothing else. Be careful about taking on too much and accept help as needed. The following are a few questions to ask:

- Can my baby be brought to me in the recovery room?
- What are the best positions for me to breastfeed?[2]

---

[2] Office on Women's Health (OWH), "Labor and Birth," U.S. Department of Health and Human Services (HHS), February 22, 2021. Available online. URL: www.womenshealth.gov/pregnancy/childbirth-and-beyond/labor-and-birth. Accessed May 22, 2023.

Section 62.3 | Vaginal Birth after Cesarean Delivery or Repeat Cesarean Section

WHAT IS VAGINAL BIRTH AFTER CESAREAN?

Vaginal birth after cesarean (VBAC) refers to the vaginal delivery of a baby after a previous pregnancy was delivered by cesarean delivery. In the past, pregnant women who had one cesarean delivery would automatically have another. But research shows that for many women who had prior cesarean deliveries, attempting to give birth vaginally—called a "trial of labor after cesarean delivery" (TOLAC)—and VBAC might be safe options in certain situations.

In fact, *Eunice Kennedy Shriver* National Institute of Child Health and Human Development (NICHD) research shows that among appropriate candidates, about 75 percent of VBAC attempts are successful. A 2010 National Institutes of Health (NIH) Consensus Development Conference on VBAC evaluated available data and determined that VBAC was a reasonable option for many women.

The NICHD-supported researchers also developed a way to calculate a woman's chances of a successful VBAC. Access the calculator (https://mfmunetwork.bsc.gwu.edu/web/mfmunetwork/vaginal-birth-after-cesarean-calculator). It is to be noted that this calculator only determines the likelihood of successful VBAC; it does not guarantee success.

Women should discuss VBAC and TOLAC with their healthcare providers early in pregnancy to learn whether these options are appropriate for them. Providers are encouraged to discuss plans for VBAC or refer women to a facility that can support VBAC when it is medically safe to consider.

WHEN IS VAGINAL BIRTH AFTER CESAREAN APPROPRIATE?

Vaginal birth after cesarean may be safe and appropriate for some women, including those:

- whose prior cesarean incision was across the uterus toward its base (called a "low-transverse incision")—the most common type of incision (Note that the

incision on the uterus is different than the incision on the skin.)
- with two previous low-transverse cesarean incisions
- who are carrying twins
- with an unknown type of uterine incision

Benefits of VBAC include the following:
- no abdominal surgery
- lower risk of hemorrhage and infection compared with a cesarean section (C-section)
- faster recovery
- potential to avoid the risks of many cesarean deliveries, such as hysterectomy, bowel and bladder injury, blood transfusion, infection, and abnormal placenta conditions
- greater likelihood of being able to have more children in the future

If labor fails to progress or if there is another problem, a woman may need a C-section after trying TOLAC. Most risks associated with a C-section after TOLAC are similar to those associated with choosing a repeat cesarean. They include the following:
- uterine rupture
- maternal hemorrhage and infection
- blood clots
- need for a hysterectomy[3]

---

[3] "What Is Vaginal Birth after Cesarean (VBAC)?" *Eunice Kennedy Shriver* National Institute of Child Health and Human Development (NICHD), September 1, 2017. Available online. URL: www.nichd.nih.gov/health/topics/labor-delivery/topicinfo/vbac. Accessed May 22, 2023.

Chapter 63 | **Pain Relief during Labor**

The amount of pain felt during labor and delivery is different for every woman. The level of pain depends on many factors, including the size and position of the baby, the woman's level of comfort with the process, and the strength of her contractions. There are two general ways to relieve pain during labor and delivery: using medications and using "natural" methods (no medications). Some women choose one way or another, while other women rely on a combination of the two. A woman should discuss the many aspects of labor with her health-care provider well before labor begins to ensure that she understands all of the options, risks, and benefits of pain relief during labor and delivery before making a decision. It might also be helpful to put all the decisions in writing to clarify things for all those who might be involved with delivering the baby.

PAIN-RELIEVING MEDICATIONS

Pain-relief drugs fall into two categories: analgesics and anesthetics. Each category has different forms of medications. Some of these medications carry risks. It is important for women to discuss medications with their health-care provider before going into labor to ensure that they are making informed decisions about pain relief.

Analgesics

Analgesics relieve pain without causing total loss of feeling or muscle movement. These drugs do not always stop the pain completely, but they reduce it.

- **Systemic analgesics.** These analgesics affect the whole nervous system rather than a single area. They ease the pain but do not cause the patient to go to sleep. Systemic analgesics are often used in early labor. They are not given right before delivery because they may slow the baby's breathing and reflexes. They are given in the following three ways:
  - injected into a muscle or vein
  - administered through a small tube placed in a vein (The woman can often control the amount of analgesic flowing through the tube.)
  - inhaled or breathed in with a mixture of oxygen (The woman holds a mask to her face, so she decides how much or how little analgesic she receives for pain relief.)
- **Regional analgesics.** These analgesics relieve pain in one region of the body. In the United States, regional analgesia is the most common way to relieve pain during labor. Several types of regional analgesia can be given during labor, so you should discuss your options with a health-care provider before your due date. Examples include (but are not limited to) the following:
  - **Epidural analgesia.** Also called an "epidural block" or an "epidural," this causes a loss of feeling in the lower body while the patient stays awake. The drug starts working about 10–20 minutes after it is given. A health-care provider injects the drug near the spinal cord. A small tube (catheter) is placed through the needle. The needle is then withdrawn, but the tube stays in place. Small amounts of the drug can then be given through the catheter throughout labor without the need for another injection.
  - **A spinal block.** This is an injection of a much smaller amount of the drug into the sac of spinal fluid around the spine. The drug starts working right away, but it lasts for only one to two hours. Usually,

a spinal block is given only once during labor to help with pain during delivery.

Anesthetics

Anesthetics block all feelings, including pain.

- **General anesthesia.** It causes the patient to go to sleep. The patient does not feel pain while asleep.
- **Local anesthesia.** It removes all feelings, including pain, from a small part of the body while the patient stays awake. It does not lessen the pain of contractions. Health-care providers often use it when performing an episiotomy, a surgical cut made in the region between the vagina and anus to widen the vaginal opening for delivery, or when repairing vaginal tears that happen during birth.

NATURAL PAIN-RELIEF METHODS (ALSO CALLED "NATURAL CHILDBIRTH")

Women who choose natural childbirth rely on a number of ways to ease pain without taking medication. These include the following:

- the company of others who offer reassurance, advice, or other help throughout labor, also known as "continuous labor support"
- relaxation techniques, such as deep breathing, music therapy, or biofeedback
- a soothing atmosphere
- moving and changing positions frequently
- using a birthing ball
- massage
- yoga
- taking a bath or shower
- hypnosis
- using soothing scents (aromatherapy)
- acupuncture or acupressure
- applying small doses of electrical stimulation to nerve fibers to activate the body's own pain-relieving

substances (called "transcutaneous electrical nerve stimulation" (TENS))

- injecting sterile water into the lower back, which can relieve the intense discomfort and pain in the lower back, known as "back labor"[1]

[1] "What Are the Options for Pain Relief during Labor and Delivery?" *Eunice Kennedy Shriver* National Institute of Child Health and Human Development (NICHD), April 17, 2023. Available online. URL: www.nichd.nih.gov/health/topics/labor-delivery/topicinfo/pain-relief. Accessed May 22, 2023.

Chapter 64 | **Problems during Childbirth**

WHAT ARE SOME COMMON COMPLICATIONS DURING LABOR AND DELIVERY?

Each pregnancy and delivery is different, and problems may arise. If complications occur, providers may assist by monitoring the situation closely and intervening as necessary. Some of the more common complications are as follows:

- **Labor that does not progress.** Sometimes, contractions weaken; the cervix does not dilate enough or in a timely manner; or the infant's descent into the birth canal does not proceed smoothly. If labor is not progressing, a health-care provider may give the woman medications to increase contractions and speed up labor, or the woman may need a cesarean delivery.

- **Perineal tears.** A woman's vagina and the surrounding tissues are likely to tear during the delivery process. Sometimes, these tears heal on their own. If a tear is more serious or the woman has had an episiotomy (a surgical cut between the vagina and anus), her provider will help repair the tear using stitches.

- **Problems with the umbilical cord.** The umbilical cord may get caught on an arm or leg as the infant travels through the birth canal. Typically, a provider intervenes if the cord becomes wrapped around the infant's neck, is compressed, or comes out before the infant.

- **Abnormal heart rate of the baby.** Many times, an abnormal heart rate during labor does not mean that there is a problem. A health-care provider will likely ask the woman to switch positions to help the infant get more blood flow. In certain instances, such as when test results show a larger problem, delivery might have to happen right away. In this situation, the woman is more likely to need an emergency cesarean delivery, or the health-care provider may need to do an episiotomy to widen the vaginal opening for delivery.

- **Water breaking early.** Labor usually starts on its own within 24 hours of the woman's water breaking. If not and if the pregnancy is at or near term, the provider will likely induce labor. If a pregnant woman's water breaks before 34 weeks of pregnancy, the woman will be monitored in the hospital. Infection can become a major concern if the woman's water breaks early and labor does not begin on its own.

- **Perinatal asphyxia.** This condition occurs when the fetus does not get enough oxygen in the uterus or the infant does not get enough oxygen during labor or delivery or just after birth.

- **Shoulder dystocia.** In this situation, the infant's head has come out of the vagina, but one of the shoulders becomes stuck.

- **Excessive bleeding.** If delivery results in tears to the uterus or if the uterus does not contract to deliver the placenta, heavy bleeding can result. Worldwide, such bleeding is a leading cause of maternal death. The *Eunice Kennedy Shriver* National Institute of Child Health and Human Development (NICHD) has supported studies to investigate the use of misoprostol to reduce bleeding, especially in resource-poor settings.

Delivery may also require a provider's special attention when the pregnancy lasts more than 42 weeks, when the woman had a cesarean section (C-section) in a previous pregnancy, or when she is older than a certain age.[1]

CHILDBIRTH PROBLEMS

Childbirth is the process of giving birth to a baby. It includes labor and delivery. Usually, everything goes well, but problems can happen. They may cause a risk to the mother, baby, or both. Some of the more common childbirth problems include the following:

- pre-term (premature) labor when your labor starts before 37 completed weeks of pregnancy
- premature rupture of membranes (PROM) when your water breaks too early (If labor does not start soon afterward, this can raise the risk of infection.)
- problems with the placenta, such as the placenta covering the cervix, separating from the uterus before birth, or being attached too firmly to the uterus
- labor that does not progress, meaning that labor is stalled, that can happen when:
  - your contractions weaken
  - your cervix does not dilate (open) enough or is taking too long to dilate
  - the baby is not in the right position
  - the baby is too big or your pelvis is too small for the baby to move through the birth canal
- abnormal heart rate of the baby (Often, an abnormal heart rate is not a problem. But, if the heart rate gets very fast or very slow, it can be a sign that your baby is not getting enough oxygen or that there are other problems.)
- problems with the umbilical cord, such as the cord getting caught on the baby's arm, leg, or neck, which is also a problem if the cord comes out before the baby does

---

[1] "What Are Some Common Complications during Labor and Delivery?" *Eunice Kennedy Shriver* National Institute of Child Health and Human Development (NICHD), September 1, 2017. Available online. URL: www.nichd.nih.gov/health/topics/labor-delivery/topicinfo/complications. Accessed May 22, 2023.

- problems with the position of the baby, such as breech, in which the baby is going to come out feet first.
- shoulder dystocia when the baby's head comes out, but the shoulder gets stuck
- perinatal asphyxia, which happens when the baby does not get enough oxygen in the uterus, during labor or delivery, or just after birth
- perineal tears, tearing of your vagina and the surrounding tissues
- excessive bleeding, which can happen when the delivery causes tears to the uterus or if you are not able to deliver the placenta after you give birth to the baby
- post-term pregnancy when your pregnancy lasts more than 42 weeks

If you have problems in childbirth, your health-care provider may need to give you medicines to induce or speed up labor, use tools to help guide the baby out of the birth canal, or deliver the baby by C-section.[2]

---

[2] MedlinePlus, "Childbirth Problems," National Institutes of Health (NIH), March 11, 2020. Available online. URL: https://medlineplus.gov/childbirthproblems.html. Accessed May 22, 2023.

Chapter 65 | Cord Blood Banking

Expecting a baby can be a very exciting time for soon-to-be parents. It can also be very confusing, with many decisions to make. One choice prospective parents often face is whether to donate, bank, or discard their baby's cord blood. Did you know that the U.S. Food and Drug Administration (FDA) regulates cord blood? Here is some information for expectant parents about the regulations in place designed to help ensure the safety of cord blood for transplantation.

WHAT IS CORD BLOOD?
Cord blood is the blood contained in the placental blood vessels and umbilical cord, which connects an unborn baby to the mother's womb. Cord blood contains hematopoietic progenitor cells (HPCs). At birth, cord blood can be collected (or "recovered") from the umbilical cord.

WHAT ARE HEMATOPOIETIC PROGENITOR CELLS?
Hematopoietic progenitor cells are blood-forming stem cells. HPCs are found in the bone marrow, peripheral blood, and cord blood. These types of stem cells are routinely used to treat patients with cancers such as leukemia or lymphoma and other disorders of the blood and immune systems.

HOW ARE PATIENTS AND DONATED CORD BLOOD UNITS "MATCHED" SO THAT A UNIT OF CORD BLOOD CAN BE USED FOR A PATIENT'S TRANSPLANT?

Human leukocyte antigen (HLA) typing is used to match patients and donors for cord blood transplants. HLAs are proteins found in most cells in the body. A person's immune system uses these proteins as markers to recognize which cells belong in their body and which do not. A close match between the patient's and the donor's HLA markers can reduce the risk that the patient's immune cells will attack the donor's cells or that the donor's immune cells will attack the patient's body after the transplant.

HOW ARE HPCS FROM CORD BLOOD DIFFERENT FROM HPCS FROM OTHER SOURCES?

There is evidence that cord blood HPCs may not require as exact a match as HPCs from the bone marrow or the bloodstream because the antigens in cord blood are less mature. This suggests that transplants involving compatible HPCs from cord blood may be less likely to cause adverse reactions because the donor's cells are less likely to see the patient's cells as foreign bodies and attack them.

WHAT ARE THE OPTIONS FOR CORD BLOOD BANKING?

Cord blood can be donated to a public cord blood bank, where it will be stored for potential future use by anyone who may need it. Alternatively, parents may arrange for the cord blood to be stored in a private cord bank, for potential use if it is later needed for treatment of the child from whom it was recovered, or for use in first- or second-degree relatives. You may also wish to consult your health-care provider about the options.

HOW DOES THE FDA REGULATE CORD BLOOD STORED FOR PERSONAL OR FAMILY USE?

Cord blood stored for personal use and for use in first- or second-degree relatives that also meets other criteria in the FDA's regulations does not require approval before use. Private cord banks must still comply with other FDA requirements, including establishment registration and listing, donor screening and testing for infectious diseases (except when used for the original donor), reporting and labeling requirements, and compliance with current good tissue practice regulations.

HOW DOES THE FDA REGULATE CORD BLOOD INTENDED FOR USE IN PATIENTS UNRELATED TO THE DONOR (I.E., CORD BLOOD STORED IN PUBLIC BANKS)?

Cord blood stored for potential future use by a patient unrelated to the donor meets the definition of "drug" under the Food, Drug and Cosmetic Act and "biological product" under Section 351 of the Public Health Service Act (PHSA). Cord blood in this category must meet additional requirements and be licensed under a Biologics License Application (BLA) or subject to an Investigational New Drug (IND) application before use.

ARE THERE ANY FDA-APPROVED USES FOR CORD BLOOD?

Cord blood can be used in hematopoietic stem cell transplantation procedures in patients with some disorders affecting the hematopoietic (blood-forming) system. For example, cord blood transplants have been used to treat patients with certain blood cancers and some inherited metabolic and immune system disorders.

IF A CORD BLOOD BANK IS REGISTERED WITH THE FDA, DOES THAT MEAN THAT THE CORD BANK IS FDA-APPROVED?

Establishments that perform any of the manufacturing steps for cord blood must register with the FDA and list their products and each of the manufacturing steps they perform. Registration with the FDA does not mean a firm is "endorsed" by the agency; it simply means the firm has notified the FDA that it is performing one or more manufacturing steps.

DOES THE FDA INSPECT FACILITIES THAT STORE CORD BLOOD?

Yes. Registered establishments are subject to FDA inspection to ensure they are complying with the regulations. The inspections of private banks are designed to ensure the prevention of infectious disease transmission.

WHERE CAN YOU GET MORE INFORMATION ABOUT DONATING YOUR BABY'S CORD BLOOD?

To make your baby's cord blood available for use by anyone who needs a cord blood transplant, you may donate it to a public cord blood bank.

WHERE CAN YOU GET MORE INFORMATION ABOUT BANKING YOUR BABY'S CORD BLOOD?

To make your baby's cord blood available for use by the child from whom it was recovered or for use in first- or second-degree relatives, you may bank it with a private cord blood bank.

For some diseases, such as genetically heritable diseases, in the event that your child would need treatment, it is possible that cord blood would not be recommended for such use.[1]

---

[1] "Cord Blood Banking—Information for Consumers," Centers for Disease Control and Prevention (CDC), July 23, 2012. Available online. URL: www.fda.gov/vaccines-blood-biologics/consumers-biologics/cord-blood-banking-information-consumers. Accessed May 22, 2023.

Chapter 66 | Disaster Safety for Expecting and New Parents

GET PREPARED FOR AN EMERGENCY OR DISASTER

Disasters can be scary and stressful, especially if you are expecting or have a baby. You can take the following steps now to help prepare for an emergency and better cope if an emergency happens:

- Talk to your health-care provider about where you will get prenatal care or deliver your baby if your provider's office or hospital is closed.
- If you are close to your due date, learn the signs of labor, including information on preterm birth. Talk to your health-care provider about what to do in case of an emergency.
- Be informed—check with your local emergency management agency to find out how to get emergency alerts (such as text alerts).
- Make a family emergency action plan for how you and your family will contact one another and what steps you will take in different types of situations.
- Prepare an emergency kit that includes at least a three-day supply of food and water for each person, health supplies including medications, baby care and safety supplies, and backup chargers for electronics such as a cellphone or tablet. Try to store a two-week supply of water if possible.

- Keep a copy of important family documents such as insurance policies, ID cards, copies of all prescription information, and medical supplies in a waterproof, portable container.
- Plan ahead to help your baby sleep safely if you need to leave your home. Your baby is safe sleeping on their back in their own sleep area (such as a portable crib or bassinet) that does not have pillows, blankets, or toys.

WHAT TO DO DURING AND JUST AFTER A DISASTER
If You Are Pregnant

There are special medical needs during pregnancy. If you are pregnant or think you may be pregnant, you can take the following steps to help you in the event of a disaster:

- If you have any signs of labor, call your health-care provider or 911 or go to the hospital immediately if it is safe to travel.
- If you need to leave your home, find out where to shelter. Be prepared to leave quickly and have your emergency kit that includes copies of medical records, health-care providers' information, and prenatal vitamins or medicines, ready to go. Tell the shelter staff as soon as possible that you are pregnant and if you have any health problems.
- Continue taking your prenatal vitamins or prescription medicines as directed.
- Protect yourself from infections by washing your hands often and staying away from moldy or dirty places and people who are sick. If you do get sick, talk with a health-care provider right away.
- During extreme heat, wear loose, lightweight, light-colored clothing, stay hydrated, and try to keep cool to prevent your body from overheating. Stay in air-conditioned buildings as much as you can. If your home is not air-conditioned, spend time in public facilities that are air-conditioned and use air-conditioning in vehicles. Contact your local health

department or find an air-conditioned shelter or cooling center in your area.

- Once you are out of immediate danger, continue your prenatal care, even if it is not with your regular health-care provider. Tell the health-care provider if you have any health problems and if you need help getting your prenatal vitamins or medications.
- Take care of your emotional health and practice healthy stress management. Engaging in physical activity, getting enough rest, and drinking enough water can help you reduce stress. Ask for help if you are feeling overwhelmed or stressed.

If You Are a New Parent or Caregiver of an Infant

A disaster can make it difficult to access necessary supplies and health care. Parents and caregivers of infants can take the following steps to help keep their families safe and healthy in the event of a disaster:

- If you have to leave your home, have your emergency kit that includes copies of medical records and emergency telephone numbers, health-care providers' information, medicines, and infant care supplies, such as baby food and a portable crib, ready to go. Have at least a three-day supply of water and food for each person. Try to store a two-week supply of water if possible.
- Be prepared to leave quickly.
  - Tell the shelter staff about any care needs you or your baby may have and take action to help your baby sleep safely.
  - If you or your baby use prescription medicines and you have them with you, take them with you and continue taking or giving them as directed.
- If you breastfeed your baby, continue to do so. If you feed your baby formula, use ready-to-feed formula if possible. Clean water may not be available for mixing formula or washing bottles.

- During disasters, harmful chemicals from businesses and other places may be released into the environment. Listen to announcements from emergency officials about chemical safety and actions you may need to take to protect yourself. If you have questions about exposure to harmful chemicals during pregnancy and breastfeeding, call MotherToBaby at 866-626-6847. To reach the nationwide poison control center, call 800-222-1222.
- As soon as it is safe to do so, see a health-care provider for well-baby checkups or if you are concerned about a health problem, even if it is not with your baby's usual health-care provider. Tell them if you need help getting your baby's prescription medications.

If You Recently Gave Birth

If you gave birth within the past year, you may face unique challenges during disasters. In addition to the tips for parents above, follow these tips to protect yourself in case of an emergency.

If you have given birth within the last two months, do the following:

- If you need to leave your home, prepare a kit with essential items. If you use feminine hygiene products, such as menstrual pads or tampons, consider bringing a supply, as they might not be immediately available when you need them.
- As soon as it is safe to do so, get a postpartum checkup if you are due for a visit, even if it is not with your usual health-care provider. Tell them if you need help getting your prescription medications. If you are not ready to get pregnant, you can ask for several months' supply of the pill, patch, or ring or consider using a birth control method that will prevent pregnancy for an extended period of time.

If you have given birth within the past year, do the following:
- If you think that you may be depressed, make an appointment to talk to your health-care provider as soon as possible.
- Learn the urgent maternal warning signs and symptoms (www.cdc.gov/hearher/maternal-warning-signs/index.html). Seek medical care immediately if you experience any of these signs or symptoms.[1]

---

[1] "Natural Disaster Safety for Expecting and New Parents," Centers for Disease Control and Prevention (CDC), November 29, 2022. Available online. URL: www.cdc.gov/reproductivehealth/features/disaster-planning-parents/index.html. Accessed May 22, 2023.

Part 7 | **Postpartum and Newborn Care**

Chapter 67 | Recovering from Delivery: Physical and Emotional Concerns

Right now, you are focused on caring for your new baby. But new mothers must take special care of their bodies after giving birth and while breastfeeding, too. Doing so will help you regain your energy and strength. When you take care of yourself, you are able to best care for and enjoy your baby.

GETTING REST

The first few days at home after having your baby are a time for rest and recovery—physically and emotionally. You need to focus your energy on yourself and on getting to know your new baby. Even though you may be very excited and have requests for lots of visits from family and friends, try to limit visitors and get as much rest as possible. Do not expect to keep your house perfect. You may find that all you can do is eat, sleep, and care for your baby. And that is perfectly okay. Learn to pace yourself from the first day that you arrive back home. Try to lie down or nap while the baby naps. Do not try to do too much around the house. Allow others to help you and do not be afraid to ask for help with cleaning, laundry, meals, or caring for the baby.

PHYSICAL CHANGES

After the birth of your baby, your doctor will talk with you about things you will experience as your body starts to recover.

- You will have vaginal discharge called "lochia." It is the tissue and blood that line your uterus during pregnancy. It is heavy and bright red at first, becoming lighter in flow and color until it goes away after a few weeks.
- You might also have swelling in your legs and feet. You can reduce swelling by keeping your feet elevated when possible.
- You might feel constipated. Try to drink plenty of water and eat fresh fruits and vegetables.
- Menstrual-like cramping is common, especially if you are breastfeeding. Your breast milk will come in within three to six days after your delivery. Even if you are not breastfeeding, you can have milk leaking from your nipples, and your breasts might feel full, tender, or uncomfortable.
- Follow your doctor's instructions on how much activity, such as climbing stairs or walking, you can do for the next few weeks.

Your doctor will check your recovery at your postpartum visit, about six weeks after birth. Ask about resuming normal activities, as well as eating and fitness plans to help you return to a healthy weight. Also, ask your doctor about having sex and birth control. Your period could return in six to eight weeks or sooner if you do not breastfeed. If you breastfeed, your period might not resume for many months. Still, using reliable birth control is the best way to prevent pregnancy until you want to have another baby.

Some women develop thyroid problems in the first year after giving birth. This is called "postpartum thyroiditis." It often begins with overactive thyroid, which lasts two to four months. Most women then develop symptoms of an underactive thyroid, which can last up to a year. Thyroid problems are easy to overlook as many symptoms, such as fatigue, sleep problems, low energy, and changes in weight, are common after having a baby. Talk to your doctor if you have symptoms that do not go away. An underactive thyroid needs to be treated. In most cases, thyroid function returns to normal as the thyroid heals. But some women develop permanent underactive thyroid disease, called "Hashimoto disease," and need lifelong treatment.

REGAINING A HEALTHY WEIGHT AND SHAPE
Both pregnancy and labor can affect a woman's body. After giving birth, you will lose about 10 pounds right away and a little more as body fluid levels decrease. Do not expect or try to lose additional pregnancy weight right away. Gradual weight loss over several months is the safest way, especially if you are breastfeeding. Nursing mothers can safely lose a moderate amount of weight without affecting their milk supply or their babies' growth.

A healthy eating plan, along with regular physical fitness, might be all you need to return to a healthy weight. If you are not losing weight or losing weight too slowly, cut back on foods with added sugars and fats, such as soft drinks, desserts, fried foods, fatty meats, and alcohol. Keep in mind nursing mothers should avoid alcohol. By cutting back on "extras," you can focus on healthy, well-balanced food choices that will keep your energy level up and help you get the nutrients you and your baby need for good health. Make sure to talk to your doctor before you start any type of diet or exercise plan.

FEELING BLUE
After childbirth, you may feel sad, weepy, and overwhelmed for a few days. Many new mothers have the "baby blues" after giving birth. Changing hormones, anxiety about caring for the baby, and lack of sleep all affect your emotions.

Be patient with yourself. These feelings are normal and usually go away quickly. But, if sadness lasts more than two weeks, go see your doctor. Do not wait until your postpartum visit to do so. You might have a serious but treatable condition called "postpartum depression." Postpartum depression can happen at any time within the first year after birth. Signs of postpartum depression include:

* feeling restless or irritable
* feeling sad, depressed, or crying a lot

- having no energy
- having headaches, chest pains, heart palpitations (the heart being fast and feeling like it is skipping beats), numbness, or hyperventilation (fast and shallow breathing)
- not being able to sleep, being very tired, or both
- not being able to eat and weight loss
- overeating and weight gain
- trouble focusing, remembering, or making decisions
- being overly worried about the baby
- not having any interest in the baby
- feeling worthless and guilty
- having no interest or getting no pleasure from activities such as sex and socializing
- thoughts of harming your baby or yourself

Some women do not tell anyone about their symptoms because they feel embarrassed or guilty about having these feelings at a time when they think they should be happy. Do not let this happen to you! Postpartum depression can make it hard to take care of your baby. Infants with mothers with postpartum depression can have delays in learning how to talk. They can have problems with emotional bonding. Your doctor can help you feel better and get back to enjoying your new baby. Therapy and/or medicine can treat postpartum depression.

Emerging research suggests that 1 in 10 new fathers may experience depression during or after pregnancy. Although more research is needed, having depression may make it harder to be a good father and perhaps affect the baby's development. Having depression may also be related to a mother's depression. Expecting or new fathers with emotional problems or symptoms of depression should talk to their doctors. Depression is a treatable illness.[1]

---

[1] Office on Women's Health (OWH), "Recovering from Birth," U.S. Department of Health and Human Services (HHS), February 22, 2021. Available online. URL: www.womenshealth.gov/pregnancy/childbirth-and-beyond/recovering-birth. Accessed May 23, 2023.

Chapter 68 | **Your Baby's First Hours and Newborn Screening Tests**

After months of waiting, finally, your new baby has arrived! Mothers-to-be often spend so much time in anticipation of labor; they do not think about or even know what to expect during the first hours after delivery. Read on, so you will be ready to bond with your new bundle of joy.

WHAT NEWBORNS LOOK LIKE

You might be surprised by how your newborn looks at birth. If you had a vaginal delivery, your baby entered this world through a narrow and bony passage. It is not uncommon for newborns to be born bluish, bruised, and with a misshapen head. An ear might be folded over. Your baby may have a complete head of hair or be bald. Your baby will also have a thick, pasty, whitish coating, which protects the skin in the womb. This will wash away during the first bathing.

Once your baby is placed into your arms, your gaze will go right to his or her eyes. Most newborns open their eyes soon after birth. Eyes will be brown or bluish-gray at first. Looking over your baby, you might notice that the face is a little puffy. You might notice small white bumps inside your baby's mouth or on his or her tongue. Your baby might be very wrinkly. Some babies, especially those born early, are covered in soft, fine hair, which will come off in a couple of weeks. Your baby's skin might have various

633

colored marks, blotches, or rashes, and fingernails could be long. You might also notice that your baby's breasts and penis or vulva are a bit swollen.

How your baby looks will change from day to day, and many of the early marks of childbirth go away with time. If you have any concerns about something you see, talk to your doctor. After a few weeks, your newborn will look more and more like the baby you pictured in your dreams.

BONDING WITH YOUR BABY

Spending time with your baby in those first hours of life is very special. Although you might be tired, your newborn could be quite alert after birth. Cuddle your baby skin-to-skin. Let your baby get to know your voice and study your face. Your baby can see up to about two feet away. You might notice that your baby throws his or her arms out if someone turns on a light or makes a sudden noise. This is called the "startle response." Babies are also born with grasp and sucking reflexes. Put your finger in your baby's palm and watch how he or she knows to squeeze it. Feed your baby when he or she shows signs of hunger.

MEDICAL CARE FOR YOUR NEWBORN

Right after birth, babies need many important tests and procedures to ensure their health. Some of these are even required by law. But, as long as the baby is healthy, everything but the Apgar test can wait for at least an hour. Delaying further medical care will preserve the precious first moments of life for you, your partner, and the baby. A baby who has not been poked and prodded may be more willing to nurse and cuddle. So, before delivery, talk to your doctor or midwife about delaying shots, medicine, and tests. At the same time, do not assume "everything is being taken care of." As a parent, it is your job to make sure your newborn gets all the necessary and appropriate vaccines and tests in a timely manner.

The following tests and procedures are recommended or required in most hospitals in the United States.

Apgar Evaluation

The Apgar test is a quick way for doctors to figure out if the baby is healthy or needs extra medical care. Apgar tests are usually done twice: one minute after birth and again five minutes after birth. Doctors and nurses measure the following five signs of the baby's condition:

- heart rate
- breathing
- activity and muscle tone
- reflexes
- skin color

Apgar scores range from 0 to 10. A baby who scores seven or more is considered very healthy. But a lower score does not always mean there is something wrong. Perfectly healthy babies often have low Apgar scores in the first minute of life.

In more than 98 percent of cases, the Apgar score reaches seven after five minutes of life. When it does not, the baby needs medical care and close monitoring.

Eye Care

Your baby may receive eye drops or ointment to prevent eye infections they can get during delivery. Sexually transmitted infections (STIs), including gonorrhea and chlamydia, are the main cause of newborn eye infections. These infections can cause blindness if not treated. Medicines used can sting and/or blur the baby's vision. So you may want to postpone this treatment for a little while.

Some parents question whether this treatment is really necessary. Many women at low risk for STIs do not want their newborns to receive eye medicine. But there is no evidence to suggest that this medicine harms the baby.

It is important to note that even pregnant women who test negative for STIs may get an infection by the time of delivery. Plus, most women with gonorrhea and/or chlamydia do not know it because they have no symptoms.

Vitamin K Shot

The American Academy of Pediatrics (AAP) recommends that all newborns receive a shot of vitamin K in the upper leg. Newborns usually have low levels of vitamin K in their bodies. This vitamin is needed for the blood to clot. Low levels of vitamin K can cause a rare but serious bleeding problem. Research shows that vitamin K shots prevent dangerous bleeding in newborns.

Newborns probably feel pain when the shot is given. But, afterward, babies do not seem to have any discomfort. Since it may be uncomfortable for the baby, you may want to postpone this shot for a little while.

Newborn Metabolic Screening

Doctors or nurses prick your baby's heel to take a tiny sample of blood. They use this blood to test for many diseases. All babies should be tested because a few babies may look healthy but have rare health problems. A blood test is the only way to find out about these problems. If found right away, serious problems such as developmental disabilities, organ damage, blindness, and even death might be prevented.

All 50 states and U.S. territories screen newborns for phenylketonuria (PKU), hypothyroidism, galactosemia, and sickle cell disease. But many states routinely test for up to 30 different diseases. The March of Dimes recommends that all newborns be tested for at least 29 diseases.

You can find out what tests are offered in your state by contacting your state's health department or newborn screening program. Or you can contact the National Newborn Screening and Genetics Resource Center (NNSGRC).

Hearing Test

Most babies have a hearing screening soon after birth, usually before they leave the hospital. Tiny earphones or microphones are used to see how the baby reacts to sounds. All newborns need a hearing screening because hearing defects are not uncommon and hearing loss can be hard to detect in babies and young children.

When problems are found early, children can get the services they need at an early age. This might prevent delays in speech, language, and thinking. Ask your hospital or your baby's doctor about newborn hearing screening.

Hepatitis B Vaccine

All newborns should get a vaccine to protect against the hepatitis B virus (HBV) before leaving the hospital. Sadly, one in five babies at risk of HBV infection leaves the hospital without receiving the vaccine and treatment shown to protect newborns, even if exposed to HBV at birth. HBV can cause lifelong infection, serious liver damage, and even death.

The hepatitis B vaccine (HepB) is a series of three different shots. The AAP and the Centers for Disease Control and Prevention (CDC) recommend that all newborns get the first HepB shot before leaving the hospital. If the mother has HBV, her baby should also get a hepatitis B immune globulin (HBIG) shot within 12 hours of birth. The second HepB shot should be given one to two months after birth. The third HepB shot should be given no earlier than 24 weeks of age but before 18 months of age.

Complete Checkup

Soon after delivery, most doctors or nurses also:
- measure the newborn's weight, length, and head
- take the baby's temperature
- measure the baby's breathing and heart rate
- give the baby a bath and clean the umbilical cord stump[1]

---

[1] Office on Women's Health (OWH), "Your Baby's First Hours of Life," U.S. Department of Health and Human Services (HHS), February 22, 2021. Available online. URL: www.womenshealth.gov/pregnancy/childbirth-and-beyond/your-babys-first-hours-life. Accessed May 23, 2023.

Chapter 69 | Newborn Health Concerns

If this is your first baby, you might worry that you are not ready to take care of a newborn. You are not alone. Lots of new parents feel unprepared when it is time to bring their new babies home from the hospital. You can take steps to help yourself get ready for the transition home.

NEWBORN CARE

Taking a newborn care class during your pregnancy can prepare you for the real thing. But feeding and diapering a baby doll is not quite the same. During your hospital stay, make sure to ask the nurses for help with basic baby care. Do not hesitate to ask the nurse to show you how to do something more than once. Remember, practice makes perfect. Before discharge, make sure you—and your partner—are comfortable with these newborn care basics:

- handling a newborn, including supporting your baby's neck
- changing your baby's diaper
- bathing your baby
- dressing your baby
- swaddling your baby
- feeding and burping your baby
- cleaning the umbilical cord
- caring for a healing circumcision
- using a bulb syringe to clear your baby's nasal passages

- taking a newborn's temperature
- tips for soothing your baby

Before leaving the hospital, ask about home visits by a nurse or health-care worker. Many new parents appreciate somebody checking in with them and their baby a few days after coming home. If you are breastfeeding, ask whether a lactation consultant can come to your home to provide follow-up support, as well as other resources in your community, such as peer support groups.

Many first-time parents also welcome the help of a family member or friend who has "been there." Having a support person stay with you for a few days can give you the confidence to go at it alone in the weeks ahead. Try to arrange this before delivery.

Your baby's first doctor's visit is another good time to ask about any infant care questions you might have. Ask about reasons to call the doctor. Also, ask about what vaccines your baby needs and when. Infants and young children need vaccines because the diseases they protect against can strike at an early age and can be very dangerous in childhood. This includes rare diseases and more common ones, such as the flu.

SUDDEN INFANT DEATH SYNDROME

Since 1992, the American Academy of Pediatrics (AAP) has recommended that infants be placed to sleep on their backs to reduce the risk of sudden infant death syndrome (SIDS), also called "crib death." SIDS is the sudden and unexplained death of a baby under one year of age. Even though there is no way to know which babies might die of SIDS, the following are a few things that you can do to make your baby safer:

- **Always place your baby on his or her back to sleep, even for naps**. This is the safest sleep position for a healthy baby to reduce the risk of SIDS.
- **Place your baby on a firm mattress, such as in a safety-approved crib**. For more information on crib safety, contact the Consumer Product Safety Commission at 800-638-2772. Research has shown that

placing a baby to sleep on soft mattresses, sofas, sofa cushions, waterbeds, sheepskins, or other soft surfaces raises the risk of SIDS.

- **Remove soft, fluffy, and loose bedding and stuffed toys from your baby's sleep area**. Make sure you keep all pillows, quilts, stuffed toys, and other soft items away from your baby's sleep area.
- **Do not use infant sleep positioners.** Using a positioner to hold an infant on his or her back or side for sleep is dangerous and not needed.
- **Make sure everyone who cares for your baby knows to place your baby on his or her back to sleep and about the dangers of soft bedding**. Talk to childcare providers, grandparents, babysitters, and all caregivers about SIDS risk. Remember, every sleep time counts.
- **Make sure your baby's face and head stay uncovered during sleep**. Keep blankets and other coverings away from your baby's mouth and nose. The best way to do this is to dress the baby in sleep clothing, so you will not have to use any other covering over the baby. If you do use a blanket or another covering, make sure that the baby's feet are at the bottom of the crib, the blanket is no higher than the baby's chest, and the blanket is tucked in around the bottom of the crib mattress.
- **Do not allow smoking around your baby**. Do not smoke before or after the birth of your baby and make sure no one smokes around your baby.
- **Do not let your baby get too warm during sleep**. Keep your baby warm during sleep, but not too warm. Your baby's room should be at a temperature that is comfortable for an adult. Too many layers of clothing or blankets can overheat your baby.

Some mothers worry if the baby rolls over during the night. However, by the time your baby is able to roll over by himself or herself, the risk for SIDS is much lower. During the time of the greatest risk, two to four months of age, most babies are not able to turn over from their backs to their stomachs.[1]

WHAT ARE SOME OF THE BASICS OF INFANT HEALTH?

Some physical conditions and issues are very common during the first couple of weeks after birth. Many are normal, and the infant's caregivers can deal with them if they occur. Mostly, it is a matter of the caregivers learning about what is normal for their infant and getting comfortable with the new routine in the household. New parents and caregivers often have questions about several aspects of their infant's health and well-being.

Bowel Movements

Infants' bowel movements go through many changes in color and consistency, even within the first few days after birth. It is important to keep track of your infant's bowel movements. Some things to look for are as follows:

- **Color.** A newborn's first bowel movements usually consist of a thick, black or dark green substance called "meconium." After the meconium is passed, the stools ("poop") will turn yellow-green. The stools of breastfed infants look mustard-yellow with seed-like particles.
- **Consistency.** Until the infant starts to eat solid foods, the consistency of the stool can range from very soft to loose and runny. Formula-fed infants usually have stools that are tan or yellow in color and firmer than those of a breastfed infant. Whether your baby is breastfed or bottle-fed, hard or very dry stools may be a sign of dehydration.

---

[1] Office on Women's Health (OWH), "Newborn Care and Safety," U.S. Department of Health and Human Services (HHS), February 22, 2021. Available online. URL: www.womenshealth.gov/pregnancy/childbirth-and-beyond/newborn-care-and-safety. Accessed May 23, 2023.

- **Frequency.** Infants who are eating solid foods can become constipated if they eat too many constipating foods, such as cereal or cow's milk, before their system can handle them. The U.S. Food and Drug Administration (FDA) and the AAP do not recommend cow's milk for babies under 12 months.

Also, because an infant's stools are normally soft and a little runny, it is not always easy to tell when a young infant has mild diarrhea. The main signs are a sudden increase in the number of bowel movements (more than one per feeding) and watery stools.

Diarrhea can be a sign of intestinal infection, or it may be caused by a change in diet. If the infant is breastfeeding, diarrhea can result from a change in the mother's diet. The main concern with diarrhea is the possibility that dehydration can develop. If fever is also present and your infant is less than two months old, you should call your health-care provider. If the infant is over two months old and the fever lasts more than a day, check the infant's urine output and rectal temperature and consult a health-care provider. Make sure the infant continues to feed often.

Starting around the age of three to six weeks, some breastfed babies have only one bowel movement a week. This is normal because breast milk leaves very little solid waste to pass through the digestive system. Formula-fed infants should have at least one bowel movement a day. If a formula-fed infant has fewer bowel movements than this and appears to be straining because of hard stools, constipation may be the cause. Check with your health-care provider if there are any changes in or problems with your infant's bowel movements.

Care of the Umbilicus

The umbilical cord delivers oxygen and nutrients to the fetus while it is in the womb. After delivery, the umbilical cord is cut. The remaining part of the cord dries and falls off in about 10 days, forming the belly button (navel). Follow your health-care provider's recommendations about how to care for the umbilicus. This care might include the following:

- keeping the area clean and dry
- folding down the top of the diaper to expose the umbilicus to the air
- cleaning the umbilicus gently with a baby wipe or with a cotton swab dipped in rubbing alcohol

Contact your health-care provider if there is pus or redness.

Colic

Many infants are fussy in the evenings, but if the crying does not stop and gets worse throughout the day or night, it may be caused by colic. According to the AAP, about one-fifth of all infants develop colic, usually starting between two and four weeks of age. They may cry inconsolably or scream, extend or pull up their legs, and pass gas. Their stomachs may be enlarged. The crying spells can occur anytime although they often get worse in the early evening.

The colic will likely improve or disappear by the age of three or four months. There is no definite explanation for why some infants get colic. Sometimes, in breastfeeding babies, colic is a sign of sensitivity to a food in the mother's diet. Rarely, colic is caused by sensitivity to milk protein in formula. Colic could be a sign of a medical problem, such as a hernia or some type of illness.

If your infant shows signs of colic, the first step is to consult with your health-care provider. Sometimes, changing the diet of a breastfeeding mother or changing the formula for bottle-fed infants can help. Some infants seem to be soothed by being held, rocked, or wrapped snugly in a blanket. Some like a pacifier.

Diaper Rash

A rash on the skin covered by a diaper is quite common. It is usually caused by irritation of the skin from being in contact with stool and urine. It can get worse during bouts of diarrhea. Diaper rash can

usually be prevented by frequent diaper changes. Your health-care provider can recommend care for diaper rash, which may include:
- rinsing the skin with warm water, using soap only after bowel movements (Because baby wipes may leave a film of bacteria on the skin, their use is often not recommended.)
- exposing the rash to air as much as possible by loosely attaching the diaper at the waist or removing the diaper entirely during naps
- laying the infant on a towel to absorb urine

Caregivers should contact a health-care provider if the rash is not better in three days or if the child becomes worse.

Spitting Up/Vomiting

Spitting up is a common occurrence for newborns and is usually not a sign of a more serious problem. After feeding, try to keep the infant calm and in an upright position for a little while. Keep a burp towel handy, just in case. Contact your health-care provider immediately if your infant:
- is not gaining weight
- is spitting up so forcefully that stomach contents shoot out of the infant's mouth
- spits up green or yellow liquid, blood, or a substance that looks like coffee grounds
- has blood in the stool
- shows other signs of illness, such as fever, diarrhea, or difficulty with breathing

Some parents worry that their infant will spit up and choke if they are put to sleep on their backs, but this is not the case. Healthy infants naturally swallow or cough up fluids—it is a reflex all people have. Where the opening to the windpipe is located in the body makes it unlikely for fluids to cause choking. Babies may actually clear such fluids better when on their backs.

The National Institute of Child Health and Human Development (NICHD) Safe to Sleep® campaign (formerly, the Back to Sleep campaign; https://safetosleep.nichd.nih.gov) recommends placing infants to sleep on their backs to reduce the risk for SIDS. Since the recommendation for back sleeping began in 1992, the number of fatal choking deaths has not increased. In fact, in most of the few reported cases of fatal choking, an infant was sleeping on his or her stomach.

Teething

Although newborns usually have no visible teeth, baby teeth begin to appear generally about six months after birth. During the first few years, all 20 baby teeth will push through the gums, and most children will have their full set of these teeth in place by age three.

An infant's front four teeth usually appear first, at about six months of age, although some children do not get their first tooth until 12 or 14 months. As their teeth break through the gums, some infants become fussy, sleepless, and irritable; lose their appetite; or drool more than usual. If an infant has a fever or diarrhea while teething or continues to be cranky and uncomfortable, contact your baby's health-care provider.

The FDA does not recommend gum-numbing medications with an ingredient called "benzocaine" because they can cause a potentially fatal condition in young children. Talk to your health-care provider for advice on using these products for your teething infant. Other potential forms of relief for your infant include a chilled teething ring or gently rubbing the child's gums with a clean finger.

Urination

Infants urinate as often as every one to three hours or as infrequently as every four or six hours. In case of sickness or if the weather is very hot, urine output might drop by half and still be normal.

Urination should never be painful. If you notice any signs of distress while your infant is urinating, notify your child's health-care provider because this could be a sign of infection or some other problem in the urinary tract. In a healthy child, urine is light to dark yellow in color. (The darker the color, the more concentrated the urine; the urine is more concentrated when the child is not drinking much liquid.) The presence of blood in the urine or a bloody spot on the diaper is not normal and should prompt a call to the health-care provider. If this bleeding occurs with other symptoms, such as abdominal pain or bleeding in other areas, immediate medical attention is needed.

Jaundice

Jaundice can cause an infant's skin, eyes, and mouth to turn a yellowish color. The yellow color is caused by a buildup of bilirubin, a substance that is produced in the body during the normal process of breaking down old red blood cells and forming new ones.

Normally, the liver removes bilirubin from the body. But, for many infants, in the first few days after birth, the liver is not yet working at its full power. As a result, the level of bilirubin in the blood gets too high, causing the infant's color to become slightly yellow—this is jaundice.

Although jaundice is common and usually not serious, in some cases, high levels of bilirubin could cause brain injury. All infants with jaundice need to be seen by a health-care provider. Many infants need no treatment. Their livers start to catch up quickly and begin to remove bilirubin normally, usually within a few days after birth. For some infants, health-care providers prescribe phototherapy—a treatment using a special lamp—to help break down the bilirubin in their bodies.

If your infant has jaundice, ask your health-care provider how long the child's jaundice should last after leaving the hospital and schedule a follow-up appointment as directed. If the jaundice lasts longer than expected or an infant who did not have jaundice starts to turn yellowish after going home, a health-care provider should be consulted right away. If you intend to get discharged early, particularly within 48 hours of birth, your infant's jaundice may peak later in the first week.

It is almost impossible to say how severe the jaundice level is by just looking at the baby's skin, especially for infants of color. Therefore, make every effort to keep follow-up appointments, so the health-care provider can check the level of jaundice with a simple blood test.[2]

[2] "What Are Some of the Basics of Infant Health?" *Eunice Kennedy Shriver* National Institute of Child Health and Human Development (NICHD), September 7, 2021. Available online. URL: www.nichd.nih.gov/health/topics/infantcare/conditioninfo/basics. Accessed May 23, 2023.

Chapter 70 | Infant Feeding

Chapter Contents

Section 70.1 | **Breastfeeding**

Research shows that breastfeeding provides many health benefits for you and your baby. But it can also be difficult to manage breastfeeding in today's hurried world. Learning all you can before you give birth can help. The decision to breastfeed is a personal one. As a new mom, you deserve support no matter how you decide to feed your baby.

MAKING THE DECISION TO BREASTFEED
When you breastfeed, you give your baby a healthy start that lasts a lifetime. Breast milk is the perfect food for your baby. Breastfeeding saves lives, money, and time.

WHAT HEALTH BENEFITS DOES BREASTFEEDING GIVE YOUR BABY?
The cells, hormones, and antibodies in breast milk help protect babies from illness. This protection is unique and changes every day to meet your baby's growing needs. Research shows that breastfed babies have lower risks of:
- asthma
- leukemia (during childhood)
- obesity (during childhood)
- ear infections
- eczema (atopic dermatitis)
- diarrhea and vomiting
- lower respiratory infections
- necrotizing enterocolitis, a disease that affects the gastrointestinal tract in premature babies, or babies born before 37 weeks of pregnancy
- sudden infant death syndrome (SIDS)
- type 2 diabetes

WHAT IS COLOSTRUM, AND HOW DOES IT HELP YOUR BABY?

Your breast milk helps your baby grow healthy and strong from day one.

- **Your first milk is liquid gold.** Called "liquid gold" for its deep yellow color, colostrum is the thick first milk that you make during pregnancy and just after birth. This milk is very rich in nutrients and includes antibodies to protect your baby from infections. Colostrum also helps your newborn's digestive system to grow and function. Your baby gets only a small amount of colostrum at each feeding because the stomach of a newborn infant is tiny and can hold only a small amount.
- **Your milk changes as your baby grows.** Colostrum changes into mature milk by the third to fifth day after birth. This mature milk has just the right amount of fat, sugar, water, and protein to help your baby continue to grow. It looks thinner than colostrum, but it has the nutrients and antibodies your baby needs for healthy growth.

WHAT ARE THE HEALTH BENEFITS OF BREASTFEEDING FOR MOTHERS?

Breastfeeding helps a mother's health and healing following child-birth. Breastfeeding leads to a lower risk of these health problems in mothers:

- type 2 diabetes
- certain types of breast cancer
- ovarian cancer

HOW DOES BREASTFEEDING COMPARE TO FORMULA FEEDING?

- **Formula can be harder for your baby to digest.** For most babies, especially premature babies (babies born before 37 weeks of pregnancy), breast milk substitutes such as formula are harder to digest than breast milk. Formula is

652

made from cow's milk, and it often takes time for babies' stomachs to adjust to digesting it.

- **Your breast milk changes to meet your baby's needs.** As your baby gets older, your breast milk adjusts to meet your baby's changing needs. Researchers think that a baby's saliva transfers chemicals to a mother's body through breastfeeding. These chemicals help a mother's body create breast milk that meets the baby's changing needs.
- **Life can be easier for you when you breastfeed.** Breastfeeding may seem like it takes a little more effort than formula feeding at first. But breastfeeding can make your life easier once you and your baby settle into a good routine. When you breastfeed, there are no bottles and nipples to sterilize. You do not have to buy, measure, and mix formula. And there are no bottles to warm in the middle of the night! When you breastfeed, you can satisfy your baby's hunger right away.
- **Not breastfeeding costs money.** Formula and feeding supplies can cost well over $1,500 each year. As your baby gets older, he or she will eat more formula. But breast milk changes with the baby's needs, and babies usually need the same amount of breast milk as they get older. Breastfed babies may also be sick less often, which can help keep your baby's health costs lower.
- **Breastfeeding keeps the mother and the baby close.** Physical contact is important to newborns. It helps them feel more secure, warm, and comforted. Mothers also benefit from this closeness. The skin-to-skin contact boosts your oxytocin levels. Oxytocin is a hormone that helps breast milk flow and can calm the mother.

Sometimes, formula feeding can save lives:
- Very rarely, babies are born unable to tolerate milk of any kind. These babies must have an infant formula that is hypoallergenic, dairy-free, or lactose-free. A wide selection of specialist baby formulas now on

the market include soy formula, hydrolyzed formula, lactose-free formula, and hypoallergenic formula.
- Your baby may need formula if you have a health problem that will not allow you to breastfeed and you do not have access to donor breast milk.

Talk to your doctor before feeding your baby anything besides your breast milk.

CAN BREASTFEEDING HELP YOU LOSE WEIGHT?
Besides giving your baby nourishment and helping to keep your baby from becoming sick, breastfeeding may help you lose weight. Many women who breastfed their babies said it helped them get back to their prepregnancy weight more quickly, but experts are still looking at the effects of breastfeeding on weight loss. Learn more about weight loss while breastfeeding from ChooseMyPlate. gov (www.choosemyplate.gov/moms-breastfeeding-weight-loss).

HOW DOES BREASTFEEDING BENEFIT SOCIETY?
Society benefits overall when mothers breastfeed.
- **Breastfeeding saves lives.** Research shows that if 90 percent of families breastfed exclusively for six months, nearly 1,000 deaths among infants could be prevented each year.
- **Breastfeeding saves money.** Medical costs may be lower for fully breastfed infants than for never-breastfed infants. Breastfed infants usually need fewer sick care visits, prescriptions, and hospitalizations.
- **Breastfeeding also helps make a more productive workforce.** Mothers who breastfeed may miss less work to care for sick infants than mothers who feed their infants formula. Employer medical costs may also be lower.
- **Breastfeeding is better for the environment.** Formula cans and bottle supplies create more trash and plastic waste. Your milk is a renewable resource that comes packaged and warmed.

HOW DOES BREASTFEEDING HELP IN AN EMERGENCY?

During an emergency, such as a natural disaster, breastfeeding can save your baby's life:

- Breastfeeding protects your baby from the risks of an unclean water supply.
- Breastfeeding can help protect your baby against respiratory illnesses and diarrhea.
- Your milk is always at the right temperature for your baby. It helps keep your baby's body temperature from dropping too low.
- Your milk is always available without needing other supplies.[1]

Section 70.2 | Formula Feeding

INFANT FORMULA FEEDING

If you are feeding your baby infant formula, there are some important things to know, such as how to choose an infant formula and how to prepare and store your infant's formula.

No brand of infant formula is best for all babies. You should pick an infant formula that is made especially for babies. The U.S. Food and Drug Administration (FDA) regulates commercial infant formulas to make sure they meet minimum nutritional and safety requirements. Iron-fortified infant formulas are recommended, and most commercial infant formulas sold in the United States contain iron. Commercial infant formulas come in liquid and powdered forms. When choosing an infant formula, do the following:

- Make sure it is not expired.
- Make sure the container is sealed and in good condition. If there are any leaks, puffy ends, or rust spots, do not feed it to your baby.
- Make sure it is not labeled for toddlers.

---

[1] Office on Women's Health (OWH), "Breastfeeding," U.S. Department of Health and Human Services (HHS), February 22, 2021. Available online. URL: www.womenshealth.gov/breastfeeding. Accessed May 23, 2023.

Talk with your child's doctor or nurse if you have questions about choosing an infant formula for your baby or if you are thinking of switching the infant formula brand or type.

Homemade Infant Formula

The FDA and the American Academy of Pediatrics (AAP) warn against using recipes to make homemade infant formula. Using homemade infant formula can lead to serious health problems for your baby. Your baby's nutritional needs are very specific, especially in the first year of life. Homemade infant formulas may contain too little or too much of certain components, such as vitamins and minerals (such as iron).

Homemade infant formula may also have an increased risk of contamination, which could lead to your baby getting sick or developing an infection. Commercial powdered formulas are also not guaranteed to be sterile. However, the FDA regularly inspects these products and the manufacturing facilities where they are made to help make sure these products are safe.

Imported Infant Formulas

There are some public claims that infant formulas sold in other countries and promoted as "natural" or "organic" are better for babies. However, there is no scientific evidence that these infant formulas are better for babies than commercial infant formulas sold in the United States. All infant formulas legally sold in the United States—whether made in the United States or imported from other countries—must be reviewed by the FDA. The AAP warns against using illegally imported formulas, such as products ordered online from third-party distributors. The FDA may not have reviewed these products. Illegally imported formulas may not have been shipped and stored properly.

The FDA reviews all infant formulas sold legally in the United States to make sure they meet minimum nutritional and safety requirements. The FDA also makes sure that the water used to make formulas meets safety standards set by the U.S. Environmental Protection Agency (EPA).

Toddler Milk, Drinks, or Formulas

Toddler milk, drinks, or formulas are not needed to meet the nutritional needs of young children. They typically have added sugars. At age 12 months, your child can be introduced to plain whole cow's milk or fortified unsweetened soy beverage.

Babies younger than age 12 months should be fed infant formulas specifically designed to meet their nutritional needs. They should not be fed toddler milk, drinks, or formulas labeled for toddlers.

INFANT FORMULA PREPARATION AND STORAGE

Carefully read and follow the instructions on the infant formula container. These steps will help you know how to prepare and store your infant's formula correctly. Preparing your infant's formula according to the instructions is important.

Here are additional pointers to keep in mind when preparing and storing your infant's formula.

Preparation

- Wash your hands well before preparing bottles or feeding your baby. Clean and sanitize the workspace where you will be preparing the infant formula.
- Bottles need to be cleaned and sanitized.
- Milk for babies or infant formula does not need to be warmed before feeding, but some people like to warm their baby's bottle.
  - If you do decide to warm the bottle, never use a microwave. Microwaves heat milk and food unevenly, resulting in "hot spots" that can burn your baby's mouth and throat.
  - To warm a bottle, place the bottle under running warm water, taking care to keep the water from getting into the bottle or on the nipple. Put a couple drops of infant formula on the back of your hand to see if it is too hot.
- If you use powdered infant formula, do the following:
  - Use water from a safe source to mix your infant formula. If you are not sure if your tap water is safe to

use for preparing infant formula, contact your local health department.

- Use the amount of water listed on the instructions of the infant formula container. Always measure the water first and then add the powder.

  - Too much water may not meet the nutritional needs of your baby.

  - Too little water may cause your baby's kidneys and digestive system to work too hard and may cause your baby to become dehydrated.

- If your baby is very young (younger than two months old), is born prematurely, or has a weakened immune system, you may want to take extra precautions in preparing your infant's formula to protect against *Cronobacter*.

Use Quickly or Store Safely

- Prepared infant formula can spoil if it is left out at room temperature.

  - Use prepared infant formula within two hours of preparation and within one hour from when feeding begins.

  - If you do not start to use the prepared infant formula within two hours, immediately store the bottle in the fridge and use it within 24 hours.

  - Throw out any infant formula that is left in the bottle after feeding your baby. The combination of infant formula and your baby's saliva can cause bacteria to grow. Be sure to clean and sanitize the bottle before its next use.

- Store unopened infant formula containers in a cool, dry, indoor place—not in vehicles, garages, or outdoors.

- Once a container of infant formula is opened, store it in a cool, dry place with the lid tightly closed. Do not store it in the refrigerator.

- Most infant formulas need to be used within one month of opening the container (check the label). When you first open the container, write the date on the lid to help you remember.
- Never use the formula after the "Use By" date on the container.

HOW MUCH AND HOW OFTEN TO FEED INFANT FORMULA

Every baby is different. How much and how often your baby feeds will depend on your baby's needs. Here are a few things to know about infant formula feeding during the first days, weeks, and months of your baby's life.

First Days

If you have questions about your baby's growth or how much infant formula he or she is taking, talk with your child's doctor or nurse.

- Your newborn baby's belly is tiny. He or she does not need a lot of infant formula with each feeding to be full.
- You can start by offering your baby 1–2 ounces of infant formula every two to three hours in the first days of life if your baby is only getting infant formula and no breast milk. Give your baby more if he or she is showing signs of hunger.
- Most infant-formula-fed newborns will feed 8–12 times in 24 hours. Talk with your child's doctor or nurse about how much infant formula is right for your baby.
- As your baby grows, his or her belly grows too. Your baby will be able to drink more infant formula at each feeding, and the time between feedings will get longer.

First Weeks and Months

- Over the first few weeks and months, the time between feedings will get longer—about every three to four hours for most infant-formula-fed babies. This means you may need to wake your baby to feed. You can try patting, stroking, undressing, or changing the diaper to help wake your baby to feed.

- Some feeding sessions may be long, and other feedings may be short. That is okay. Babies will generally take what they need at each feeding and stop eating when they are full.

Six to Twelve Months Old

- Continue feeding your baby when he or she shows signs of hunger. Most 6- to 12-month-olds will need infant formula or solid foods about five to six times in 24 hours.
- As your baby gradually starts eating more solid foods, the amount of infant formula he or she needs each day will likely start to decrease.

Twelve to Twenty-Four Months Old

- When your toddler is 12 months old, you can switch from infant formula to plain whole cow's milk or fortified unsweetened soy beverage. You can do this gradually. You may want to start by replacing one infant formula feeding with cow's milk to help your child transition.[2]

---

[2] "Infant Formula Feeding," Centers for Disease Control and Prevention (CDC), May 16, 2022. Available online. URL: www.cdc.gov/nutrition/infantandtoddlernutrition/formula-feeding/index.html. Accessed May 23, 2023.

Chapter 71 | Bonding with Your Baby

WHAT IS HAPPENING?

Attachment is a deep, lasting bond that develops between a caregiver and a child during the baby's first few years of life. This attachment is crucial to the growth of a baby's body and mind. Babies who have this bond and feel loved have a better chance to grow up to be adults who trust others and know how to return affection.

WHAT YOU MIGHT BE SEEING

Normal babies:

- have brief periods of sleep, crying or fussing, and quiet alertness many times each day
- often cry for long periods for no apparent reason
- love to be held and cuddled
- respond to and imitate facial expressions
- love soothing voices and respond to them with smiles and small noises
- grow and develop every day
- learn new skills quickly and can outgrow difficult behaviors in a matter of weeks

WHAT CAN YOU DO?

No one knows your child as you do, so you are in the best position to recognize and fulfill your child's needs. Parents who give lots of loving care and attention to their babies help their babies develop a strong attachment. Affection stimulates your child to grow, learn, connect with others, and enjoy life. Here are some ways to promote bonding:

- Respond when your baby cries. Try to understand what he or she is saying to you. You cannot "spoil" babies with too much attention—they need and benefit from a parent's loving care, even when they seem inconsolable.
- Hold and touch your baby as much as possible. You can keep him or her close with baby slings, pouches, or backpacks (for older babies).
- Use feeding and diapering times to look into your baby's eyes, smile, and talk to your baby.
- Read, sing, and play peek-a-boo. Babies love to hear human voices and will try to imitate your voice and the sounds you make.
- As your baby gets a little older, try simple games and toys. Once your baby can sit up, plan on spending lots of time on the floor with toys, puzzles, and books.
- If you feel you are having trouble bonding with your infant, do not wait to get help! Talk to your doctor or your baby's pediatrician as soon as you can.[1]

---

[1] Child Welfare Information Gateway, "Bonding with Your Baby," U.S. Department of Health and Human Services (HHS), February 11, 2011. Available online. URL: www.childwelfare.gov/pubPDFs/bonding.pdf. Accessed May 23, 2023.

Chapter 72 | **Bringing Your Baby Home**

Bringing a new baby home is exciting, but it can also be overwhelming. Do not worry—you will do fine! Here is what to expect during the first few days at home with your baby.

YOUR RECOVERY

Delivering a baby is hard work, and you did it! Now that you are home, it is important to care for yourself as lovingly as you care for your baby. That is especially true if you had a cesarean section (C-section). Get plenty of sleep and make healthy food choices. Have visitors only when you feel ready. Ask your partner, family, and friends for help when you need it.

You may also be having emotional highs and lows. Your hormones are changing, and while you are in love with your new baby, being a new parent is exhausting!

If you have deep feelings of sadness, difficulty sleeping, irritability, changes in appetite, and trouble concentrating, these may be a sign of depression. If you are worried about the way you have been feeling, it is important to tell your doctor about your concerns. The National Helpline is available 24 hours a day at 800-662-HELP to refer you to local support networks and resources.

YOUR BABY

After you return from the hospital or birthing center, continue cuddling your baby to help them adjust to life outside the womb. Skin-to-skin time with your baby will also help regulate your hormones and help with breastfeeding. You will take your baby to their first checkups this week. Your doctor or nurse will answer any questions you have about your baby and breastfeeding.

BREASTFEEDING

In the first few days at home, it will seem like all you are doing is caring for your baby. As your milk transitions from colostrum to mature milk, your baby should nurse early and often, about 8–12 times every 24 hours. Since babies do not feed on a schedule, it is best to watch your baby for hunger signs and not the clock.

You can see if your baby is getting plenty of milk by tracking the color, texture, and frequency of poops and wet diapers. If it seems like your baby is too sleepy to eat, not making enough wet or dirty diapers, or not eating at least eight times a day, talk to your baby's doctor.

In the first or second week at home, your baby may go through a period of rapid growth, referred to as a growth spurt. If this occurs, your baby will need to eat more often—probably every hour. If you are worried about your milk supply, just follow your baby's lead. Your body will adjust to the baby's needs.

Remember, while this seems like a lot, it is only temporary. Asking your family and friends for support can help you get through it. They can change diapers, run errands, and snuggle with your baby while you get some rest. That way, you only need to focus on feeding your baby.

Feeding your baby in those early days is not easy. If you face challenges, you are not alone. New moms often ask the following questions:

- How do I know if my baby is getting enough milk?
- What should I do if my breasts feel too full or uncomfortable?
- What if my baby does not latch well?
- What should I do if my nipples hurt?
- How can I tell when my baby is hungry?
- What if my baby wants to eat around the clock?[1]

---

[1] Food and Nutrition Service (FNS), "Bringing Baby Home," U.S. Department of Agriculture (USDA), April 23, 2023. Available online. URL: https://wicbreastfeeding.fns.usda.gov/bringing-baby-home. Accessed May 24, 2023.

Chapter 73 | Making Your Home Safe for the Baby

Your baby is on the way, and there is a lot to think about. Besides making sure that you have baby furniture and clothing for your new daughter or son, you will want to check that your home is safe. The following tips can help you cover all the safety bases.

BEFORE YOU BRING THE BABY HOME
Before you bring the baby home, do the following:
- Check the safety of your baby's crib and other baby items. Many new parents welcome hand-me-down baby items from family and friends. Although it is wise to save money, some products could be unsafe if recalled or if parts are missing or loose. Unsafe cribs and other items can put your baby's life in danger. Most brand-new cribs and mattresses purchased in the United States are safe. Make sure the crib conforms to the current government safety standards. Also, check to see if hand-me-down items, such as bassinets or portable cribs, have been recalled. Check for recalls and get information on buying a safe crib and mattress at the U.S. Consumer Product Information Safety Commission website (www.cpsc.gov). Or call them at 800-638-2772.
- Remove pillows, blankets, and stuffed animals from the crib to prevent your baby from suffocation.
- Check to see that smoke detectors and carbon monoxide detectors in your home are working. Place

at least one smoke detector on each level of your home
and in halls outside of bedrooms. Have an escape plan
in case of fire.

- Put emergency numbers, including poison control,
  near each phone. Have at least one phone in your home
  connected by landline. Cordless phones do not work
  when the power is out, and cell phone batteries can run
  out.
- Make sure your home or apartment number is easy
  to see, so fire or rescue can locate you quickly in an
  emergency.
- Make sure handrails are installed and secure in
  stairways. Always hold the handrail when using stairs,
  especially when holding your baby.

BEFORE YOUR BABY STARTS CRAWLING

Your baby will be crawling before you know it. Most babies begin
crawling around six to nine months. Crawling on their hands and
knees will reveal many dangers to your baby. Thinking ahead to
the toddler years will help you take care of other hazards before
your baby grows and finds them first. Here are some things to do
before your baby is crawling:

- Cover all unused electrical sockets with outlet plugs.
- Keep cords out of the baby's reach. Tack up cords
  to vertical blinds and move furniture, lamps, or
  electronics to hide cords.
- Secure furniture and electronics, such as bookcases
  and TVs, so they cannot be pulled down on top of your
  baby.
- Use protective padding to cover sharp edges and
  corners, such as from a coffee table or fireplace hearth.
- Install safety gates at the bottom and top of stairwells or
  block entry to unsafe rooms.
- Use safety latches on cabinets and doors.
- Store all medicines, cleaning products, and other
  poisons out of the baby's reach.

Making Your Home Safe for the Baby

- Remove rubber tips from doorstops or replace them with one-piece doorsteps.
- Look for and remove all small objects. Objects that can easily pass through the center of a toilet paper roll might cause choking.
- Keep houseplants out of the baby's reach. Some plants can poison or make your baby sick.
- Set your water heater temperature to no higher than 125 °F (51.67 °C). Water that is hotter can cause bad burns.
- Closely supervise your baby around a family pet. Pets need time to adjust to a new baby.[1]

[1] Office on Women's Health (OWH), "Making Your Home Safe for Baby," U.S. Department of Health and Human Services (HHS), February 22, 2021. Available online. URL: www.womenshealth.gov/pregnancy/getting-ready-baby/making-your-home-safe-baby. Accessed May 24, 2023.

Chapter 74 | Working after Birth: Parental Leave Considerations

Chapter Contents

Section 74.1 | Family and Medical Leave Act

The Family and Medical Leave Act (FMLA) entitles eligible employees of covered employers to take unpaid, job-protected leave for specified family and medical reasons with continuation of group health insurance coverage under the same terms and conditions as if the employee had not taken leave. Eligible employees are entitled to the following:

- twelve workweeks of leave in a 12-month period:
  - for the birth of a child and to care for the newborn child within one year of birth
  - for the placement with the employee of a child for adoption or foster care and to care for the newly placed child within one year of placement
  - to care for the employee's spouse, child, or parent who has a serious health condition
  - for a serious health condition that makes the employee unable to perform the essential functions of his or her job
  - for any qualifying exigency arising out of the fact that the employee's spouse, son, daughter, or parent is a covered military member on "covered active duty"
- twenty-six workweeks of leave during a single 12-month period to care for a covered service member with a serious injury or illness if the eligible employee is the service member's spouse, son, daughter, parent, or next of kin (military caregiver leave)

COVERAGE

The FMLA applies to all:

- public agencies, including local, state, and federal employers, and local education agencies (schools)
- private sector employers who employ 50 or more employees for at least 20 workweeks in the current or preceding calendar year—including joint employers and successors of covered employers

ELIGIBILITY

In order to be eligible to take leave under the FMLA, an employee must:

- work for a covered employer
- have worked 1,250 hours during the 12 months prior to the start of leave (Special hours of service rules apply to airline flight crew members: www.dol.gov/agencies/whd/fact-sheets/28j-fmla-airline-crew.)
- work at a location where the employer has 50 or more employees within 75 miles
- have worked for the employer for 12 months (The 12 months of employment are not required to be consecutive in order for the employee to qualify for FMLA leave. In general, only employment within seven years is counted unless the break in service is due to an employee's fulfillment of military obligations or governed by a collective bargaining agreement or other written agreement.)[1]

Section 74.2 | Breastfeeding and Going Back to Work

Planning ahead for your return to work can help ease the transition. Learn as much as you can before the baby's birth and talk with your employer about your options. Planning ahead can help you continue to enjoy breastfeeding your baby long after your maternity leave is over.

WHAT CAN YOU DO DURING YOUR PREGNANCY TO PREPARE FOR BREASTFEEDING AFTER RETURNING TO WORK?

- Take a breastfeeding class, which may be offered at the hospital where you plan to deliver your baby. These

---

[1] "Family and Medical Leave Act," U.S. Department of Labor (DOL), October 30, 2009. Available online. URL: www.dol.gov/agencies/whd/fmla. Accessed May 24, 2023.

classes offer tips on returning to work and continuing to breastfeed.

- Join a breastfeeding support group to talk with other moms about breastfeeding while working.
- Watch the videos of moms who successfully breastfed, including after returning to work, at www.womenshealth. gov/its-only-natural/ fitting-breastfeeding-yourlife?from=breastfeeding.
- Talk with your boss about your plans to breastfeed before you go out on maternity leave.
- Encourage your boss to visit the Supporting Nursing Moms at Work: Employer Solutions site (www.womenshealth.gov/blog/work-and-breastfeeding?from=breastfeeding) to get tips and solutions for supporting nursing mothers at work in all different types of workplaces.
- Discuss different types of schedules with your boss, such as starting back part-time at first or taking split shifts. For tips on talking to your boss, read the Business Case for Breastfeeding (www.womenshealth.gov/ breastfeeding/breastfeeding-home-work-and-public/ breastfeeding-and-going-back-work/business-case).
- Learn about your rights under the federal Break Time for Nursing Mothers law (www.dol.gov/whd/ nursingmothers). The law requires some employers to provide reasonable break time for employees to express milk for their nursing child for one year after their child's birth. These include a functional space and time for women to express milk each time they need to.
- Find out if your company offers a lactation support program for employees.
- Talk to other women at your company. Ask the lactation program director, your supervisor, the wellness program director, the employee human resources office, or other coworkers if they know of other women who breastfed after returning to work.

- Explore childcare options. Find out whether a childcare facility close to where you work is available so that you can visit and breastfeed your baby during lunch or other breaks. Ask whether the facility has a place set aside for breastfeeding mothers. Make sure the facility will feed your baby with your pumped breast milk.

WHAT CAN YOU DO WHILE ON MATERNITY LEAVE TO MAKE BREASTFEEDING MORE SUCCESSFUL AFTER YOU RETURN TO WORK?

- Take as many weeks off as you can. Taking at least 6 weeks of leave can help you recover from childbirth and settle into a good breastfeeding routine.
- Practice expressing your milk by hand or with a breast pump several days or weeks before you have to go back to work. It can feel very different to pump breast milk compared to breastfeeding your baby. Some women find it helpful to get comfortable with their breast pump or hand expression while they are at home in a stress-free environment.
- A breast pump may be the best method for quickly removing milk during work. A hands-free breast pump may even allow you to work while pumping if you do office work.
- Pump breast milk while your baby is napping or being looked after by others. Build up a supply of breast milk for caregivers to give your baby while you are at work.
- Help your baby adjust to taking breast milk from a bottle or cup. It may be helpful to have someone else give the bottle or cup to your baby at first. Wait at least a month after birth before introducing a bottle to your infant. Your baby may be able to drink from a cup at three or four months old.
- Talk with your family and your childcare provider about your desire to breastfeed for as long as possible. Let them know you will need their support and how they can best help you. Follow the suggestions on how

people in your network can support your breastfeeding goals at www.womenshealth.gov/itsonlynatural/finding-support/building-your-support-network.html?from=breastfeeding.

WHAT CAN YOU DO WHEN YOU RETURN TO WORK TO HELP EASE THE TRANSITION?

- Keep talking with your boss about your schedule and what is or is not working for you. Under the Patient Protection and Affordable Care Act (ACA), most employers, with few exceptions, must offer a breastfeeding employee reasonable break times to pump for up to one year after her baby is born and a place other than a bathroom to comfortably, safely, and privately express breast milk.
- When you arrive to pick up your baby from childcare, see if you can take time to breastfeed your baby right away. This will give you and your baby time to reconnect before going home.

HOW OFTEN SHOULD YOU PUMP AT WORK?

At work, you will need to pump during the times you would feed your baby if you were at home. As a general rule, in the first few months of life, babies need to breastfeed 8–12 times in 24 hours. As the baby gets older, the number of feedings may go down.

Pumping can take about 10–15 minutes once you are used to using your breast pump. Sometimes, it may take longer. Many women use their regular breaks and lunch break to pump. Some women come to work early or stay late to make up the time needed to pump.

WHERE SHOULD YOU STORE YOUR BREAST MILK?

Breast milk is food, so it is safe to keep it in an employee refrigerator or a cooler with ice packs. Talk to your boss about keeping your milk in an employee refrigerator if you think anyone will be concerned. If you work in a medical department, do not store milk in the same refrigerators where medical specimens are kept.

Label the milk container with your name and the date you expressed the milk. Try to keep the milk in the back of the refrigerator where the temperature is the most constant and coldest.

HOW MUCH BREAST MILK SHOULD YOU SEND WITH YOUR BABY DURING THE DAY?

You may need to pump two to three times each day at work to make enough milk for your baby while he or she is with a caregiver.

Research shows that breastfed babies between one and six months old take in an average of 2–3 ounces per feeding. As your baby gets older, your breast milk changes to meet your baby's needs. So your baby will get the nutrition he or she needs from the same number of ounces at nine months as he or she did at three months.

Some babies eat less during the day when they are away from their mothers and then nurse more often at night. This is called "reverse cycling." Or babies may eat during the day and still nurse more often at night. This may be more for the closeness with you that your baby craves. If your baby reverse cycles, you may find that you do not need to pump as much milk for your baby during the day.[2]

Section 74.3 | Understanding Childcare Options

Before you start your childcare search, you may find it helpful to learn about all the childcare options that may be available. You want what is best for your child, so it is important to find a provider that fits your child's and family's needs. This means considering things like the size of the program, the type of physical environment it provides (such as a home environment versus a classroom setting), the hours when it is available, and so on.

---

[2] Office on Women's Health (OWH), "Breastfeeding and Going Back to Work," U.S. Department of Health and Human Services (HHS), February 22, 2021. Available online. URL: www.womenshealth.gov/breastfeeding/breast-feeding-home-work-and-public/breastfeeding-and-going-back-work. Accessed May 24, 2023.

This section provides an overview of the types of childcare options, including how each option may be regulated to ensure your child's health and safety. These include the following:

- childcare centers
- family childcare homes
- Head Start and Early Head Start programs
- prekindergarten programs
- school-age childcare programs
- childcare options for military families
- informal in-home childcare

MORE RESOURCES

If you have questions or want to talk with someone about the types of childcare available in your community, the following additional resources can help you learn more about your state or territory's childcare options.

State and Territory Childcare Consumer Education Websites

Every state and territory has a childcare consumer education website, which should be your "go-to" resource for learning about and finding quality childcare in your area. Your state or territory's website offers information to help you choose the right kind of care for your child. It also includes an online search to find licensed, regulated childcare where you live. To find your state or territory's childcare consumer education website, select your state or territory on the "See Your State's Resources" page (www.childcare.gov/state-resources-home) and select the "Understanding and Finding Child Care" tab.

Childcare Resources and Referral Agencies

Many states have childcare resource and referral agencies that can provide you with information about childcare options by phone, in person, online, or via email. Most of these agencies also have websites with childcare information and resources. To find your state or territory's childcare resource and referral agencies, select your state or territory on the "See Your State's Resources" page (www.

childcare.gov/state-resources-home) and select the "Understanding and Finding Child Care" tab.

THINGS TO CONSIDER
Is the Provider or Program Licensed?
Licensing is the main way the United States and its territories regulate childcare. States and territories set minimum childcare licensing requirements to ensure children stay healthy and safe while they are in care. Childcare providers must meet these requirements to operate legally. In addition to childcare licensing, some states may offer certification or registration to help ensure basic health and safety standards in certain home-based childcare programs. Not all childcare options are licensed, so it is important to check to see if the childcare program you are considering is licensed.

- To learn more about what childcare licensing is and why it is important, see the "How Is Child Care Regulated to Ensure Children's Health and Safety?" section (www.childcare.gov/consumer-education/how-is-child-care-regulated).
- To learn about your state or territory's specific childcare licensing requirements, select your state or territory on the "See Your State's Resources" page (www.childcare.gov/state-resources-home) and select the "Understanding and Finding Child Care" tab.

Tip: Your state or territory's online childcare search includes licensed childcare programs. The licensing status is usually clearly marked in your childcare search results. For instance, search tools may show the provider's license number and licensing status. To go to your state or territory's online childcare search, go to "Find Child Care" (www.childcare.gov/home) and select your state or territory. To learn more about how to choose quality childcare, visit the "How Do I Find and Choose Quality Child Care?" (www.childcare.gov/consumer-education/choosing-quality-childcare) section.

Which Type of Childcare Option May Be Best for Your Child?

There are many things to consider when choosing a childcare option that will meet your child's and family's needs. For instance, some children may respond best to a home setting with a small group of children, while others may thrive in a larger group setting with several children of a similar age. When it comes to choosing a childcare provider for your child, think about which setting would best support your child's specific learning and social needs. For more information and tips on how to choose the best childcare program for your child, see the "How Do I Find and Choose Quality Child Care?" section (www.childcare.gov/consumer-education/choosing-quality-childcare).

Does the Program Accept Childcare Financial Assistance?

Every state and territory has a childcare financial assistance program to help families with low incomes "pay for childcare." Each state and territory also has its own guidelines for who is eligible for this assistance. Your state or territory's childcare financial assistance program can offer you a list of childcare providers that participate in this program. If you are eligible to receive help, you should make sure that your childcare provider accepts childcare financial assistance.[3]

---

[3] ChildCare.gov, "What Are My Child Care Options?" Administration for Children and Families (ACF), December 26, 2022. Available online. URL: www.childcare.gov/consumer-education/childcare-options. Accessed May 24, 2023.

Part 8 | Additional Help and Information

Chapter 75 | Glossary of Terms Related to Pregnancy and Birth

absorption: The process of taking in. For a person or an animal, absorption is the process of a substance getting into the body through the eyes, skin, stomach, intestines, or lungs.

acquired immunodeficiency syndrome (AIDS): A disease caused by the human immunodeficiency virus (HIV). People with AIDS are at an increased risk of developing certain cancers and infections that usually occur only in individuals with a weak immune system.

adverse effect: An unexpected medical problem that happens during treatment with a drug or other therapy. Also called "adverse event."

amino acid: One of several molecules that join together to form proteins. There are 20 common amino acids found in proteins.

anemia: A condition in which the number of red blood cells is below normal.

anesthetic: A drug that causes insensitivity to pain and is used for surgeries and other medical procedures.

antibiotic: A drug used to treat infections caused by bacteria and other microorganisms.

antibody: A protein made by plasma cells (a type of white blood cell) in response to an antigen (a substance that causes the body to make a specific immune response). Each antibody can bind to only one specific antigen.

This glossary contains terms excerpted from documents produced by several sources deemed reliable.

antigen: Any substance that causes the body to make an immune response against that substance. Antigens include toxins, chemicals, bacteria, viruses, or other substances that come from outside the body.

anxiety: Feelings of fear, dread, and uneasiness that may occur as a reaction to stress. A person with anxiety may sweat, feel restless and tense, and have a rapid heartbeat.

assessment: The process of gathering evidence and documentation of a student's learning.

asthma: A chronic disease in which the bronchial airways in the lungs become narrowed and swollen, making it difficult to breathe.

autoimmune disease: A condition in which the body recognizes its own tissues as foreign and directs an immune response against them.

bacteria: A large group of single-cell microorganisms. Some cause infections and diseases in animals and humans.

bacterial vaginosis (BV): The most common vaginal infection in women of childbearing age, which happens when the normal bacteria (germs) in the vagina get out of balance, such as from douching or from sexual contact.

birth control: The use of drugs, devices, or surgery to prevent pregnancy. There are many different types of birth control.

bladder: The organ in the human body that stores urine. It is found in the lower part of the abdomen.

body mass index (BMI): A measure of body fat based on a person's height and weight.

breast cancer: Cancer that forms in tissues of the breast. The most common type of breast cancer is ductal carcinoma, which begins in the lining of the milk ducts (thin tubes that carry milk from the lobules of the breast to the nipple).

calcium: A mineral that is an essential nutrient for bone health. It is also needed for the heart, muscles, and nerves to function properly and for blood to clot.

calorie: A measurement of the energy content of food. The body needs calories to perform its functions, such as breathing, circulating the blood, and physical activity.

cancer: A term for diseases in which abnormal cells in the body divide without control. Cancer cells can invade nearby tissues and can spread to other parts of the body through the blood and lymphatic system, which is a network of tissues that clears infections and keeps body fluids in balance.

carbohydrate: A sugar molecule. Carbohydrates can be small and simple (e.g., glucose), or they can be large and complex (e.g., polysaccharides such as starch, chitin, or cellulose).

cervix: The lower, narrow part of the uterus (womb). The cervix forms a canal that opens into the vagina, which leads to the outside of the body.

childbearing age: Range of ages during which a woman may become pregnant. For example, it can be defined as 16–49 years of age.

chromosome: A chromosome is an organized package of deoxyribonucleic acid (DNA) found in the nucleus of the cell. Different organisms have different numbers of chromosomes. Humans have 23 pairs of chromosomes—22 pairs of numbered chromosomes, called "autosomes," and one pair of sex chromosomes, X and Y.

chronic disease: A disease that has one or more of the following characteristics: is permanent; leaves residual disability; is caused by nonreversible pathological alternation; requires special training of the patient for rehabilitation; or may be expected to require a long period of supervision, observation, or care.

chronic pain: Pain that can range from mild to severe and persists or progresses over a long period of time.

computed tomography (CT): A procedure for taking x-ray images from many different angles and then assembling them into a cross-section of the body.

constipation: A decrease in the frequency of stools or bowel movements with hardening of the stool.

diabetes: A disease in which blood glucose (blood sugar) levels are above normal. There are two main types of diabetes. Type 1 diabetes is caused by a problem with the body's defense system, called the "immune system."

ectopic pregnancy: A pregnancy that is not in the uterus. It happens when a fertilized egg settles and grows in a place other than the inner lining of the uterus. Most happen in the fallopian tube but can happen in the ovary, cervix, or abdominal cavity.

endometriosis: A condition in which tissue that normally lines the uterus grows in other areas of the body, usually inside the abdominal cavity, but acts as if it were inside the uterus. Bloodshed monthly from the misplaced tissue has no place to go, and tissues surrounding the area of endometriosis may become inflamed or swollen.

enzyme: A protein that speeds up chemical reactions in the body.

estrogen: A group of female hormones that are responsible for the development of breasts and other secondary sex characteristics in women. Estrogen is produced by the ovaries and other body tissues. Estrogen, along with progesterone, is important in preparing a woman's body for pregnancy.

exercise: A type of physical activity that involves planned, structured, and repetitive bodily movement done to maintain or improve one or more components of physical fitness.

fallopian tube(s): Part of the female reproductive system, one of a pair of tubes connecting the ovaries to the uterus.

gynecologist: A doctor who diagnoses and treats conditions of the female reproductive system and associated disorders.

hormone: A substance produced by one tissue and conveyed by the bloodstream to another to affect a function of the body, such as growth or metabolism.

human immunodeficiency virus (HIV): The virus that infects and destroys the body's immune cells and causes a disease called "AIDS," or "acquired immunodeficiency syndrome."

hypertension: Also called "high blood pressure," it is having blood pressure greater than 140 over 90 millimeters of mercury (mm Hg). Long-term high blood pressure can damage blood vessels and organs, including the heart, kidneys, eyes, and brain.

immune system: A complex system of cellular and molecular components having the primary function of distinguishing self from not self and defense against foreign organisms or substances.

infertility: A condition in which a couple has problems conceiving, or getting pregnant, after one year of regular sexual intercourse without using any birth control methods. Infertility can be caused by a problem with the man or the woman, or both.

intestines: Also known as the "bowels," or the long, tube-like organ in the human body that completes digestion or the breaking down of food. They consist of the small intestine and the large intestine.

lesion: An area of abnormal tissue. A lesion may be benign (not cancer) or malignant (cancer).

Glossary of Terms Related to Pregnancy and Birth

low birth weight: Having a weight at birth that is less than 2,500 grams, or 5 pounds, 8 ounces.

lupus: A chronic inflammatory disease that occurs when the body's immune system attacks its own tissues and organs. It is also called "systemic lupus erythematosus" (SLE).

magnetic resonance imaging (MRI): A noninvasive procedure that uses magnetic fields and radio waves to produce three-dimensional (3D) computerized images of areas inside the body.

menopause: The cessation of menstruation in women.

menstruating: The blood flow from the uterus that happens about every four weeks in a woman.

metabolism: The chemical changes that take place in a cell or an organism. These changes make energy and the materials cells and organisms need to grow, reproduce, and stay healthy. Metabolism also helps get rid of toxic substances.

miscarriage: An unplanned loss of a pregnancy. Also called a "spontaneous abortion."

nipple: The protruding part of the breast that extends and becomes firmer upon stimulation. In breastfeeding, milk travels from the milk sinuses through the nipple to the baby.

nutrition: The taking in and use of food and other nourishing material by the body. Nutrition is a three-part process. First, food or drink is consumed. Second, the body breaks down the food or drink into nutrients. Third, the nutrients travel through the bloodstream to different parts of the body where they are used as "fuel" and for many other purposes.

organ: A part of the body that performs a specific function. For example, the heart is an organ.

ovary (ovaries): Part of a woman's reproductive system, the ovaries produce her eggs. Each month, through the process called "ovulation," the ovaries release eggs into the fallopian tubes, where they travel to the uterus, or womb. If an egg is fertilized by a man's sperm, a woman becomes pregnant, and the egg grows and develops inside the uterus. If the egg is not fertilized, the egg and the lining of the uterus are shed during a woman's monthly menstrual period.

over-the-counter (OTC): Refers to a medicine that can be bought without a prescription (doctor's order). Also called "nonprescription" and "OTC."

overweight: Overweight refers to an excessive amount of body weight that includes muscle, bone, fat, and water. A person who has a body mass index (BMI) of 25 to 29.9 is considered overweight.

ovulation: The release of a single egg from a follicle that developed in the ovary. It usually occurs regularly, around day 14 of a 28-day menstrual cycle.

penis: An external male reproductive organ. It contains a tube called the "urethra," which carries semen and urine to the outside of the body.

perinatal: The time period immediately before and after birth.

physical activity: Any bodily movement that is produced by the contraction of skeletal muscle and that substantially increases energy expenditure.

physical fitness: A set of attributes that people possess or achieve that relates to the ability to perform physical activity and is comprised of skill-related, health-related, and physiological components.

pica: A craving to eat nonfood items, such as dirt, paint chips, and clay. Some children exhibit pica-related behavior.

placenta: During pregnancy, a temporary organ joins the mother and fetus. The placenta transfers oxygen and nutrients from the mother to the fetus and permits the release of carbon dioxide and waste products from the fetus.

placental abruption: When the placenta separates from the uterine wall before delivery, which can mean the fetus does not get enough oxygen.

postpartum depression (PPD): A serious condition that requires treatment from a health-care provider. With this condition, feelings of the baby blues (feeling sad, anxious, afraid, or confused after having a baby) do not go away or get worse.

preconception health: A woman's health before she becomes pregnant. It involves knowing how health conditions and risk factors could affect a woman or her unborn baby if she becomes pregnant.

pregnancy: The condition between conception (fertilization of an egg by a sperm) and birth, during which the fertilized egg develops in the uterus. In humans, pregnancy lasts about 288 days.

premature birth: The birth of a baby before 37 weeks of pregnancy. In humans, a normal pregnancy lasts about 40 weeks. The risk of premature birth may be increased by certain health problems in the mother, such as diabetes, heart disease, and kidney disease, or problems during pregnancy and also called "preterm birth."

Glossary of Terms Related to Pregnancy and Birth

prevention: Actions that reduce exposure or other risks, keep people from getting sick, or keep the disease from getting worse.

progesterone: A female hormone produced by the ovaries. Progesterone, along with estrogen, prepares the uterus (womb) for a possible pregnancy each month and supports the fertilized egg if conception occurs. Progesterone also helps prepare the breasts for milk production and breastfeeding.

prognosis: The likely outcome or course of a disease; the chance of recovery or recurrence.

puberty: Time when the body is changing from the body of a child to the body of an adult. This process begins earlier in girls than in boys, usually between the ages of 8 and 13, and lasts two to four years.

risk reduction: Actions that can decrease the likelihood that individuals, groups, or communities will experience disease or other health conditions.

saliva: The watery fluid in the mouth made by the salivary glands. Saliva moistens food to help digestion, and it helps protect the mouth against infections.

semen: The fluid (which contains sperm) a male releases from his penis when he becomes sexually aroused or has an orgasm.

serum: The liquid part of blood that remains after clotting proteins and blood cells are removed.

sexually transmitted infections (STIs): Diseases that are spread by sexual activity. Also called "sexually transmitted diseases" (STDs).

sickle cell anemia: A blood disorder passed down from parents to children. It involves problems in the red blood cells. Normal red blood cells are round and smooth and move through blood vessels easily. Sickle cells are hard and have a curved edge.

stillbirth: When a fetus dies during birth or when the fetus dies during the late stages of pregnancy when it would have been otherwise expected to survive.

sudden infant death syndrome (SIDS): The diagnosis given for the sudden death of an infant under one year of age that remains unexplained after a complete investigation. Because most cases of SIDS occur when a baby is sleeping in a crib, SIDS is also commonly known as "crib death." Most SIDS deaths occur when a baby is between one and four months of age.

testicle (testis): The male sex gland. There are a pair of testes behind the penis in a pouch of skin called the "scrotum." The testes make and store sperm and make the male hormone testosterone.

umbilical cord: Connected to the placenta and provides the transfer of nutrients and waste between the woman and the fetus.

urinary tract infection (UTI): An infection anywhere in the urinary tract or organs that collect and store urine and release it from your body (the kidneys, ureters, bladder, and urethra).

uterine contractions: During the birthing process, a woman's uterus tightens, or contracts. Contractions can be strong and regular (meaning that they can happen every five minutes, every three minutes, and so on) during labor until the baby is delivered. Women can have contractions before labor starts; these are not regular and do not progress or increase in intensity or duration.

uterine fibroids: Common, benign (noncancerous) tumors that grow in the muscle of the uterus or womb. Fibroids often cause no symptoms and need no treatment, and they usually shrink after menopause.

uterus: A woman's womb, or the hollow, pear-shaped organ, located in a woman's lower abdomen between the bladder and the rectum.

vagina: The muscular canal that extends from the cervix to the outside of the body. Its walls are lined with mucus membranes and tiny glands that make vaginal secretions.

vulva: The external female genital organ. It has five parts, including the urinary opening and the opening to the vagina.

withdrawal: Symptoms that occur after chronic use of a drug is reduced abruptly or stopped.

X-ray: A type of high-energy radiation. In low doses, x-rays are used to diagnose diseases by making pictures of the inside of the body.

yoga: A mind and body practice with origins in ancient Indian philosophy. The various styles of yoga typically combine physical postures, breathing techniques, and meditation or relaxation.

Chapter 76 | Directory of Organizations That Provide Help and Information about Pregnancy and Birth

GOVERNMENT AGENCIES THAT PROVIDE INFORMATION ABOUT PREGNANCY AND RELATED CONCERNS

Agency for Healthcare Research and Quality (AHRQ)
5600 Fishers Ln.
7th Fl. Rockville, MD 20857
Phone: 301-427-1104
Website: www.ahrq.gov

Centers for Disease Control and Prevention (CDC)
1600 Clifton Rd.
Atlanta, GA 30329-4027
Toll-Free: 800-232-4636
Toll-Free TTY: 888-232-6348
Website: www.cdc.gov
Email: cdcinfo@cdc.gov

Centers for Medicare & Medicaid Services (CMS)
7500 Security Blvd.
Baltimore, MD 21244
Toll-Free: 800-633-4227
Toll-Free TTY: 877-486-2048
Website: www.cms.gov

Resources in this chapter were compiled from several sources deemed reliable; all contact information was verified and updated in July 2023.

Eunice Kennedy Shriver National Institute of Child Health and Human Development (NICHD)
P.O. Box 3006
Rockville, MD 20847
Toll-Free: 800-370-2943
Toll-Free Fax: 866-760-5947
Website: www.nichd.nih.gov
Email:
NICHDInformationResource
Center@mail.nih.gov

National Cancer Institute (NCI)
9609 Medical Center Dr.
Rockville, MD 20850
Toll-Free: 800-422-6237
Website: www.cancer.gov
Email: NCIinfo@nih.gov

National Center for Complementary and Integrative Health (NCCIH)
9000 Rockville Pike
Bethesda, MD 20892
Toll-Free: 888-644-6226
Toll-Free TTY: 866-464-3615
Website: nccih.nih.gov
Email: info@nccih.nih.gov

National Heart, Lung, and Blood Institute (NHLBI)
31 Center Dr. Bldg. 31
Bethesda, MD 20892
Toll-Free: 877-645-2448
Website: www.nhlbi.nih.gov/about/
divisions/division-lung-diseases/
national-center-sleep-disorders-
research
Email: nhlbiinfo@nhlbi.nih.gov

National Human Genome Research Institute (NHGRI)
9000 Rockville Pike, Bldg. 31,
Rm. 4B09
31 Center Dr., MSC 2152
Bethesda, MD 20892-2152
Phone: 301-402-0911
Fax: 301-402-2218
Website: www.genome.gov

National Institute of Arthritis and Musculoskeletal and Skin Diseases (NIAMS)
1 AMS Cir.
Bethesda, MD 20892-3675
Toll-Free: 877-226-4267
Phone: 301-495-4484
TTY: 301-565-2966
Fax: 301-718-6366
Website: www.niams.nih.gov
Email: NIAMSinfo@mail.nih.gov

National Institute of Diabetes, Digestive, and Kidney Diseases (NIDDK)
9000 Rockville Pike
Bethesda, MD 20892
Toll-Free: 800-860-8747
Website: www.niddk.nih.gov
Email: healthinfo@niddk.nih.gov

National Institute of Environmental Health Sciences (NIEHS)
P.O. Box 12233 MD K3-16
Research Triangle Park, NC 27709
Phone: 919-541-3345
Fax: 919-541-4395
Website: www.niehs.nih.gov
Email: webcenter@niehs.nih.gov

National Institute of Mental Health (NIMH)

6001 Executive Blvd.
Rm. 6200, MSC 9663
Bethesda, MD 20892-9663
Toll-Free: 866-615-6464
Website: www.nimh.nih.gov
Email: nimhinfo@nih.gov

National Institute of Neurological Disorders and Stroke (NINDS)

P.O. Box 5801
Bethesda, MD 20824
Toll-Free: 800-352-9424
Website: www.ninds.nih.gov

National Institutes of Health (NIH)

9000 Rockville Pike
Bethesda, MD 20892
Phone: 301-496-4000
TTY: 301-402-9612
Website: www.nih.gov

National Library of Medicine (NLM)

8600 Rockville Pike
Bethesda, MD 20894
Toll-Free: 888-346-3656
(888-FIND-NLM)
Phone: 301-594-5983
Website: www.nlm.nih.gov
Email: NLMCommunications@nih.gov

Office of Minority Health (OMH)

1101 Wootton Pkwy.
Tower Oaks Bldg., Ste. 100
Rockville, MD 20852
Toll-Free: 800-444-6472
TDD: 301-251-1432
Fax: 301-251-2160
Website: www.minorityhealth.hhs.gov
Email: info@minorityhealth.hhs.gov

U.S. Department of Health and Human Services (HHS)

200 Independence Ave., S.W.
Hubert H. Humphrey Bldg.
Washington, DC 20201
Toll-Free: 877-696-6775
Website: www.hhs.gov

U.S. Food and Drug Administration (FDA)

10903 New Hampshire Ave.
Silver Spring, MD 20993-0002
Toll-Free: 888-463-6332
Website: www.fda.gov

PRIVATE AGENCIES THAT PROVIDE INFORMATION ABOUT PREGNANCY AND RELATED CONCERNS

American Academy of Family Physicians (AAFP)
11400 Tomahawk Creek Pkwy.
Leawood, KS 66211
Toll-Free: 800-274-2237
Website: www.aafp.org
Email: aafp@aafp.org

American Academy of Pediatrics (AAP)
345 Park Blvd.
Itasca, IL 60143
Toll-Free: 800-433-9016
Fax: 847-434-8000
Website: www.aap.org
Email: mcc@aap.org

American Association of Birth Centers (AABC)
3123 Gottschall Rd.
Perkiomenville, PA 18074
Phone: 215-234-8068
Website: www.birthcenters.org

American College of Allergy, Asthma and Immunology (ACAAI)
85 W. Algonquin Rd., Ste. 550
Arlington Heights, IL 60005
Phone: 847-427-1200
Fax: 847-427-9656
Website: college.acaai.org
Email: mail@acaai.org

American College of Nurse-Midwives (ACNM)
8403 Colesville Rd., Ste. 1230
Silver Spring, MD 20910
Phone: 240-485-1800
Fax: 240-485-1818
Website: www.midwife.org
Email: membership@acnm.org

The American College of Obstetricians and Gynecologists (ACOG)
409 12th St., S.W.
P.O. Box 96920 Washington,
DC 20024-9998
Toll-Free: 800-673-8444
Phone: 202-638-5577
Website: www.acog.org
Email: communications@acog.org

American College of Surgeons (ACS)
633 N. Saint Clair St.
Chicago, IL 60611-3295
Toll-Free: 800-621-4111
Phone: 312-202-5000
Fax: 312-202-5001
Website: www.facs.org
Email: postmaster@facs.org

American Diabetes Association (ADA)

2451 Crystal Dr., Ste. 900
Arlington, VA 22202
Toll-Free: 800-342-2383
(800-DIABETES)
Website: www.diabetes.org
Email: askada@diabetes.org

American Institute of Ultrasound in Medicine (AIUM)

14750 Sweitzer Ln., Ste. 100
Laurel, MD 20707-5906
Toll-Free: 800-638-5352
Phone: 301-498-4100
Fax: 301-498-4450
Website: www.aium.org

American Medical Association (AMA)

AMA Plz., 330 N. Wabash Ave.,
Ste. 39300
Chicago, IL 60611-5885
Toll-Free: 800-262-3211
Phone: 312-464-4782
Website: www.ama-assn.org

American Pregnancy Association (APA)

Toll-Free: 800-672-2296
Website: www.americanpregnancy.org
Email: info@americanpregnancy.org

American Public Human Services Association (APHSA)

1300 17th. St., N., Ste. 340
Arlington, VA 22209-3801
Phone: 202-682-0100
Fax: 202-289-6555
Website: www.aphsa.org
Email: memberservice@aphsa.org

American Society for Reproductive Medicine (ASRM)

1209 Montgomery Hwy.
Birmingham, AL 35216-2809
Phone: 205-978-5000
Fax: 205-978-5005
Website: www.asrm.org
Email: asrm@asrm.org

American Society of Anesthesiologists (ASA)

1061 American Ln.
Schaumburg, IL 60173-4973
Phone: 847-825-5586
Fax: 847-825-1692
Website: www.asahq.org
Email: info@asahq.org

Association of Maternal and Child Health Programs (AMCHP)

1825 K St., N.W., Ste. 250
Washington, DC 20006
Phone: 202-775-0436
Fax: 202-478-5120
Website: www.amchp.org

Association of Women's Health, Obstetric and Neonatal Nurses (AWHONN)
1800 M St., N.W., Ste. 740S
Washington, DC 20036
Toll-Free: 800-673-8499
Phone: 202-261-2400
Fax: 202-728-0575
Website: www.awhonn.org
Email: customerservice@awhonn.org

Center for Health Care Strategies (CHCS)
200 American Metro Blvd., Ste. 119
Hamilton, NJ 08619
Phone: 609-528-8400
Fax: 609-586-3679
Website: www.chcs.org
Email: hr@chcs.org

Center for Research on Reproduction and Women's Health (CRRWH)
1355 Biomedical Research Bldg.
II/III, 421 Curie Blvd.
Philadelphia, PA 19104-6160
Phone: 215-898-0147
Website: www.med.upenn.edu/crrwh
Email: adamoli@pennmedicine.upenn.edu

Childbirth and Postpartum Professional Association (CAPPA)
P.O. Box 340
Hoschton, GA 30548
Phone: 770-965-9777
Website: www.cappa.net
Email: info@cappa.net

Childbirth Connection
1725 Eye St., N.W., Ste. 950
Washington, DC 20006
Phone: 202-986-2600
Fax: 202-986-2539
Website: nationalpartnership.org/childbirthconnection
Email: info@nationalpartnership.org

Cleveland Clinic
9500 Euclid Ave.
Cleveland, OH 44195
Toll-Free: 800-223-2273
Phone: 216-444-220
Website: my.clevelandclinic.org

DONA International
35 E. Wacker Dr., Ste. 850
Chicago, IL 60601-2106
Toll-Free: 888-788-3662
Website: www.dona.org
Email: DONA@dona.org

Guttmacher Institute
1301 Connecticut Ave., N.W., Ste. 700
Washington, DC 20036
Toll-Free: 877-823-0262
Phone: 202-296-4012
Fax: 202-223-5756
Website: www.guttmacher.org
Email: info@guttmacher.org

HER Foundation
10117 S.E. Sunnyside Rd., Ste. F8
Clackamas, OR 97015
Toll-Free: 888-264-2914
Website: www.hyperemesis.org
Email: info@hyperemesis.org

Institute for Women's Policy Research (IWPR)
1200 18th St., N.W., Ste. 301
Washington, DC 20036
Phone: 202-785-5100
Fax: 202-629-3611
Website: www.iwpr.org
Email: iwpr@iwpr.org

International Childbirth Education Association (ICEA)
110 Horizon Dr., Ste. 210
Raleigh, NC 27615
Phone: 919-674-4183
Fax: 919-459-2075
Website: www.icea.org
Email: info@icea.org

International Council on Infertility Information Dissemination (INCIID)
5765 F Burke Centre Pkwy.
P.O. Box 330
Burke, VA 22015
Phone: 703-379-9178
Fax: 703-379-1593
Website: www.inciid.org
Email: INCIIDinfo@inciid.org

La Leche League International (LLLI)
110 Horizon Dr., Ste. 210
Raleigh, NC 27615
Toll-Free: 800-525-3243
Phone: 919-459-2167
Fax: 919-459-2075
Website: www.llli.org
Email: info@llli.org

Lamaze International
2001 K St., N.W.
3rd Fl., N.
Washington, DC 20006
Phone: 202-367-1128
Website: www.lamaze.org
Email: info@lamaze.org

March of Dimes (MOD)
1550 Crystal Dr., Ste. 1300
Arlington, VA 22202
Toll-Free: 888-663-4637
(888-MODIMES)
Website: www.marchofdimes.org
Email: support@marchofdimes.org

Midwives Alliance of North America (MANA)
P.O. Box 83
Milaca, MN 56353
Toll-Free: 844-626-2674
Website: www.mana.org
Email: contact@mana.org

National Coalition on Health Care (NCHC)
4306 Pkwy Centre Dr.
Grove City, OH 43123
Phone: 614-820-8081
Website: www.nchc.org

National Rural Health Association (NRHA)
7015 College Blvd., Ste. 150
Overland Park, KS 66211
Phone: 816-756-3140
Fax: 816-756-3144
Website: www.ruralhealthweb.org
Email: mail@ruralhealth.us

The Organization of Teratology Information Specialist (OTIS)
5034A Thoroughbred Ln.
Brentwood, TN 37027
Toll-Free: 866-626-6847
(866-626-OTIS)
Phone: 615-649-3082
Website: www.mothertobaby.org
Email: ContactUs@mothertobaby.org

Planned Parenthood Federation of America, Inc. (PPFA)
123 William St.
New York, NY 10038
Toll-Free: 800-230-7526
(800-230-PLAN)
Phone: 212-541-7800
Website: www.plannedparenthood.org
Email: dmca@ppfa.org

Power to Decide
1776 Massachusetts Ave., N.W., Ste. 200
Washington, DC 20036
Phone: 202-478-8500
Fax: 202-478-8588
Website: www.thenationalcampaign.org
Email: info@powertodecide.org

Preeclampsia Foundation
3840 W. Eau Gallie Blvd., Ste. 104
Melbourne, FL 32934
Toll-Free: 800-665-9341
Phone: 321-421-6957
Website: www.preeclampsia.org
Email: info@preeclampsia.org

RESOLVE: The National Infertility Association
1660 International Dr., Ste. 600
McLean, VA 22102
Phone: 703-556-7172
Fax: 703-506-3266
Website: www.resolve.org
Email: info@resolve.org

Robert Wood Johnson Foundation (RWJF)
50 College Rd., E.
Princeton, NJ 08540-6614
Toll-Free: 877-843-7953
Phone: 609-627-6000
Website: www.rwjf.org
Email: mail@rwjf.org

Urban Institute
500 L'Enfant Plz., S.W.
Washington, DC 20024
Phone: 202-833-7200
Website: www.urban.org
Email: devoffice@urban.org

INDEX

INDEX

Page numbers followed by "n" refer to citation information; by "t" indicate tables; and by "f" indicate figures.

Index

Index

Index

Index

Index

Index

Index

Index

overweight
eating disorders 376
gestational diabetes 413
high-risk pregnancy 291
nutrition and pregnancy 206
overdue pregnancy 559
overview 381–383
pelvic floor disorder (PFD) 120
preconception health 47
preeclampsia 479
pregnancy 29, 239
stillbirth 538
ovulation
contraception 60
female reproductive system 6
fertility 33
obesity and overweight 381
overview 49–54
oxytocin
breastfeeding 653
doula 169
overdue pregnancy 559

P

pain
carpal tunnel syndrome (CTS) 110
chickenpox 437
doula 169
ectopic pregnancy 393, 528
gestational hypertension 418
gestational trophoblastic disease
(GTD) 326
group B *Streptococcus* (GBS) 451
herpes simplex virus (HSV) 515
iron deficiency anemia 211
labor 582
lupus 350
menstrual cycle 34
molar pregnancy 544
nonsteroidal anti-inflammatory
drugs (NSAIDs) 199

overview 609–612
pelvic floor disorder (PFD) 121
placental complications 496
postpartum depression 158
preeclampsia 476
pregnancy and oral health 147
pregnancy exercises 235
recovering from delivery 632
second trimester 93
stress incontinence 137
substance use 268
travel during pregnancy 255
vaginal (natural) childbirth 597
parvovirus B19
fifth disease 429
thalassemia 358
PCOS *see* polycystic ovary syndrome
PDA *see* Pregnancy Discrimination
Act
PE *see* pulmonary embolism
pelvic examination, ectopic
pregnancy 528
pelvic floor disorder (PFD),
overview 119–126
pelvic floor muscles
pelvic floor disorder (PFD) 120
pregnancy exercises 237
stress incontinence 136
urinary frequency 106
urinary incontinence 127
pelvic inflammatory disease (PID)
menstrual cycle 34
trichomoniasis 517
pelvic organ prolapse *see* pelvic floor
disorder (PFD)
pelvic pain
ectopic pregnancy 528
pregnancy back pain 107
penicillin, group B *Streptococcus*
(GBS) 455
perinatal depression,
overview 153–157

Index

Index